Advances in Cancer Drug Targets
(Volume 1)

Editor

Atta-ur-Rahman
Honorary Life Fellow
Kings College
University of Cambridge
UK

CONTENTS

FOREWORD

Cancer drug therapy has evolved significantly in the last two decades. Progress in the synthesis and isolation of organic compounds as well as our understanding of the structure and nature of DNA have also contributed to advances in anti-cancer drug development. Contemporary biochemical strategies to combat cancers range from cytotoxic and DNA damaging mechanisms to regulating programmed cell death (apoptosis). This eBook is the first volume of the series ***Advances in Cancer Drug Targets*** and is a compilation of recent expert reviews published in ***Current Cancer Drug Targets*** on the subject with a focus on these strategies. The reference work serves to give readers a brief yet comprehensive overview of current theory and practice behind employing chemical compounds for tackling tumor suppression, DNA site specific drug targeting and the inhibition of enzymes involved in growth control pathways. The reviews, written by experts in pharmaceutical sciences and molecular biology, have been carefully selected and represent an attempt to collect and current research on anti-cancer drug development for interested researchers and pharmaceutical scientists. ***Advances in Cancer Drug Targets*** should also provide insights into development of new approaches to anti-cancer therapy. I hope that the articles contained in this volume will be greatly enjoyed by the readers.

I would like to thank Mr. Mahmood Alam, Mr. Taimur Khan, Ms. Nazia Kamran and Ms. Humaira Hashmi for their help and support.

Atta-ur-Rahman, FRS

Honorary Life Fellow
Kings College
University of Cambridge
Cambridge
UK

List of Contributors

Alonso-González, Carolina

Department of Physiology and Pharmacology
School of Medicine
University of Cantabria
Spain

Alvarez-García, Virginia

Department of Physiology and Pharmacology
School of Medicine
University of Cantabria
Spain

Bruserud, Øystein

Institute of Medicine
University of Bergen
Haukeland University Hospital
Norway

Cavaletti, Guido

Department of Neuroscience and Biomedical Technologies
University of Milano-Bicocca
Italy

Cidado, Justin

The Sidney Kimmel Comprehensive Cancer Center
School of Medicine
The Johns Hopkins University
USA

Cos, Samuel

Department of Physiology and Pharmacology
School of Medicine
University of Cantabria
Spain

Cosgrove, David

Division of Medical Oncology
The Johns Hopkins University
School of Medicine
USA

Croessmann, Sarah

The Sidney Kimmel Comprehensive Cancer Center
School of Medicine
The Johns Hopkins University
USA

Ersvær, Elisabeth

Institute of Medicine
University of Bergen
Norway

Finn, Greg

Cancer Biology Program
Division of Hematology/Oncology
Department of Medicine
Beth Israel Deaconess Medical Center
Harvard Medical School
USA

Gjertsen, Bjørn Tore

Section for Hematology
Department of Medicine
Haukeland University Hospital
Norway

González, Alicia

Department of Physiology and Pharmacology
School of Medicine
University of Cantabria
Spain

Gustin, John P.

The Sidney Kimmel Comprehensive Cancer Center
School of Medicine
The Johns Hopkins University
USA

Jiang, Bing-Hua

Department of Pathology
Anatomy and Cell Biology
Thomas Jefferson University
USA

Kittang, Astrid Olsnes

Section for Hematology

Department of Medicine
Haukeland University Hospital
Norway

Liu, Ling-Zhi

Department of Pathology
Anatomy and Cell Biology
Thomas Jefferson University
USA

Lu, Kun Ping

Cancer Biology Program
Division of Hematology/Oncology
Department of Medicine
Beth Israel Deaconess Medical Center
Harvard Medical School
USA

Luo, Man-Li

Cancer Biology Program
Division of Hematology/Oncology
Department of Medicine
Beth Israel Deaconess Medical Center
Harvard Medical School
USA

Martínez-Campa, Carlos

Department of Physiology and Pharmacology
School of Medicine
University of Cantabria
Spain

Melve, Guro Kristin

Department of Immunology and Transfusion Medicine
Haukeland University Hospital
Norway

Park, Ben Ho

Department of Oncology
The Sidney Kimmel Comprehensive Cancer Center
The Johns Hopkins University
USA

Reikvam, Håkon

Institute of Medicine

University of Bergen
Haukeland University Hospital
Norway

Rodriguez-Menendez, Virginia

Department of Neuroscience and Biomedical Technologies
University of Milano-Bicocca
Italy

Safa, Ahmad R.

Department of Pharmacology and Toxicology
Indiana University Simon Cancer Center,
Indiana University School of Medicine
USA

Sharma, Pooja S.

Department of Chemistry
C.S.S.S. (P.G.) College
India

Sharma, Rajan

Department of Chemistry
C.S.S.S. (P.G.) College
India

Tremolizzo, Lucio

Department of Neuroscience and Biomedical Technologies
University of Milano-Bicocca
Italy

Zhou, Xiao Zhen

Cancer Biology Program
Division of Hematology/Oncology
Department of Medicine
Beth Israel Deaconess Medical Center
Harvard Medical School
USA

Send Orders of Reprints at bspsaif@emirates.net.ae
Advances in Cancer Drug Targets, Vol. 1, **2013, 3-21**

CHAPTER 1

The *PIK3CA* Gene as a Mutated Target for Cancer Therapy

Sarah Croessmann, Justin Cidado, John P. Gustin, David Cosgrove and Ben Ho Park[1,2,*]

[1]The Sidney Kimmel Comprehensive Cancer Center, The Johns Hopkins University School of Medicine, Baltimore, MD 21231, USA and [2]The Johns Hopkins University, Department of Chemical and Biomolecular Engineering, Baltimore, MD 21218, USA

Abstract: The development of targeted therapies with true specificity for cancer relies upon exploiting differences between cancerous and normal cells. Genetic and genomic alterations including somatic mutations, translocations, and amplifications have served as recent examples of how such differences can be exploited as effective drug targets. Small molecule inhibitors and monoclonal antibodies directed against the protein products of these genetic anomalies have led to cancer therapies with high specificity and relatively low toxicity. Our group and others have demonstrated that somatic mutations in the *PIK3CA* gene occur at high frequency in breast and other cancers. Moreover, the majority of mutations occur at three hotspots, making these ideal targets for therapeutic development. Here we review the literature on *PIK3CA* mutations in cancer, as well as existing data on p110α inhibitors and inhibitors of downstream effectors for potential use as targeted cancer therapeutics.

Keywords: *PIK3CA*, mutation, oncogene, PI3 kinase, AKT, mTOR.

INTRODUCTION

Insults to the genome are a hallmark of cancer and a driving force in carcinogenesis. These genomic alterations are an obvious difference between normal and cancerous cells, and provide an opportunity for exploitation as potential targets for therapeutics. Over the past decade, successful clinical trials of imatinib, gefitinib, erlotinib, and trastuzumab, which are specific for *BCR-ABL* translocations [1], epidermal growth factor receptor (*EGFR)* mutations [2, 3], and HER2/neu amplifications [4-6] respectively, have illustrated the ability to develop drugs that target genetic abnormalities in human malignancies. This has opened

[*]**Address correspondence to Ben Ho Park:** Department of Oncology, The Sidney Kimmel Comprehensive Cancer Center, The Johns Hopkins University, 1650 Orleans Street, Room 151, Baltimore, MD, 21287, USA; Tel: 410-502-7399; Fax: 410-614-8397; E-mail: bpark2@jhmi.edu

the possibility for future streamlined therapies based on the genomic landscape of an individual's cancer.

Phosphatidylinositol 3-kinases (PI3K)s are heterodimeric proteins consisting of a regulatory subunit (p85) and a catalytic component (p110), and there are several isoforms and classes of known PI3Ks. The p110α catalytic subunit of the Class I PI3Kα, encoded by the gene *PIK3CA*, is one of the most highly mutated oncogenes in human cancers. High mutational frequencies of *PIK3CA* have been reported in colorectal [7], breast [8] and liver cancers [9] while lower rates of mutation have been described in many other human malignancies including ovarian [10, 11], lung [7, 9], gastric [7, 9, 12, 13], and brain cancers [7, 9, 14-21]. In breast cancer, *PIK3CA* has a reported overall mutational rate of 25%, with more than 80% being attributed to "hot spot" regions within exon 9 of the helical domain and exon 20 of the catalytic domain [8]. These three mutations, E542K and E545K in exon 9 and H1047R in exon 20 lead to increased PI3K catalytic activity. This increased activity results in cellular transformation through growth factor- and anchorage-independent cellular proliferation [22-24]. Studying the effects of these mutations in colorectal cells [25-27], breast epithelial cells [28, 29], and chicken embryo fibroblasts [30, 31] have illustrated a direct connection between these mutations and carcinogenesis. Through crystallographic and biochemical methods, it has been determined that the probable oncogenic mechanism of the E545K mutation is the disruption of an inhibitory charge-charge interaction between p110α and the N-terminal SH2 domain of the p85 regulatory subunit [32] (Fig. **1**). It has been previously proposed that the oncogenic mechanism of the E542K mutation is similar to E545K, exhibiting a change in the interaction of p110α with the p85 regulatory subunit. The proposed oncogenic mechanism of the H1047R mutation differs from the exon 9 mutations. The H1047R mutation increases the binding affinity of p110α for the negatively charged phosphatidylinositol substrate leading to increased activity and transforming potential [33]. Furthermore, aberrant PI3K signaling has also been linked to resistance of cells in preclinical models to a number of targeted and cytotoxic cancer therapies, including trastuzumab and paclitaxel resistance in human breast epithelial cells harboring *PIK3CA* mutations [28, 34]. Clinically, the presence of *PIK3CA* mutations has been linked to both favorable [35, 36] and unfavorable [37, 38] patient prognosis, and it has also been reported that exon 9 mutations have a less favorable prognosis than exon 20 mutations in breast cancer [39]. The reasons for these conflicting data are not clear, but likely reflect limited sample sizes and difference in treatment regimens between the various studies.

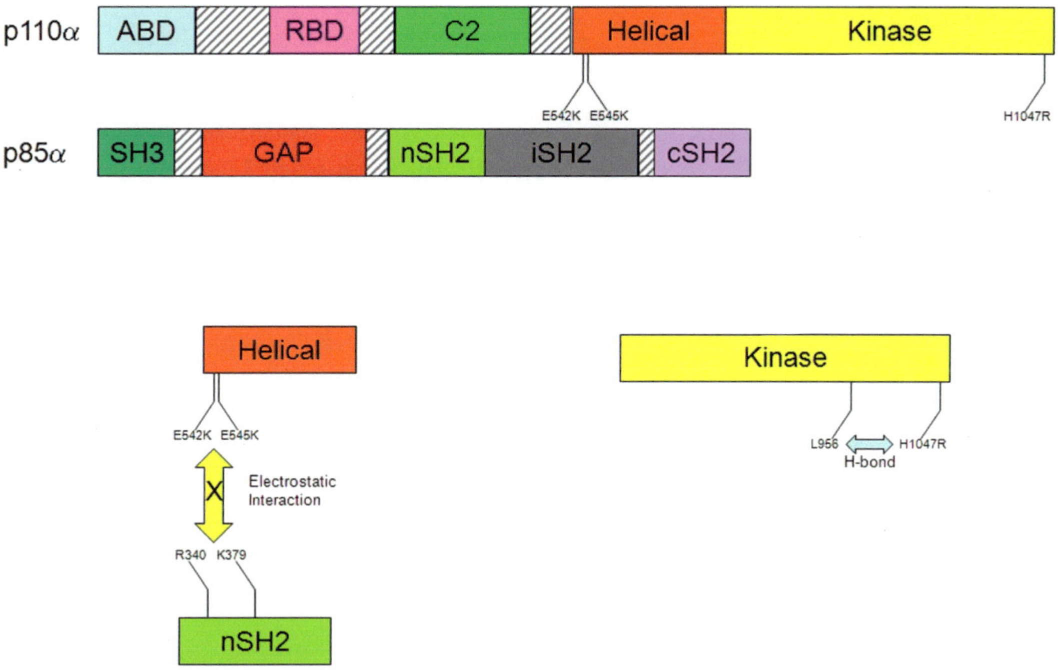

Figure 1: A representation of the Domains of the PI3K Subunits p110α and p85α. The p110α catalytic subunit has 5 domains including adaptor-binding domain (ABD), the Ras-binding domain (RBD), a calcium binding domain (C2), a helical domain and a kinase domain. The p85α regulatory subunit contains 5 domains as well, which include a Src homology 3 domain (SH3), a GTPase activating protein domain (GAP), an N-terminal Src homology 2 domain (nSH2), an inter- Src homology 2 domain (iSH2), and a C-terminal Src homology 2 domain (cSH2). The exon 9 hotspot mutations, E542K and E545K, occur in the helical domain of the catalytic subunit p110α, and the charge reversal caused by these mutations inhibits electrostatic interactions between those amino acids on the p110α helical domain and R340 and K379 on the nSH2 domain of p85α. The exon 20 hotspot mutation, H1047R, is in the kinase domain of p110α, and this mutation has been proposed to form a hydrogen bond with L956 of p110α, which in turn leads to catalytic activity of p110α.

TARGETING *PIK3CA* MUTATIONS

With the recent success of biologics and small molecular inhibitors for anti-cancer therapy, the identification and validation of additional therapeutic targets is of great importance and interest. *PIK3CA* somatic mutations would be ideal for targeting due to their high rate of occurrence and the fact that 80% to 90% of these mutations are in one of the three previously discussed hotspots. Below, we review several classes of targeted compounds that may have clinical utility for the treatment of cancers harboring *PIK3CA* mutations.

PI3K Inhibitors

The most direct method of targeting cancers that have *PIK3CA* mutations would be to develop inhibitors that have high specificity for mutant p110α but not its wild type counterpart. The ability to create relatively mutation-specific small molecule inhibitors is exemplified by erlotinib and gefitinib, which were initially developed as EGFR inhibitors but were found to be most effective in patients whose tumors contained specific EGFR mutations [40, 41]. This finding is attributed to oncogene addiction [40], which is the phenomenon whereby cancer cells become dependent on particular alterations for survival as well as preservation of the malignant state. Thus, specific genetic changes within cancer cells, such as the *PIK3CA* hotspot mutations, result in increased growth signals from aberrantly activated pathways, and therefore removal of these signals leads to decreased cellular growth and apoptosis [42]. Recent structural data demonstrate that rational design of mutation specific inhibitors is feasible [43], and therefore the emergence of targeted mutant *PIK3CA* therapies is likely to be imminent.

Prior to the discovery of somatic *PIK3CA* mutations in human cancers, the PI3K enzyme was already recognized as being an important molecule in mediating carcinogenesis. As such, inhibitors of PI3K were developed with the hope that a therapeutic window could be achieved. The earliest and best characterized PI3K inhibitors are wortmannin and LY294002. Both of these compounds have been shown to be effective anti-tumor agents in *in vitro* cell culture models, as well as in *in vivo* animal models [44-46]. LY294002 has been shown to inhibit both *in vitro* PI3K activity and phosphorylation of downstream effectors of *PIK3CA* in breast epithelial [28] and colorectal cancer cells [27]. However, due to their poor pharmacological properties and marked cytotoxicity, LY294002 and wortmannin do not have clinical utility as reviewed by Workman [47]. Additionally, they are not ideal for specifically targeting *PIK3CA* mutants because they can inhibit other kinases of the PI-3 kinase-like kinase (PIKK) family, and several other kinases such as the mammalian target of rapamycin (mTOR) [48-52]. Despite having limited preclinical studies due to poor solubility, instability and high toxicity, both the structures of LY294002 and wortmannin have served as templates for derivatives and prodrugs with better pharmacological properties [53, 54]. The prodrug, SF-1126, is a vasculature-targeting Arg-Gly-Asp peptide conjugated to LY294002 that exhibits increased stability and tolerance in murine models [55]. Similarly, wortmannin has served as an analog template for a pan-PI3K inhibitor, PX-866, which demonstrated increased cell permeability and a prolonged serum half-life [56]. Recently, a number of groups have reported developing p110α selective inhibitors [57-63], and some have demonstrated efficacy *in vitro* and *in vivo* [57-59, 61, 62, 64]. The development of subsequent generations of PI3K pathway inhibitors and combined therapies have aided in circumventing the limitations of first generation inhibitors [65].

Class-specific and isoform-specific PI3K inhibitors are attractive target options, providing the opportunity for global inhibition of downstream components. It is important to note, however, that PI3K inhibitors have the potential for greater toxicity due to their importance for normal cellular processes. Class I PI3Ks inhibitors, such as GDC-0941[66], XL-147 [67], BKM120 [68], GSK1059615, CAL-101[69], and PX-866[70], are currently in clinical development. Despite significant homology between the different p110 catalytic subunits (α, β, δ, γ), recent structural data supports the potential for success of current Class I PI3K p110 isoform-specific inhibitors [43], with a particular interest in p110α specific inhibitors due to the possibility of oncogenic *PIK3CA* mutations being predictors of response [71]. BYL719, GDC-0032, and INK-1117, are three p110α-specific inhibitors currently in early clinical development [72]. Initial studies have identified other p110 isoform-specific inhibitors TGX-221[73], CAL-101, and AS-252424 [74] for p110β, p110δ, and p110γ, respectively. Isoform-specific inhibitors demonstrate the ability to target particular alterations in the PI3K pathway with theoretically less off target effects. In addition to isoform specific inhibitors, Class specific inhibitors in pre-clinical studies have shown the possibility of preferential responses to tumors harboring *PIK3CA* mutations. For example the novel Class I PI3K inhibitor, CH5132799, is particularly selective for cancer cells harboring *PIK3CA* mutations [75]. In addition, other PI3K isoforms may also prove to be attractive targets for breast cancer therapy. For example, studies have demonstrated that expression of *PIK3CB* in conjunction with *HER2* amplification, can lead to a worse overall prognosis [76]. The future development of isoform specific PI3K inhibitors may allow for novel therapeutic development and targeting of breast cancers based upon the genetic alterations that drive the PI3K pathway.

Buttressed against these exciting developments, specific targeting of *PIK3CA* may be problematic, because as previously mentioned, *PIK3CA* is involved in a number of signaling pathways associated with normal cellular function, such as insulin signaling [63, 77]. This may result in *PIK3CA* inhibitors that are prohibitively cytotoxic, thus limiting their clinical benefit. To illustrate this point, some *PIK3CA* inhibitors have been shown to abrogate the effects of insulin in mice [63]. Similarly, *PIK3CA* deficient mice have recently been shown to have an increased rate of heart failure in response to cardiac stress [78]. Thus, the possibility of a significant side effect profile has led to the development of compounds designed to target downstream effectors within the PI3K pathway with the hope that this may be a more effective strategy to target cancers containing *PIK3CA* mutations.

AKT Inhibitors

AKT, also known as protein kinase B, is a serine threonine kinase directly downstream of PI3K, and due to its central role in signal transduction, the dysregulation of AKT is commonly associated with many different cancers [79]. More specifically, constitutive activation of AKT has been associated with *PIK3CA* mutations in several *in vitro* cell models [26-30]. Therefore, AKT inhibitors may prove to be useful in targeting cancers with *PIK3CA* mutations.

AKT was identified as an oncogene over two decades ago [80], and multiple AKT inhibitors have been developed and used successfully to inhibit AKT activation and cellular growth in *in vitro* and *in vivo* tumor models [81-108]. Unlike PI3K, development of isoform-specific AKT inhibitors has proven difficult due to the high degree of homology among the three AKT isoforms. Perifosine is the most studied AKT inhibitor, proving efficacious at inhibiting the growth of various cancer cell types [105]. As a single agent, Perifosine has not shown therapeutic benefit in several phase II trials, however, Perifosine may have some therapeutic potential when used in combination with radiation or other standard cytotoxic agents, as evidenced by *in vitro* studies [109-111]. Another AKT inhibitor, Miltefosine, has shown efficacy in clinical trials for the topical treatment of cutaneous lymphoma and breast cancer skin metastases [112-115]. API-2, another early AKT inhibitor [102], had shown some efficacy in early phase trials, but was abandoned due to excessive toxicity [116, 117]. These early AKT specific compounds aided in directing the investigation of more specific AKT inhibitors at lower doses than those used previously, thus potentially avoiding detrimental side effects. Recent strategies for developing AKT inhibitors have included ATP-competitive inhibitors, phosphotidylinositol analogs, and allosteric inhibitors. GSK690693 and A-443654, two pan-AKT ATP-competitive agents, have demonstrated anti-tumor activity in preclinical models and are currently in early Phase trials [118, 119]. Allosteric inhibitors, such as MK-2205, have demonstrated relatively high selectivity and shown marked suppression of breast cancer growth, and are currently in late Phase II clinical trials [120]. These compounds interact with the pleckstrin homology (PH) domain or hinge region, promoting an inactive form of the enzyme by preventing localization to the membrane or access to the PDK-1-dependent phosphorylation site.

Additional studies are needed to further elucidate the relationship between *PIK3CA* mutations and AKT as there are three distinct isoforms (AKT1, AKT2, and AKT3) and each may have different effects on tumor growth and/or cytotoxicity. To date, *PIK3CA* mutations have been most closely linked to AKT1 in *in vitro* cell models [26, 28-30], with a single study examining all three isoforms revealing that AKT1 may be most affected by *PIK3CA* mutations [27]. However, isoform specific functions have been delineated through various laboratory studies. For example, RNA interference (RNAi) mediated gene knockdown of *AKT1* in breast cancer cell lines has been shown to increase cell motility [121], and *AKT1* knockout mice are small in size and infertile [122]. In addition, *AKT2* knockout mice develop diabetes mellitus [123], while *AKT3* knockout mice exhibit abnormal brain development [124]. Although AKT isoforms are highly homologous, selective AKT1 and 2 inhibitors have been developed and have shown promise *in vitro* [97]. Further study of the relative effects of inhibiting different AKT isoforms in cancers harboring *PIK3CA* mutations will be required, as the potential for significant toxicities remains obstacle challenge for using AKT inhibitors as effective targeted therapies for these cancers.

mTOR Inhibitors

mTOR is a downstream effector of *PIK3CA* and is very important for many cellular processes, including cell proliferation [125] and angiogenesis [126]. The mTOR pathway has been shown to be activated by *PIK3CA* mutations in both chicken embryo fibroblasts [30] and colorectal cancer cells [26]. Therefore, blocking the mTOR pathway may prove to be an effective strategy for targeting aberrant growth signaling in cancers with *PIK3CA* mutations.

mTOR inhibitors are the most mature in terms of their development and clinical use of potential compounds targeting cancers harboring *PIK3CA* mutations. Rapamycin, the prototypical mTOR inhibitor, was initially developed in the early 1970's as an antifungal agent [127] and was later FDA approved as an immunosuppressive therapy [128]. As seen with most first generation inhibitors, rapamycin exhibited undesirable pharmacological properties. More reliable rapamycin analogs, or "rapalogs", were developed and have shown cytostatic activity in preclinical models and anti-tumor activity when used in combination with chemotherapies [71]. RAD001 (everolimus), CCI-779 (temsirolimus), and AP-23573 (deferolimus), are three rapalogs that have exhibited variable and moderate success. Previously, the best evidence of response was shown in the treatment of advanced renal cancers with temsirolimus [129]. More recently, the BOLERO-2 trial demonstrated that in metastatic breast cancer patients refractory to hormone therapies, the addition of everolimus to exemestane lead to improved progression free survival compared to women taking exemestane alone [130].

The proposed mechanism of action of rapamycin and its analogs is the formation of a complex with the FK506-binding protein (FKBP12). This complex can then bind the C-terminal region of mTOR, interfering with the kinase activity of the multimeric mTORC1 complex but not with mTORC2 [131]. Furthermore, identifying biomarkers that predict for response to mTOR inhibitors is paramount for the development of these agents, as response to mTOR inhibitors has been highly variable. Theoretically, *PIK3CA* mutations may lend themselves as predictive biomarkers for response to mTOR inhibitors. For example, rapamycin and its analogs prevent the transformation of chicken embryo fibroblasts expressing *PIK3CA* mutations [30], inhibit *PIK3CA* induced tumor growth in chicken embryos [31], and reduce the formation of abnormal human breast epithelial cell acini induced by mutant *PIK3CA* overexpression [28].

Despite the clinical potential of mTOR inhibitors, significant hurdles for their further development still exist. mTOR forms two complexes within cells, mTORC1 and mTORC2 [132]. mTORC1 is known to mediate a negative feedback loop with PI3K/AKT signaling, and therefore inhibiting mTOR pharmacologically causes a paradoxical upregulation of PI3K/AKT growth promoting signaling [133]. Additionally, mTORC2 directly phosphorylates AKT [134] but is only rarely inhibited by rapamycin and its analogs in a cell/tissue type dependent manner [135]. Despite the initial promise of the previously mentioned mTORC1 allosteric inhibitors, feedback activation of PI3K and AKT persists *via* mTORC2. This suggests a potential shift in the focus of compound development to ATP-competitive compounds that can inactivate both complexes and completely abrogate mTOR signaling. PP242, its derivative INK128, as well as several other pan-mTOR inhibitors such as AZD-8055 and OSI-027, are ATP-competitive compounds in early phase clinical trials for solid malignancies including breast cancers [136, 137]. Other effective strategies for targeting this complex signaling pathway in the future may include combining current mTOR inhibitors with either newer PI3K/AKT inhibitors or more traditional therapies, such as chemotherapy and endocrine therapy. In addition, it is possible that the current development of new inhibitors capable of blocking mTORC2, or alternatively both mTORC1 and mTORC2, could provide a more effective therapeutic regimen.

Possibilities of Novel Dual Inhibition

Due to the genetic instability of most human cancers, it can be expected that any targeted therapy when used as a single agent will ultimately succumb to drug resistance. However, the development of targeted therapies with minimal side effects would hopefully enable the combinatorial use of multiple drugs with nonoverlapping toxicities, to effectively treat and eradicate the disease. Recently, it was demonstrated that the combination of p110α and mTOR inhibitors could prevent the increase in AKT signaling caused by mTOR inhibition alone [138]. A single molecule, PI-103, was found to effectively inhibit both p110α and mTOR, and its efficacy has been shown in gliomas, ovarian cancer, and breast cancer in *in vitro* and *in vivo* models [138, 139]. This class of molecules, capable of inhibiting multiple targets within the PI3K pathway, may prove to be an effective strategy for targeting cancer cells containing *PIK3CA* mutations.

In addition, combination therapies with existing anti-neoplastic drugs are also being explored. For example, *PIK3CA* mutations have been positively correlated with increased expression of both estrogen receptor alpha (ERα) and HER2 in the NCI 60 panel of cancer cell lines [140] as well breast tumor samples [141]. Hormonal therapies and trastuzumab are currently used to target ERα and HER2 respectively. However, it has been shown that increased AKT signaling is associated with resistance to both of these therapies [142-145], and it is therefore possible that *PIK3CA* mutations may actually confer resistance to these drugs. Recently, a study demonstrated that estrogen deprivation in ER (+) breast tumors increased the apoptotic effects of the PI3K and dual-PI3K/mTOR inhibitors, BKM120 and BGT226 respectively. Increased drug efficacy was observed when used in combination with fulvestrant, a selective estrogen receptor down-regulator (SERD) [146]. Recently, correlations have been made between the presence of mutant *PIK3CA* and activation of the MAPK pathway [147, 148]. While the development of combination therapies is still in its infancy, recent studies suggest that dual inhibition of both the PI3K and MAPK pathways presents the best strategy for targeting cancer with *PIK3CA* mutations, a testable hypothesis currently the focus of clinical trials.

CONCLUSIONS

Due to their high frequency in many cancers, *PIK3CA* mutations are a prime candidate for targeted therapeutics. However given the fact that these mutations have only recently been accurately characterized, much work lies ahead to fully elucidate their biological and clinical significance. The process of discovery for developing targeted *PIK3CA* therapies remains in its infancy. However, the wealth of potential targets along the PI3K pathway is certainly enticing from a developmental therapeutics viewpoint, and the opportunity exists to significantly impact cancer care with future success in this arena.

CONFLICT OF INTEREST

S.C., J.C., J.P.G. and D.P.C. declare no conflict of interests. B.H.P. is a member of the scientific advisory board of Horizon Discovery, LTD and receives royalties and payments for services provided and licensed reagents. B.H.P. is also a paid consultant for GlaxoSmithKline. The terms of these agreements are regulated by The Johns Hopkins University policies on conflicts of interest.

ACKNOWLEGMENTS

This work was supported by The Flight Attendant's Medical Research Institute (FAMRI), NIH/NCI CA109274, the Summer Running Fund, The Susan G. Komen for the Cure Foundation, Mary Kay Ash Charitable Foundation and the Avon Foundation. J.P.G. is a past recipient of a Department of Defense Breast Cancer Research Program Predoctoral Fellowship Award W81XWH-06-1-0325. S.C., J.C. and D.P.C. were previously supported on NIH Institutional Training Grants CA067751, GM008752, CA09071 and an American Cancer Society Young Investigator Award (D.P.C.).

DISCLOSURE

The chapter submitted for the eBook Series entitled **"Advances in Cancer Drug Targets, Volume 1"** is an update of our article in **Current Cancer Drug Targets, Volume 8, Issue 8, 2008,** with additional text and references.

ABBREVIATIONS

EGFR = epidermal growth factor receptor

PI3K = phosphatidylinositol 3-kinase

mTOR = mammalian target of rapamycin

PIKK = PI-3 kinase-like kinase

RNAi = RNA interference

ERα = estrogen receptor alpha

REFERENCES

[1] O'Brien, S.G., *et al.,* Imatinib compared with interferon and low-dose cytarabine for newly diagnosed chronic-phase chronic myeloid leukemia. New England Journal of Medicine, 2003. **348**(11): p. 994-1004.

[2] Paez, J.G., *et al.,* EGFR mutations in lung cancer: correlation with clinical response to gefitinib therapy. Science, 2004. **304**(5676): p. 1497-500.

[3] Lynch, T.J., *et al.,* Activating mutations in the epidermal growth factor receptor underlying responsiveness of non-small-cell lung cancer to gefitinib. N Engl J Med, 2004. **350**(21): p. 2129-39.

[4] Romond, E.H., *et al.,* Trastuzumab plus adjuvant chemotherapy for operable HER2-positive breast cancer. New England Journal of Medicine, 2005. **353**(16): p. 1673-1684.

[5] Piccart-Gebhart, M.J., *et al.,* Trastuzumab after adjuvant chemotherapy in HER2-positive breast cancer. New England Journal of Medicine, 2005. **353**(16): p. 1659-1672.

[6] Mass, R.D., *et al.,* Evaluation of clinical outcomes according to HER2 detection by fluorescence *in situ* hybridization in women with metastatic breast cancer treated with trastuzumab. Clinical Breast Cancer, 2005. **6**(3): p. 240-246.

[7] Samuels, Y., *et al.,* High frequency of mutations of the *PIK3CA* gene in human cancers. Science, 2004. **304**(5670): p. 554-554.

[8] Bachman, K.E., *et al.,* The *PIK3CA* gene is mutated with high frequency in human breast cancers. Cancer Biology & Therapy, 2004. **3**(8): p. 772-775.

[9] Lee, J.W., *et al., PIK3CA* gene is frequently mutated in breast carcinomas and hepatocellular carcinomas. Oncogene, 2005. **24**(8): p. 1477-1480.

[10] Levine, D.A., *et al.,* Frequent mutation of the *PIK3CA* gene in ovarian and breast cancers. Clinical Cancer Research, 2005. **11**(8): p. 2875-2878.

[11] Campbell, I.G., *et al.,* Mutation of the *PIK3CA* gene in ovarian and breast cancer. Cancer Research, 2004. **64**(21): p. 7678-7681.

[12] Velho, S., *et al.,* The prevalence of *PIK3CA* mutations in gastric and colon cancer. European Journal of Cancer, 2005. **41**(11): p. 1649-1654.

[13] Li, V.S.W., *et al.,* Mutations of *PIK3CA* in gastric adenocarcinoma. Bmc Cancer, 2005. **5**.

[14] Kita, D., *et al., PIK3CA* alterations in primary (de novo) and secondary glioblastomas. Acta Neuropathologica, 2007. **113**(3): p. 295-302.

[15] Gallia, G.L., *et al., PIK3CA* gene mutations in pediatric and adult glioblastoma multiforme. Molecular Cancer Research, 2006. **4**(10): p. 709-714.

[16] Dam, V., *et al.,* Mutations in *PIK3CA* are infrequent in neuroblastoma. Bmc Cancer, 2006. **6**.

[17] Pang, J.C.S., *et al.,* Rare mutation of *PIK3CA* in meningiomas. Acta Neuropathologica, 2006. **111**(3): p. 284-285.

[18] Hartmann, C., *et al., PIK3CA* mutations in oligodendroglial tumours. Neuropathology and Applied Neurobiology, 2006. **32**(2): p. 209-212.

[19] Hartmann, C., *et al., PIK3CA* mutations in glioblastoma multiforme. Acta Neuropathologica, 2005. **109**(6): p. 639-642.

[20] Mueller, W., *et al.,* Mutations of the *PIK3CA* gene are rare in human glioblastoma. Acta Neuropathologica, 2005. **109**(6): p. 654-655.

[21] Broderick, D.K., *et al.,* Mutations of *PIK3CA* in anaplastic oligodendrogliomas, high-grade astrocytomas, and medulloblastomas. Cancer Research, 2004. **64**(15): p. 5048-5050.

[22] Campbell, I.G., *et al.,* Mutation of the *PIK3CA* gene in ovarian and breast cancer. Cancer Res, 2004. **64**(21): p. 7678-81.

[23] Gustin, J.P., D.P. Cosgrove, and B.H. Park, The *PIK3CA* gene as a mutated target for cancer therapy. Curr Cancer Drug Targets, 2008. **8**(8): p. 733-40.

[24] Isakoff, S.J., *et al.,* Breast cancer-associated *PIK3CA* mutations are oncogenic in mammary epithelial cells. Cancer Res, 2005. **65**(23): p. 10992-1000.

[25] Guo, X.N., *et al.,* Mutant *PIK3CA*-bearing colon cancer cells display increased metastasis in an orthotopic model. Cancer Research, 2007. **67**(12): p. 5851-5858.

[26] Ikenoue, T., *et al.,* Functional analysis of *PIK3CA* gene mutations in human colorectal cancer. Cancer Research, 2005. **65**(11): p. 4562-4567.

[27] Samuels, Y., *et al.,* Mutant *PIK3CA* promotes cell growth and invasion of human cancer cells. Cancer Cell, 2005. **7**(6): p. 561-573.

[28] Isakoff, S.J., *et al.,* Breast cancer-associated *PIK3CA* mutations are oncogenic in mammary epithelial cells. Cancer Research, 2005. **65**(23): p. 10992-11000.

[29] Zhao, J.J., *et al.,* The oncogenic properties of mutant p110 alpha and p110 beta phosphatidylinositol 3-kinases in human mammary epithelial cells. Proceedings of the National Academy of Sciences of the United States of America, 2005. **102**(51): p. 18443-18448.

[30] Kang, S.Y., A.G. Bader, and P.K. Vogt, Phosphatidylinositol 3-kinase mutations identified in human cancer are oncogenic. Proceedings of the National Academy of Sciences of the United States of America, 2005. **102**(3): p. 802-807.

[31] Bader, A.G., S.Y. Kang, and P.K. Vogt, Cancer-specific mutations in *PIK3CA* are oncogenic *in vivo*. Proceedings of the National Academy of Sciences of the United States of America, 2006. **103**(5): p. 1475-1479.

[32] Miled, N., *et al.,* Mechanism of two classes of cancer mutations in the phosphoinositide 3-kinase catalytic subunit. Science, 2007. **317**(5835): p. 239-242.

[33] Kang, S., *et al.,* Mutated PI 3-kinases - Cancer targets on a silver platter. Cell Cycle, 2005. **4**(4): p. 578-581.

[34] Berns, K., *et al.,* A functional genetic approach identifies the PI3K pathway as a major determinant of trastuzumab resistance in breast cancer. Cancer Cell, 2007. **12**(4): p. 395-402.

[35] Maruyama, N., *et al.,* Clinicopathologic analysis of breast cancers with *PIK3CA* mutations in Japanese women. Clinical Cancer Research, 2007. **13**(2): p. 408-414.

[36] Pérez-Tenorio, G., *et al., PIK3CA* mutations and PTEN loss correlate with similar prognostic factors and are not mutually exclusive in breast cancer. Clinical Cancer Research, 2007. **13**(12): p. 3577-3584.

[37] Li, S.Y., *et al., PIK3CA* mutations in breast cancer are associated with poor outcome. Breast Cancer Research and Treatment, 2006. **96**(1): p. 91-95.

[38] Kato, S., *et al., PIK3CA* mutation is predictive of poor survival in patients with colorectal cancer. International Journal of Cancer, 2007. **121**(8): p. 1771-1778.

[39] Barbareschi, M., *et al.,* Different Prognostic Roles of Mutations in the Helical and Kinase Domains of the *PIK3CA* Gene in Breast Carcinomas. Clinical Cancer Research, 2007. **13**(20): p. 6064-6069.

[40] Davies, M., B. Hennessy, and G.B. Mills, Point mutations of protein kinases ion and individualised cancer therapy. Expert Opinion on Pharmacotherapy, 2006. 7(16): p. 2243-2261.

[41] Pao, W., *et al.*, EGF receptor gene mutations are common in lung cancers from "never smokers" and are associated with sensitivity of tumors to gefitinib and erlotinib. Proceedings of the National Academy of Sciences of the United States of America, 2004. **101**(36): p. 13306-13311.

[42] Weinstein, I.B., Cancer: Addiction to oncogenes - The Achilles heal of cancer. Science, 2002. **297**(5578): p. 63-64.

[43] Huang, C.H., *et al.*, The structure of a human p110alpha/p85alpha complex elucidates the effects of oncogenic PI3Kalpha mutations. Science, 2007. **318**(5857): p. 1744-8.

[44] Schultz, R.M., *et al.*, *In vitro* and *in vivo*_Antitumor-Activity of the Phosphatidylinositol-3-Kinase Inhibitor, Wortmannin. Anticancer Research, 1995. **15**(4): p. 1135-1139.

[45] Semba, S., *et al.*, The *in vitro* and *in vivo* effects of 2-(4-morpholinyl)-8-phenyl-chromone (LY294002), a specific inhibitor of phosphatidylinositol 3 '-kinase, in human colon cancer cells. Clinical Cancer Research, 2002. **8**(6): p. 1957-1963.

[46] Hu, L.M., *et al.*, *In vivo* and *in vitro* ovarian carcinoma growth inhibition by a phosphatidylinositol 3-kinase inhibitor (LY294002). Clinical Cancer Research, 2000. **6**(3): p. 880-886.

[47] Workman, P., Inhibiting the phosphoinositide 3-kinase pathway for cancer treatment. Biochemical Society Transactions, 2004. **32**: p. 393-396.

[48] Gharbi, S.I., *et al.*, Exploring the specificity of the PI3K family inhibitor LY294002. Biochemical Journal, 2007. **404**: p. 15-21.

[49] Sarkaria, J.N., *et al.*, Inhibition of phosphoinositide 3-kinase related kinases by the radiosensitizing agent wortmannin. Cancer Research, 1998. **58**(19): p. 4375-4382.

[50] Banin, S., *et al.*, Enhanced phosphorylation of p53 by ATN in response to DNA damage. Science, 1998. **281**(5383): p. 1674-1677.

[51] Brunn, G.J., *et al.*, Direct inhibition of the signaling functions of the mammalian target of rapamycin by the phosphoinositide 3-kinase inhibitors, wortmannin and LY294002. Embo Journal, 1996. **15**(19): p. 5256-5267.

[52] Hartley, K.O., *et al.*, DNA-Dependent Protein-Kinase Catalytic Subunit - a Relative of Phosphatidylinositol 3-Kinase and the Ataxia-Telangiectasia Gene-Product. Cell, 1995. **82**(5): p. 849-856.

[53] Arcaro, A. and M.P. Wymann, Wortmannin is a potent phosphatidylinositol 3-kinase inhibitor: the role of phosphatidylinositol 3,4,5-trisphosphate in neutrophil responses. Biochem J, 1993. **296 (Pt 2)**: p. 297-301.

[54] Vlahos, C.J., *et al.*, A specific inhibitor of phosphatidylinositol 3-kinase, 2-(4-morpholinyl)-8-phenyl-4H-1-benzopyran-4-one (LY294002). J Biol Chem, 1994. **269**(7): p. 5241-8.

[55] Garlich, J.R., *et al.*, A vascular targeted pan phosphoinositide 3-kinase inhibitor prodrug, SF1126, with antitumor and antiangiogenic activity. Cancer Res, 2008. **68**(1): p. 206-15.

[56] Ihle, N.T., *et al.*, Molecular pharmacology and antitumor activity of PX-866, a novel inhibitor of phosphoinositide-3-kinase signaling. Mol Cancer Ther, 2004. **3**(7): p. 763-72.

[57] Hayakawa, M., *et al.*, Synthesis and biological evaluation of sulfonylhydrazone-substituted imidazo 1,2-a pyridines as novel PI3 kinase p110 alpha inhibitors. Bioorganic & Medicinal Chemistry, 2007. **15**(17): p. 5837-5844.

[58] Hayakawa, M., *et al.*, Synthesis and biological evaluation of pyrido 3 ',2': 4,5 furo 3,2-d pyrimidine derivatives as novel PI3 kinase p110 alpha inhibitors. Bioorganic & Medicinal Chemistry Letters, 2007. **17**(9): p. 2438-2442.

[59] Hayakawa, M., *et al.,* Synthesis and biological evaluation of imidazo 1,2-a pyridine derivatives as novel PI3 kinase p110 alpha inhibitors. Bioorganic & Medicinal Chemistry, 2007. **15**(1): p. 403-412.

[60] Hayakawa, M., *et al.,* Synthesis and biological evaluation of 4-morpholino-2-phenylquinazolines and related derivatives as novel PI3 kinase p110 alpha inhibitors. Bioorganic & Medicinal Chemistry, 2006. **14**(20): p. 6847-6858.

[61] Marion, F., *et al.,* Liphagal, a selective inhibitor of PI3 kinase alpha isolated from the sponge Aka coralliphaga: Structure elucidation and biomimetic synthesis. Organic Letters, 2006. **8**(2): p. 321-324.

[62] Ihle, N.T., *et al.,* The phosphatidylinositol-3-kinase inhibitor PX-866 overcomes resistance to the epidermal growth factor receptor inhibitor gefitinib in A-549 human non-small cell lung cancer xenografts. Molecular Cancer Therapeutics, 2005. **4**(9): p. 1349-1357.

[63] Knight, Z.A., *et al.,* A pharmacological map of the PI3-K family defines a role for p110 alpha in insulin signaling. Cell, 2006. **125**(4): p. 733-747.

[64] Ihle, N.T., *et al.,* Molecular pharmacology and antitumor activity of PX-866, a novel inhibitor of phosphoinositide-3-kinase signaling. Molecular Cancer Therapeutics, 2004. **3**(7): p. 763-772.

[65] Garcia-Echeverria, C. and W.R. Sellers, Drug discovery approaches targeting the PI3K/Akt pathway in cancer. Oncogene, 2008. **27**(41): p. 5511-26.

[66] O'Brien, C., *et al.,* Predictive biomarkers of sensitivity to the phosphatidylinositol 3' kinase inhibitor GDC-0941 in breast cancer preclinical models. Clin Cancer Res, 2010. **16**(14): p. 3670-83.

[67] Chakrabarty, A., *et al.,* Feedback upregulation of HER3 (ErbB3) expression and activity attenuates antitumor effect of PI3K inhibitors. Proc Natl Acad Sci U S A, 2012. **109**(8): p. 2718-23.

[68] Maira, S.M., *et al.,* Identification and characterization of NVP-BKM120, an orally available pan class I PI3-Kinase inhibitor. Mol Cancer Ther, 2012.

[69] Castillo, J.J., M. Furman, and E.S. Winer, CAL-101: a phosphatidylinositol-3-kinase p110-delta inhibitor for the treatment of lymphoid malignancies. Expert Opin Investig Drugs, 2012. **21**(1): p. 15-22.

[70] Howes, A.L., *et al.,* The phosphatidylinositol 3-kinase inhibitor, PX-866, is a potent inhibitor of cancer cell motility and growth in three-dimensional cultures. Mol Cancer Ther, 2007. **6**(9): p. 2505-14.

[71] Miller, T.W., *et al.,* Mutations in the phosphatidylinositol 3-kinase pathway: role in tumor progression and therapeutic implications in breast cancer. Breast Cancer Res, 2011. **13**(6): p. 224.

[72] Arteaga, C.L., Abstracts of the IX Madrid Breast Cancer Conference. Madrid, Spain. November 16-17, 2011. Breast Cancer Res, 2011. **13 Suppl 2**: p. O1-15, P1-12.

[73] Lin, H., *et al.,* Synthesis and structure-activity relationships of imidazo[1,2-a]pyrimidin-5(1H)-ones as a novel series of beta isoform selective phosphatidylinositol 3-kinase inhibitors. Bioorg Med Chem Lett, 2012.

[74] Guerreiro, A.S., *et al.,* A sensitized RNA interference screen identifies a novel role for the PI3K p110gamma isoform in medulloblastoma cell proliferation and chemoresistance. Mol Cancer Res, 2011. **9**(7): p. 925-35.

[75] Tanaka, H., *et al.,* The selective class I PI3K inhibitor CH5132799 targets human cancers harboring oncogenic *PIK3CA* mutations. Clin Cancer Res, 2011. **17**(10): p. 3272-81.

[76] Carvalho, S., *et al.,* PIKing the right isoform: the emergent role of the p110beta subunit in breast cancer. Virchows Arch, 2010. **456**(3): p. 235-43.

[77] Engelman, J.A., J. Luo, and L.C. Cantley, The evolution of phosphatidylinositol 3-kinases as regulators of growth and metabolism. Nature Reviews Genetics, 2006. **7**(8): p. 606-619.

[78] McMullen, J.R. and P.Y. Jay, PI3K(p110 alpha) inhibitors as anti-cancer agents - Minding the heart. Cell Cycle, 2007. **6**(8): p. 910-913.

[79] Altomare, D.A. and J.R. Testa, Perturbations of the AKT signaling pathway in human cancer. Oncogene, 2005. **24**(50): p. 7455-7464.

[80] Staal, S.P., Molecular-Cloning of the Akt Oncogene and Its Human Homologs Akt1 and Akt2 - Amplification of Akt1 in a Primary Human Gastric Adenocarcinoma. Proceedings of the National Academy of Sciences of the United States of America, 1987. **84**(14): p. 5034-5037.

[81] Lin, X.D., *et al.,* Discovery of 2-pyrimidyl-5-amidothiophenes as potent inhibitors for AKT: Synthesis and SAR studies. Bioorganic & Medicinal Chemistry Letters, 2006. **16**(16): p. 4163-4168.

[82] Zhu, G.D., *et al.,* Isoquinoline-pyridine-based protein kinase B/Akt antagonists: SAR and *in vivo* antitumor activity. Bioorganic & Medicinal Chemistry Letters, 2006. **16**(12): p. 3150-3155.

[83] Hideshima, T., *et al.,* Perifosine, an oral bioactive novel alkylphospholipid, inhibits Akt and induces *in vitro* and *in vivo* cytotoxicity in human multiple myeloma cells. Blood, 2006. **107**(10): p. 4053-4062.

[84] Mandal, M., *et al.,* The Akt inhibitor KP372-1 inhibits proliferation and induces apoptosis and anoikis in squamous cell carcinoma of the head and neck. Oral Oncology, 2006. **42**(4): p. 430-439.

[85] Zeng, Z.H., *et al.,* Simultaneous inhibition of PDK1/AKT and Fms-like tyrosine kinase 3 signaling by a small-molecule KP372-1 induces mitochondrial dysfunction and apoptosis in acute myelogenous leukemia. Cancer Research, 2006. **66**(7): p. 3737-3746.

[86] Koul, D., *et al.,* Inhibition of Akt survival pathway by a small-molecule inhibitor in human glioblastoma. Molecular Cancer Therapeutics, 2006. **5**(3): p. 637-644.

[87] Gills, J.J., *et al.,* Spectrum of activity and molecular correlates of response to phosphatidylinositol ether lipid analogues, novel lipid-based inhibitors of Akt. Molecular Cancer Therapeutics, 2006. **5**(3): p. 713-722.

[88] Li, Q., *et al.,* Synthesis and structure-activity relationship of 3,4 '-bispyridinylethylenes: Discovery of a potent 3-isoquinolinylpyridine inhibitor of protein kinase B (PKB/Akt) for the treatment of cancer. Bioorganic & Medicinal Chemistry Letters, 2006. **16**(7): p. 2000-2007.

[89] Li, Q., *et al.,* Discovery of trans-3,4 '-bispyridinylethylenes as potent and novel inhibitors of protein kinase B (PKB/Akt) for the treatment of cancer: Synthesis and biological evaluation. Bioorganic & Medicinal Chemistry Letters, 2006. **16**(6): p. 1679-1685.

[90] Tang, H.J., *et al.,* A small molecule compound inhibits AKT pathway in ovarian cancer cell lines. Gynecologic Oncology, 2006. **100**(2): p. 308-317.

[91] Georgakis, G.V., *et al.,* Inhibition of the phosphatidylinositol-3 kinase/Akt promotes G1 cell cycle arrest and apoptosis in Hodgkin lymphoma. British Journal of Haematology, 2006. **132**(4): p. 503-511.

[92] Shi, Y., *et al.,* Optimal classes of chemotherapeutic agents sensitized by specific small-molecule inhibitors of Akt *in vitro* and *in vivo*. Neoplasia, 2005. **7**(11): p. 992-1000.

[93] Luo, Y., *et al.,* Potent and selective inhibitors of Akt kinases slow the progress of tumors *in vivo*. Molecular Cancer Therapeutics, 2005. **4**(6): p. 977-986.

[94] Mandal, M., *et al.,* The Akt inhibitor KP372-1 suppresses Akt activity and cell proliferation and induces apoptosis in thyroid cancer cells. British Journal of Cancer, 2005. **92**(10): p. 1899-1905.

[95] Shin, I., *et al.,* Proapoptotic activity of cell-permeable anti-Akt single-chain antibodies. Cancer Research, 2005. **65**(7): p. 2815-2824.

[96] Lindsley, C.W., *et al.,* Allosteric Akt (PKB) inhibitors: discovery and SAR of isozyme selective inhibitors. Bioorganic & Medicinal Chemistry Letters, 2005. **15**(3): p. 761-764.

[97] Barnett, S.F., *et al.,* Identification and characterization of pleckstrin-homology-domain-dependent and isoenzyme-specific Akt inhibitors. Biochemical Journal, 2005. **385**: p. 399-408.

[98] Hiromura, M., *et al.,* Inhibition of Akt kinase activity by a peptide spanning the beta A strand of the proto-oncogene TCL1. Journal of Biological Chemistry, 2004. **279**(51): p. 53407-53418.

[99] Meuillet, E.J., *et al., In vivo* molecular pharmacology and antitumor activity of the targeted Akt inhibitor PX-316. Oncology Research, 2004. **14**(10): p. 513-527.

[100] Jin, X., *et al.,* Inhibition of AKT survival pathway by a small molecule inhibitor in human endometrial cancer cells. British Journal of Cancer, 2004. **91**(10): p. 1808-1812.

[101] Shaw, Y.J., *et al.,* Pharmacological exploitation of the alpha 1-adrenoreceptor antagonist doxazosin to develop a novel class of antitumor agents that block intracellular protein kinase B/Akt activation. Journal of Medicinal Chemistry, 2004. **47**(18): p. 4453-4462.

[102] Yang, L., *et al.,* Akt/protein kinase B signaling inhibitor-2, a selective small molecule inhibitor of Akt signaling with antitumor activity in cancer cells overexpressing Akt. Cancer Research, 2004. **64**(13): p. 4394-4399.

[103] Castillo, S.S., *et al.,* Preferential inhibition of Akt and killing of Akt-dependent cancer cells by rationally designed phosphatidylinositol ether lipid analogues. Cancer Research, 2004. **64**(8): p. 2782-2792.

[104] Luo, Y., *et al.,* Pseudosubstrate peptides inhibit Akt and induce cell growth inhibition. Biochemistry, 2004. **43**(5): p. 1254-1263.

[105] Kondapaka, S.B., *et al.,* Perifosine, a novel alkylphospholipid, inhibits protein kinase B activation. Molecular Cancer Therapeutics, 2003. **2**(11): p. 1093-1103.

[106] Meuillet, E.J., *et al.,* Specific inhibition of the Akt1 pleckstrin homology domain by D-3-deoxy-phosphatidyl-myo-inositol analogues. Molecular Cancer Therapeutics, 2003. **2**(4): p. 389-399.

[107] Ruiter, G.A., *et al.,* Anti-cancer alkyl-lysophospholipids inhibit the phosphatidylinositol 3-kinase-Akt/PKB survival pathway. Anti-Cancer Drugs, 2003. **14**(2): p. 167-173.

[108] Reuveni, H., *et al.,* Toward a PKB inhibitor: Modification of a selective PKA inhibitor by rational design. Biochemistry, 2002. **41**(32): p. 10304-10314.

[109] Vink, S.R., *et al.,* Radiosensitization of squamous cell carcinoma by the alkylphospholipid perifosine in cell culture and xenografts. Clinical Cancer Research, 2006. **12**(5): p. 1615-1622.

[110] Li, X., *et al.,* Enhancement of antitumor activity of the anti-EGF receptor monoclonal antibody cetuximab/C225 by perifosine in PTEN-deficient cancer cells. Oncogene, 2006. **25**(4): p. 525-535.

[111] Rahmani, M., *et al.,* Coadministration of histone deacetylase inhibitors and perifosine synergistically induces apoptosis in human leukemia cells through Akt and ERK1/2 inactivation and the generation of ceramide and reactive oxygen species. Cancer Research, 2005. **65**(6): p. 2422-2432.

[112] Smorenburg, C.H., *et al.,* Phase II study of miltefosine 6% solution as topical treatment of skin metastases in breast cancer patients. Anti-Cancer Drugs, 2000. **11**(10): p. 825-828.

[113] Clive, S., J. Gardiner, and R.C.F. Leonard, Miltefosine as a topical treatment for cutaneous metastases in breast carcinoma. Cancer Chemotherapy and Pharmacology, 1999. **44**: p. S29-S30.

[114] Terwogt, J.M.M., *et al.,* Phase II trial of topically applied miltefosine solution in patients with skin-metastasized breast cancer. British Journal of Cancer, 1999. **79**(7-8): p. 1158-1161.

[115] Dummer, R., *et al.,* Topical Administration of Hexadecylphosphocholine in Patients with Cutaneous Lymphomas - Results of a Phase-I/Ii Study. Journal of the American Academy of Dermatology, 1993. **29**(6): p. 963-970.

[116] Feun, L.G., *et al.,* A Phase-Ii Trial of Tricyclic Nucleoside Phosphate in Patients with Advanced Squamous-Cell Carcinoma of the Cervix - a Gynecologic-Oncology-Group Study. American Journal of Clinical Oncology-Cancer Clinical Trials, 1993. **16**(6): p. 506-508.

[117] Feun, L.G., *et al.,* Phase-1 Study of Tricyclic Nucleoside Phosphate Using a 5-Day Continuous Infusion Schedule. Cancer Research, 1984. **44**(8): p. 3608-3612.

[118] Carol, H., *et al.,* Initial testing (stage 1) of the Akt inhibitor GSK690693 by the pediatric preclinical testing program. Pediatr Blood Cancer, 2010. **55**(7): p. 1329-37.

[119] Chan, T.O., *et al.,* Resistance of Akt kinases to dephosphorylation through ATP-dependent conformational plasticity. Proc Natl Acad Sci U S A, 2011. **108**(46): p. E1120-7.

[120] Yap, T.A., *et al.,* First-in-man clinical trial of the oral pan-AKT inhibitor MK-2206 in patients with advanced solid tumors. J Clin Oncol, 2011. **29**(35): p. 4688-95.

[121] Yoeli-Lerner, M., *et al.,* Akt blocks breast cancer cell motility and invasion through the transcription factor NFAT. Molecular Cell, 2005. **20**(4): p. 539-550.

[122] Chen, W.S., *et al.,* Growth retardation and increased apoptosis in mice with homozygous disruption of the *akt1* gene. Genes & Development, 2001. **15**(17): p. 2203-2208.

[123] Cho, H., *et al.,* Insulin resistance and a diabetes mellitus-like syndrome in mice lacking the protein kinase Akt2 (PKB beta). Science, 2001. **292**(5522): p. 1728-1731.

[124] Tschopp, O., *et al.,* Essential role of protein kinase B gamma (PKB gamma/Akt3) in postnatal brain development but not in glucose homeostasis. Development, 2005. **132**(13): p. 2943-2954.

[125] Wullschleger, S., R. Loewith, and M.N. Hall, TOR signaling in growth and metabolism. Cell, 2006. **124**(3): p. 471-484.

[126] Bernardi, R., *et al.,* PML inhibits HIF-1 alpha translation and neoangiogenesis through repression of mTOR. Nature, 2006. **442**(7104): p. 779-785.

[127] Sehgal, S.N., H. Baker, and C. Vezina, Rapamycin (Ay-22,989), a New Antifungal Antibiotic.2. Fermentation, Isolation and Characterization. Journal of Antibiotics, 1975. **28**(10): p. 727-732.

[128] Neuhaus, P., J. Klupp, and J.M. Langrehr, mTOR inhibitors: An overview. Liver Transplantation, 2001. **7**(6): p. 473-484.

[129] Hudes, G., *et al.,* Temsirolimus, interferon alfa, or both for advanced renal-cell carcinoma. N Engl J Med, 2007. **356**(22): p. 2271-81.

[130] Baselga, J., *et al.,* Everolimus in Postmenopausal Hormone-Receptor-Positive Advanced Breast Cancer. N Engl J Med, 2011.

[131] Wiederrecht, G.J., *et al.,* Mechanism of action of rapamycin: new insights into the regulation of G1-phase progression in eukaryotic cells. Prog Cell Cycle Res, 1995. **1**: p. 53-71.

[132] Sarbassov, D.D., S.M. Ali, and D.M. Sabatini, Growing roles for the mTOR pathway. Current Opinion in Cell Biology, 2005. **17**(6): p. 596-603.

[133] Manning, B.D., Balancing Akt with S6K: implications for both metabolic diseases and tumorigenesis. Journal of Cell Biology, 2004. **167**(3): p. 399-403.

[134] Sarbassov, D.D., *et al.,* Phosphorylation and regulation of Akt/PKB by the rictor-mTOR complex. Science, 2005. **307**(5712): p. 1098-1101.

[135] Sarbassov, D.D., *et al.,* Prolonged rapamycin treatment inhibits mTORC2 assembly and Akt/PKB. Molecular Cell, 2006. **22**(2): p. 159-168.

[136] Benjamin, D., *et al.,* Rapamycin passes the torch: a new generation of mTOR inhibitors. Nat Rev Drug Discov, 2011. **10**(11): p. 868-80.

[137] O'Regan, R. and N.N. Hawk, mTOR inhibition in breast cancer: unraveling the complex mechanisms of mTOR signal transduction and its clinical implications in therapy. Expert Opin Ther Targets, 2011. **15**(7): p. 859-72.

[138] Fan, Q.W., *et al.,* A dual PI3 kinase/mTOR inhibitor reveals emergent efficacy in glioma. Cancer Cell, 2006. **9**(5): p. 341-349.

[139] Raynaud, F.I., *et al.,* Pharmacologic characterization of a potent inhibitor of class I phosphatidylinositide 3-kinases. Cancer Research, 2007. **67**(12): p. 5840-5850.

[140] Whyte, D.B. and S.L. Holbeck, Correlation of *PIK3Ca* mutations with gene expression and drug sensitivity in NCI-60 cell lines. Biochemical and Biophysical Research Communications, 2006. **340**(2): p. 469-475.

[141] Saal, L.H., *et al., PIK3CA* mutations correlate with hormone receptors, node metastasis, and ERBB2, and are mutually exclusive with PTEN loss in human breast carcinoma. Cancer Research, 2005. **65**(7): p. 2554-2559.

[142] Chan, C.T., M.Z. Metz, and S.E. Kane, Differential sensitivities of trastuzumab (Herceptin (R))-resistant human breast cancer cells to phosphoinositide-3 kinase (PI-3K) and epidermal growth factor receptor (EGFR) kinase inhibitors. Breast Cancer Research and Treatment, 2005. **91**(2): p. 187-201.

[143] Jordan, N.J., *et al.,* Increased constitutive activity of PKB/Akt in tamoxifen resistant breast cancer MCF-7 cells. Breast Cancer Research and Treatment, 2004. **87**(2): p. 167-180.

[144] Yakes, F.M., *et al.,* Herceptin-induced inhibition of phosphatidylinositol-3 kinase and Akt is required for antibody-mediated effects on p27, cyclin D1, and antitumor action. Cancer Research, 2002. **62**(14): p. 4132-4141.

[145] Perez-Tenorio, G. and O. Stal, Activation of AKT/PKB in breast cancer predicts a worse outcome among endocrine treated patients. British Journal of Cancer, 2002. **86**(4): p. 540-545.

[146] Sanchez, C.G., *et al.,* Preclinical modeling of combined phosphatidylinositol-3-kinase inhibition with endocrine therapy for estrogen receptor-positive breast cancer. Breast Cancer Res, 2011. **13**(2): p. R21.

[147] Gupta, S., *et al.,* Binding of ras to phosphoinositide 3-kinase p110alpha is required for ras-driven tumorigenesis in mice. Cell, 2007. **129**(5): p. 957-68.

[148] Higgins, M.J., *et al., PIK3CA* mutations and EGFR overexpression predict for lithium sensitivity in human breast epithelial cells. Cancer Biol Ther, 2011. **11**(3): p. 358-67.

CHAPTER 2

AKT Signaling in Regulating Angiogenesis

Bing-Hua Jiang* **and Ling-Zhi Liu***

Department of Pathology, Anatomy and Cell Biology, Thomas Jefferson University, Philadelphia, PA 19107, USA

Abstract: AKT is a central signaling molecule in regulating cell survival, proliferation, tumor growth and angiogenesis. Upstream components of AKT signaling pathway such as PI3K, PTEN, and Ras are commonly mutated in many human cancers. Some miRNAs are also involved in regulating PI3K/AKT signaling pathway. Recently it is found that AKT plays an important role in regulating normal vascularization and pathological angiogenesis. Angiogenesis is required for tumor growth and metastasis when tumor reaches more than 1 mm in diameter. This review focuses on the role and potential mechanism of AKT signaling in regulating angiogenesis. Recent studies have shown that AKT activation is necessary and sufficient to regulate VEGF and HIF-1α expression in human cancer cells. VEGF and HIF-1α are potent inducers of angiogenesis. It was found that AKT activation induces VEGF and HIF-1α expression through its two downstream molecules HDM2 and p70S6K1. On the other hand, AKT transmits the upstream signals from growth factors, cytokines, heavy metals, and oncogenes for regulating VEGF and HIF-1α expression in human cancer cells. AKT activation and VEGF expression can be inhibited by different natural products used for cancer prevention. Thus, inhibition of AKT and its downstream targets offers a new approach for targeting angiogenesis, which could be important for the development of new cancer therapeutics in the future.

Keywords: AKT, VEGF, HIF-1, tumor growth, vascularization, and angiogenesis.

INTRODUCTION

AKT is the cellular homolog of AKT8 retroviral oncogene [1]. AKT is also known as protein kinase B (PKB) that transmits survival signals from growth factors [2-4]. Human AKT has three isoforms: AKT1, AKT2, and AKT3 (also known as PKBα, PKBβ, and PKBγ). AKT is involved in the regulation of cell survival, migration, proliferation, metabolism, tumor growth, and angiogenesis [2, 3, 5, 6]. Activation of AKT requires two events to occur: the binding of a lipid second messenger to its intact pleckstrin homology (PH) domain and phosphorylation of the

***Address corresponding to Bing-Hua Jiang and Ling-Zhi Liu:** Department of Pathology, Anatomy and Cell Biology, Thomas Jefferson University, Philadelphia, PA 19107; E-mails: binghjiang@yahoo.com; Ling-Zhi.Liu@jefferson.edu

PH domain by phosphoinositide-dependent kinase [3, 7]. AKT can be activated by phosphatidylinositol 3-kinase (PI3K), oncogenes Src and Ras [1]. The schematic representation of AKT activation is shown in Fig. **1**. PI3K is a heterodimeric enzyme composed of a 110-kD catalytic subunit and an 85-kD regulatory subunit [8]. PI3K phosphorylates the D3 hydroxyl of phosphoinositide resulting in the production of phosphatidyl-inositol-3-phosphate. PI3K binds to and is activated by several receptor and nonreceptor protein tyrosine kinases (PTKs) [9-11]. As a general rule, PTKs interact with the p85 regulatory subunit of PI3K, while Ras protein interacts directly with the p110 catalytic subunit in a GTP-dependent manner. AKT1 and AKT2 were found to be amplified in several kinds of human cancers, indicating the relationship between AKT and carcinogenesis [12-14]. PI3K and AKT have many other targets including nitric oxide synthase (NOS) [15, 16], nuclear factor-kappaB (NF-κB) [17-19], BAD [20], p70/85 S6 kinase [21, 22], glycogen synthase kinase 3 [23], and Jun N-terminal kinase [24]. AKT activity is negatively regulated by the tumor suppressor phosphatase and tensin homolog deleted on chromosome ten (PTEN), a phospholipid phosphatase that antagonizes PI3K activity by dephosphorylating PIP3 [25].

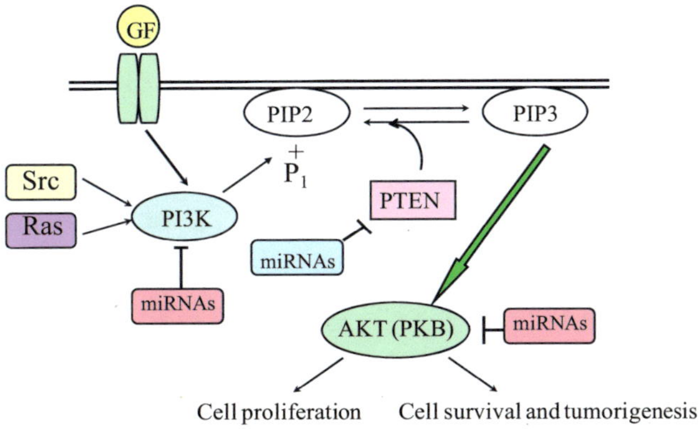

Figure 1: The schematic representation of PI3K/AKT activation. Growth factors (GF), Src, and Ras induce PI3K activation. PI3K phosphorylates phophatidylinositol-4,5- bisphosphate (PIP2) at the 3' position to generate phophatidylinositol-3,4,5-trisphosphate (PIP3), which in turn activates AKT for regulating cell proliferation, survival, and tumorigenesis. PTEN reverses this process by removing the phosphate group. MiRNAs may directly target PI3K and AKT for decreasing their expression levels.

AKT is activated by cytokines and growth factors including vascular endothelial growth factor (VEGF) [26], fibroblast growth factor (FGF) [27, 28], epidermal growth factor (EGF) [29, 30], hepatocyte growth factor (HGF) [31, 32], insulin-like growth factor (IGF) [33,34], and angiopoietin [35], by oncogenes such as Ras and Src [36], by amplification or activated mutations of PI3K [37, 38]; and by the mutations or deletions of tumor suppressor such as PTEN, which frequently occurs in human cancers [25]. AKT gene amplification has been observed in a subset of human cancers. For example, *AKT 1* gene amplification has been detected in a single gastric carcinoma and glioblastoma [14, 39], *AKT 2* gene amplification has been reported in human ovarian, pancreatic and breast cancers [13, 40], and AKT 3 mRNA was overexpressed in breast and prostate cancers [41]. *AKT 1* amplification is also involved in drug resistance of lung cancer cells against cisplatin [42].

Angiogenesis is the process by which new blood capillaries are generated from the pre-existing vasculature. The process involves multiple steps including dissolution of the basement membrane of the vessel, endothelial cell migration and proliferation, formation of a new vessel lumen and vessel branches, and maturation of the new vessel by the recruitment of pericytes, and the formation of basement membrane [43, 44]. AKT is activated by VEGF and agiopoietin 1 in endothelial cells, which is implicated in regulating angiogenesis. The first direct evidence of AKT in regulating angiogenesis was observed by the forced expression of AKT in chicken chorioallantoic membrane (CAM) by RCAS retroviral vector [5]. AKT regulates multiple downstream targets, however, the specific targets of AKT in inducing angiogenesis remain to be defined. Tumor growth and metastasis require angiogenesis when the tumor reaches 1-2 mm in diameter [45]. Inhibition of angiogenesis specifically suppresses tumor growth and invasion, while normal mature vessels in human body are not affected. Thus, there are growing interests in developing anti-angiogenesis approaches for human cancer therapy. In this review, we highlight recent findings and potential mechanisms of AKT in regulating angiogenesis.

ANGIOGENESIS AND CANCER

Angiogenesis is essential for female reproduction, embryo development, tissue repair, tumor growth and metastasis. Tumor angiogenesis occurs *via* the sprouting of new vessels from pre-existing blood vessels or *via* the insertion of interstitial tissue columns into the lumen of pre-existing vessels (*i.e.*, intussusception) [46].

Although various kinds of growth factors and cytokines are inducers of angiogenesis, recent studies have demonstrated that the VEGF/VEGF receptor (VEGFR) and angiopoietin/Tie2 signaling systems are central regulators of embryonic angiogenesis [47-49]. VEGF and its receptors are the major regulators of the vessel morphogenesis phase of angiogenesis, angiopoietin 1(Ang-1) and its receptor, Tie-2, are implicated in the vascular maturation phase [48]. Angiogenesis is important in cancer development and growth, invasion, and metastasis since tumors cannot grow larger than 1-2 millimeters in diameter without sufficient blood supply provided by angiogenesis [50].

Tumor angiogenesis can be triggered by extracellular signals, such as growth factors including FGF, EGF, VEGF, HGF, and IL-8; and by genetic alterations such as activation of oncogenes, or mutation of tumor suppressor genes including lost function of retinoblastoma protein, PTEN, and p53 [46, 50-53]. Antiangiogenic therapy is designed to inhibit signaling pathways or molecules that regulate angiogenesis during the cancer therapy. The advantages of this therapy is that some of the antiangiogenic agents have low toxicity, and can be administered long-term without interruptions during the therapeutic process [45]. More than 30 angiogenesis inhibitors are currently in clinical trials for cancer, macular degeneration and diabetic retinopathy [45]. Avastin is the first anti-angiogenesis inhibitor approved by FDA, the United States for the colorectal cancer therapy [54]. Since then, a few other angiogenesis inhibitors have been approved [45]. However, continued clinical and preclinical investigations have identified some challenges associated with the application of anti-angiogenesis agents, including inherent/acquired resistance [55], induction of tumor invasiveness [56], and lack of thoroughly validated predictive biomarkers [57]. Anti-angiogenesis therapy has demonstrated efficacy in a variety of human malignancies, in particular when added to conventional cytotoxic chemotherapy and some of the agents are ongoing clinical trials [58]. For example, most trials of anti-angiogenic agents in breast cancer have reported improved response rates and progression-free survival, but no increase of overall survival when compared to chemotherapy alone [59]. Optimizing the therapeutic strategies of antiangiogenic agents is a focus of ongoing research which would be critical to the future success of drug development

AKT SIGNALING IS ACTIVATED BY VEGF AND ANGIOPOIETINS

VEGFR family and the Tie [(tyrosine kinase with immunoglobulin (Ig) and EGF homology domains)] receptor family are two receptor tyrosine kinase subfamilies that are expressed specifically in endothelium [60]. There are three forms of VEGF receptors, VEGFR-1 (fms-like tyrosine kinase, Flt-1), VEGFR-2 (Flk-1/KDR), and VEGFR-3 (Flt-4). These receptors play a critical role in promoting vasculogenesis and angiogenesis during normal embryogenesis and pathologic angiogenesis [61-64]. Recent studies demonstrate that the p85 regulatory subunit of PI3K, is constitutively associated with and phosphorylated by Flk-1/KDR, resulting in increased PI3K and AKT activities *in vitro* [65, 66]. VEGF-induced endothelial cell survival was blocked by PI3K inhibitors, wortmannin and LY294002, and by overexpression of a dominant-negative form of AKT [65-67].

The Tie receptor family comprises of Tie1 and Tie2/Tek. Knockout of Tie1 or Tie2 is lethal because of severe defects in embryonic vasculature [68, 69]. Tie2 receptor has also been shown to play an important role in endothelial cell survival, vascular morphogenesis, and tumor angiogenesis [70-72]. The angiopoietins are a family of secreted proteins including three human angiopoietins (Ang-1, Ang-2, and Ang-4), and one mouse angiopoietin Ang-3 [73-75]. Angiopoietins and their receptor Tie2 have been reported to play a major role in angiogenesis. Ang-1 and Ang-4 activate the Tie2 receptor, whereas Ang-2 and Ang-3 inhibit Ang-1-induced Tie2 phosphorylation and activation [74-76]. Several lines of evidence suggest that PI3K/AKT signaling plays a major role in Ang-1-mediated cell migration and tube formation *in vitro*: 1) Ang-1 was shown to induce phosphorylation of the p85 subunit of PI3K which increased PI3K activities and in turn activated AKT in cultured human endothelial cells [77, 78]; 2) Ang-1 induced survival of cultured endothelial cells, which was abolished by the inhibition of PI3K and AKT activities in cultured endothelial cells [77, 78]; 3) Ang-1 was shown to induce migration and sprouting of endothelial cells *via* PI3K activation [77-79]. Ang-2 was reported to enhance endothelial cell survival through PI3K/AKT signaling pathway, while the release of Ang-2 in lung microvascular endothelial cells is regulated by PI3K/AKT signaling [80, 81]. The biological functions of Ang-4 are contradictory. While some studies found that Ang-4 induced survival and migration in primary cultured endothelial cells and increased corneal angiogenesis extending from the limbus across the mouse cornea *in vivo* [82], other studies showed that Ang-4 inhibited tumor cell-induced angiogenesis [83].

MiRNAs AND PI3K/AKT SIGNALING PATHWAY

MicroRNAs are a class of small noncoding RNAs that have been identified as a new kind of gene expression regulators through targeting mRNAs for translational repression or degradation [84-86]. MiRNAs regulate various cellular functions such as cell apoptosis, cell proliferation, neural development, and stem cell differentiation [87-89]. MiRNAs are also found to play pivotal roles in tumorigenesis, cancer invasion, and metastasis [90, 91]. Growing lines of evidence have demonstrated that some miRNAs target signaling molecules in PI3K/AKT pathway and regulate angiogenesis. For instance, miR-494 [92], miR-93 [93], miR-22 [94], miR-29a [95], miR-29b [96], miR-221/222 [97], miR-301 [98], miR-214 [99], miR-486 [100], miR-205 [101], miR-141 [102], miR-216, miR-217 [103], and miR-21 [104] target PTEN, leading to the activation of AKT. It has been demonstrated that miR-7 inhibits liver tumor growth and metastasis by targeting PI3K catalytic subunit delta (PIK3CD), miR-126 targets PIK3R2, thus inhibiting PI3K/AKT pathway [105, 106]. *AKT1* is a direct target of miR-149*, which induces apoptosis as a pro-apoptotic miRNA [107]. MiR-150 and miR-184 are demonstrated to target *AKT2*, reduce levels of phosphorylated AKT to inhibit cancer cell survival [108, 109]. On the other hand, AKT isoform can also regulate some miRNAs such as miR-210 family [110].

MiRNAs can also indirectly activate AKT pathway. A recent study has shown that miR-320 is a crucial component of a PTEN-controlled tumor-suppressive axis in stromal fibroblasts. Loss of PTEN and miR-320 promotes invasion and angiogenesis [111]. MiR-17~92 cluster mediates chemoresistance and enhances tumor growth in mantle cell lymphoma *via* PI3K/AKT pathway activation by targeting the protein phosphatase PHLPP2 [112]. Suppression of membrane-associated guanylate kinase by miR-101 reduces PTEN activity, leading to AKT activation [113]. Other recent study showed that miR-218 targets the mTOR component Rictor and inhibits AKT S473 phosphorylation in oral cancer [114]. In addition, some miRNAs can target the upstream molecules of PI3K/AKT signaling pathway, such as IGF-1R, IRS-1, and EGFR, to regulate PI3K/AKT signaling activation.

Mammalian target of rapamycin (mTOR), the downstream target of AKT, is a direct target of miR-520c, miR-373, miR-99a, miR-99b, miR-100, miR-199-3p [115-119]. P70S6K1, the downstream molecule of mTOR, plays an important role in protein synthesis, cell cycle, cell growth, cell survival and angiogenesis. Our recent studies have demonstrated that miR-145 and miR-128 directly target p70S6K1 to suppress tumor growth and angiogenesis [120, 121]. Thus, the identification of miRNAs in targeting or regulating PI3K/AKT pathway may reveal a novel field of cancer research, which will be helpful to shed light on the mechanisms of carcinogenesis and angiogenesis.

ROLE OF AKT IN TUMOR ANGIOGENESIS

The initial observation of the role of AKT in regulating angiogenesis was performed by the forced expression of AKT by the avian retroviral vector RCAS in the CAM [5]. We showed that forced expression of active forms of AKT or PI3K by RCAS vector greatly increased the number of the sprouting vessels and size of the vessels to induce angiogenesis *in vivo*, suggesting that AKT activation is sufficient for inducing angiogenesis [5]. The activation of PI3K/AKT signaling is commonly observed in different human cancers, partly due to the amplification of PI3K and AKT, or due to the activation mutations of PI3K and AKT [122]. To specifically down-regulate PI3K and AKT expression in cancer cells, we designed small interference RNA (siRNA) against p110α subunit of PI3K and AKT, and found that the downregulation of PI3K or AKT by their siRNA constructs in human ovarian cancer cells greatly decreased tumor growth and angiogenesis [123]. A recent study has shown that blocking activation of PI3K/AKT pathway during anti-angiogenesis therapy exhibits an enhanced antitumor efficacy [124]. These data suggest that the expression of PI3K and AKT in cancer cells is required for tumor angiogenesis [123]. In a different system, treatment of the cells by PI3K inhibitor LY294002 decreased glioma tumor growth and tumor-induced angiogenic response [125]. Similarly, several other compounds such as RY10-4, ON-III (2',4'-dihydroxy-6'-methoxy-3',5'-dimethylchalcone), capsaicin, SU5416, and apigenin were observed to inactivate PI3K/AKT pathway in several different kinds of cancer cells including lung, fibrosarcoma, melanoma, hepatocarcinoma, and ovarian cancer cells. These compounds were shown to decrease tumor-induced angiogenesis [126-130]. These results further support an important role of AKT in regulating tumor angiogenesis.

Oxidative stress (OS) plays an important role in the progression of chronic diseases including cancer. We found that compared to the immortalized normal ovarian surface epithelial cells, ovarian cancer cells generated higher reactive oxygen species (ROS). Similar results were found in prostate cancer cells. The increased levels of endogenous ROS in ovarian cancer cells were due to increased expression of NOX4 subunit of NADPH oxidase. ROS promotes HIF-1 and VEGF expression through the activation of PI3K/AKT pathway, leading to the induction of tumor angiogenesis and tumor growth [131]. In agree with our results, Jo M, *et al.* found that ROS enhances the malignant potential of hepatocellular carcinoma through the stimulation of angiogenesis by activation of the AKT-VEGF pathway [132]. Given that ROS have been demonstrated as mediators of angiogenesis [133-135], AKT is one of the important signaling pathways in oxidative stress-induced tumor growth and angiogenesis.

ROLE OF AKT IN NORMAL VASCULARIZATION

The tumor suppressor PTEN is a phospholipid phosphatase which dephophosphorylates phosphatidylinositol (3,4,5)-trisphosphate for inhibiting AKT activation. Forced expression of PTEN inhibited embryonic vascularization and angiogenesis, indicating that PTEN may inhibit AKT activation for decreasing angiogenesis [5]. Forced expression of a constitutively active form of AKT caused abnormal vascularization in mice, suggesting that on the other hand, appropriate down-regulation of AKT is also an essential aspect of normal vascularization [136]. In mammals, there are three isoforms of AKT: AKT-1/PKBα, AKT-2/PKBβ, and AKT-3/ PKBγ that are encoded by separate genes. These three isoforms have a similar domain structure with approximately 80% amino acid identity [137]. *Akt1-/-* mice have defects in both fetal and postnatal growth into adulthood [138, 139]. The *AKT1* deficient mice display a conspicuous impairment in organism growth. Since *AKT1* is widely expressed in placenta including all types of trophoblast and vascular endothelial cells, *Akt1-/-* mice exhibited smaller litter size, reduced fetal weight, and a higher fetal mortality due to the impaired extraembryonic vascularization and placental hypotrophy [140], indicating the significant role of AKT1 in fetal development and vascularization. AKT1 is the predominant isoform in vascular cells. Recently, impaired vascular maturation due to lower activation of endothelial nitric oxide synthase (eNOS) and the major phenotypic changes in vascular permeability and angiogenesis are linked to lower expression of two endogenous vascular inhibitors, thrombospondins 1 and 2 (TSP-1 and TSP-2) that were also found in *Akt1-/-* mice [141]. AKT1 was also shown to be critical for ischemic- and VEGF-induced angiogenesis. The *Akt1-/-* mice have defective ischemia- and VEGF-induced angiogenesis and severe peripheral vascular disease. *Akt1-/-* mice have much less endothelial progenitor cell (EPC) mobilization in response to ischemia, and reintroduction of wild-type EPCs, but not EPCs isolated from *Akt1-/-* mice, into mice improved limb blood flow after ischemia. Reconstitution of *Akt1-/-* EPCs with Akt1 construct rescued the defects, increased the migration of fibroblasts and endothelial cells [142]. Thus, these data indicate that AKT1 is sufficient and essential for regulating ischemia-induced angiogenesis. In mice, AKT2 is shown to be required for insulin signaling and for maintaining normal glucose homeostasis. In the absence of AKT2, insulin-stimulated glucose uptake in muscle and fat was significantly reduced [143]. In contrast to *Akt1-/-* mice, which have smaller sizes of all organs, *Akt3-/-* mice have a specific 20% decrease in brain size than the wild-type mice [144].

AKT REGULATES VEGF EXPRESSION

Angiogenesis is regulated by the increase of angiogenesis inducers or decrease of angiogenesis inhibitors. VEGF is a major angiogenesis inducer associated with tumor angiogenesis and growth in numerous solid malignancies [47, 145]. The VEGF has four major isoforms: VEGF 121, VEGF 165, VEGF 189, and VEGF 206 that are derived from the splicing variance of VEGF. VEGF 165 is the dominant isoform with the most potent effect in inducing angiogenesis [146]. Lines of evidence show that PI3K/AKT signaling are important for regulating VEGF expression: 1) Ras expression was shown to increase VEGF expression and PI3K was a downstream target of Ras to mediate Ras-induced VEGF expression [147]; 2) insulin induced VEGF expression through PI3K/AKT signaling [5]; and 3) hepatocyte growth factor induced VEGF expression through

AKT activation [31]. These studies indicate that PI3K/AKT signaling is required for growth factor-induced VEGF expression. Forced expression of PI3K or AKT alone directly increased VEGF mRNA expression, suggesting that PI3K and AKT are sufficient to regulate VEGF expression [5]. PI3K and AKT activation is commonly observed in cancer cells. In prostate and ovarian cancer cells, the inhibition of PI3K signaling by LY294002 decreased VEGF expression [148-150], suggesting that PI3K and AKT signaling is required for elevated levels of VEGF expression in cancer cells. The siRNA technology was used as additional approach for specifically inhibiting PI3K or AKT. Similarly, VEGF expression was decreased by PI3K and AKT down-regulation using their siRNA constructs [123]. In different cell system, it was shown that activation of AKT is required for benzo(a) pyrene diol-epoxide-induced VEGF transcriptional activation [151]. Other study showed malignant hematopoietic cells increased expression of VEGFR-1 and VEGFR-3 in bone marrow endothelial cells through activation of AKT and mTOR signaling pathways, indicating that AKT may be a key regulator for VEGF and VEGF receptor expression. It is possible that VEGF activates PI3K and AKT signaling pathway, which in turn regulates VEGF and VEGF receptor expression in the cells [152]. VEGFR-2 can maintain the hematopoietic progenitor population in mouse bone marrow and increase cell survival mediated by activation of PI3K/AKT pathway [153]. Thus, AKT and VEGF may form an autocrine loop in the cells for regulating tumor growth and angiogenesis.

AKT REGULATES HIF-1α EXPRESSION

Hypoxia-inducable factor 1 (HIF-1) is a heterodimeric transcription factor composed of HIF-1α and HIF-1β subunits [154, 155]. HIF-1α, originally cloned by our group at the Johns Hopkins University, is induced by hypoxia, growth factors, and oncogenes. In contrast, HIF-1β protein is constitutively expressed in human cells. Levels of HIF-1α protein are a rate-limiting factor for HIF-1 activity in the cells. HIF-1α regulates the expression of many genes, including VEGF, heme oxygenase 1, inducible nitric oxide synthase (iNOS), and several glycolytic enzymes [156, 157]. HIF-1α expression is important for tumor growth and angiogenesis [158-160]. HIF-1α knockout mice showed defects in embryonic vascularization [160, 161]. Under normoxic conditions, prolyl hydroxylases (PHDs) hydroxylate proline residues of HIF-1α at 402 and 564 within the oxygen-dependent degradation (ODD) domain [162-164], which triggers the binding of von Hipple-Lindau (VHL) protein to HIF-1α, and the degradation of HIF-1α through the ubiquitin-mediated proteasome degradation pathway [162-164]. In contrast, under the hypoxia condition, proline residues of HIF-1 are not hydroxylated by PHDs, preventing HIF-1α from the degradation by proteasome pathway [165].

HIF-1α expression in cancer cells was shown to be regulated by PI3K/AKT signaling by using LY294002 and wortmannin [30], indicating that AKT activation is required for HIF-1α expression. PTEN deletion increased hypoxia- and IGF-I-induced gene expression regulated by HIF-1 in glioblastoma cell lines, and overexpression of wild-type PTEN decreased the gene expression through AKT activation [166]. Similarly, we found that PTEN mutation in cancer cells exhibited much higher HIF-1α levels than those in other cancer cells with wild-type PTEN expression, and the reconstitution of PTEN expression in the cells decreased HIF-1α levels [167]. PI3K/AKT activation is required for insulin- and EGF-induced HIF-1α, but not HIF-1β expression [167]. In human ovarian cancer cells, we also found that AKT activation mediated HIF-1α expression and HIF-1-mediated VEGF transcriptional activation [150]. AKT regulated HIF-1α expression and transcriptional activation through two downstream targets, HDM2 and p70S6K1 [150]. The oncoprotein HDM2 was shown to be phosphorylated on serine 166 and serine 186 which is necessary for translocation of HDM2 from the cytoplasm into the nucleus through AKT activation [168]. Inhibition of PI3K/AKT signaling by PI3K inhibitor or expression of dominant negative PI3K and AKT mutants inhibited nuclear entry of HDM2, increased cellular levels of p53, and augmented p53 transcriptional activity [168]. It was reported that AKT overexpression, IGF-I stimulation, or loss of PTEN caused increased expression of HDM2 and HIF-1α. Moreover, transient expression of a dominant negative form of AKT or LY294002 inhibited IGF-I-induced HIF-1α expression through HDM2 expression [169]. These results demonstrate that AKT activation is required for regulating HIF-1α expression and HDM2 function.

HEAVY METALS REGULATE VEGF AND HIF-1α EXPRESSION *VIA* AKT PATHWAY

Some heavy metals such as vanadate, arsenite, and nickel are strong carcinogens for inducing tumor growth and angiogenesis [170, 171]. Vanadate is a widely distributed trace metal. The burning of fossil fuels (petroleum, coal, and oil) in power and heat producing plants causes widespread discharge of vanadate into the environment. Vanadate induced VEGF and HIF-1α expression through the activation of PI3K and AKT [172, 173], suggesting that vanadate-induced HIF-1 and VEGF expression may be important in regulating vanadate-induced carcinogenesis. Vanadate was also shown to induce HIF-1α and VEGF expression through AMP-activated protein kinase [174, 175]. Arsenite is widely distributed environmental toxicant in water, food and air. High levels of arsenite are strongly associated with human cancers originated from liver, nasal cavity, lung, skin, bladder, kidney, and prostate [176-178]. Arsenite treatment induced VEGF expression through the induction of HIF-1α, but not HIF-1β expression in human prostate cancer cells [173, 179]. AKT activation and p70S6K1 phosphorylation are required for arsenite-induced expression of HIF-1α and VEGF [173, 179]. These results are similar to other study demonstrating that arsenite induced VEGF and HIF-1α expression in a different cell system [180]. We found that arsenite induced angiogenesis through increasing HIF-1 and VEGF expression *via* AKT and ERK1/2 pathways [181]. Similar results were obtained by cadmium treatment [182]. Chronic treatment with arsenite caused cell transformation by activating EGFR, AKT and ERK1/2 pathways [182-184]. Nickel compounds exerted carcinogenic effects through alterations in gene expressions that may be mediated by increasing the expression of transcription factors [185]. Exposure of mouse epithelial cells to nickel compound Ni_3S_2 or $NiCl_2$ activated PI3K/AKT signaling pathway. Inhibition of PI3K or AKT by dominant-negative mutants of PI3K and AKT, respectively, impaired nickel-induced HIF-1α transcriptional activation [186]. These data indicate that heavy metals have a common mechanism to increase HIF-1α and VEGF expression through PI3K and AKT activation, which may account for the carcinogenic effects of heavy metals.

AKT IS THE COMMON TARGET INHIBITED BY DIFFERENT NATURAL PRODUCTS WITH POTENTIAL CHEMOPREVENTION EFFECTS

Recent studies show that some natural products from daily diets have anti-cancer effects. A few examples of these compounds include resveratrol, apigenin, capsaicin, and luteolin. Resveratrol is present in many plant species and especially abundant in grapes, peanuts, and mulberries. Apigenin (4',5,7,-trihydroxyflavone) is a common dietary flavonoid which is widely present in many fruits and vegetables including parsley, onions, oranges, tea, chamomile, wheat sprouts, and in some seasonings. Apigenin is used as a healthy food supplement and has recently been shown to possess anti-tumor properties by inhibiting cell proliferation and tube formation [187]. It was reported that apigenin inhibited skin tumorigenesis initiated by 7,12-dimethylbenz(a)anthracene (DMBA) and promoted by 2-O-tetradecanoylphorbol-13-acetate (TPA) in SENCAR mice [188]. Our recent data showed that resveratrol and apigenin inhibited HIF-1α and VEGF expression through inhibiting AKT signaling pathway [126, 148, 149]. Apigenin also inhibited tumor growth and tumor angiogenesis *in vivo* [126, 189]. Capsaicin, the major pungent ingredient in red pepper, has long been used in food additives. It inhibited VEGF-induced cell proliferation, DNA synthesis, chemotactic motility, and capillary-like tube formation *in vitro*. It was shown to inhibit tumor angiogenesis *in vivo* by CAM model [127]. Luteolin, a bioactive flavonoid, inhibited tumor growth and angiogenesis in a murine xenograft model, and inhibited VEGF-induced angiogenesis in the rabbit corneal assay [190]. It was shown that the anti-tumor effect of luteolin was through inhibiting PI3K/AKT signaling pathway [190]. Our recent study indicated that luteolin inhibited insulin-like growth factor I (IGF-I)-induced activation of IGF-IR and AKT, which may in turn suppress cell proliferation and induce apoptosis [191]. Knockdown of IGF-IR by siRNA led to inhibition of prostate cancer cell proliferation. Luteolin also inhibited tumor growth and angiogenesis *in vivo*, potentially through IGF-IR/AKT signaling [191]. Similar chemoprevention effects are observed in other natural compounds such as linoleic acid (CLA) [192], lycopene [193], and genistein [194]. These compounds commonly inhibit AKT activation in the cells. These results suggest that natural products in normal diets may inhibit AKT activation in cancer cells, which is useful for cancer prevention.

THERAPEUTIC PERSPECTIVES FOR TARGETING AKT AND MTOR

AKT plays a key role in transmitting the signals from growth factors and cytokines for regulating cell survival and proliferation. Recently it is known that AKT regulates angiogenesis and the expression of VEGF and HIF-1α. The role and mechanism of AKT in tumor growth and angiogenesis are summarized in Fig.

2. Thus, understanding the mechanism of AKT signaling pathway in regulating angiogenesis is important for potential cancer intervention and therapy. AKT is a potential target of choice for anti-angiogenesis therapy. Furthermore, mutations of

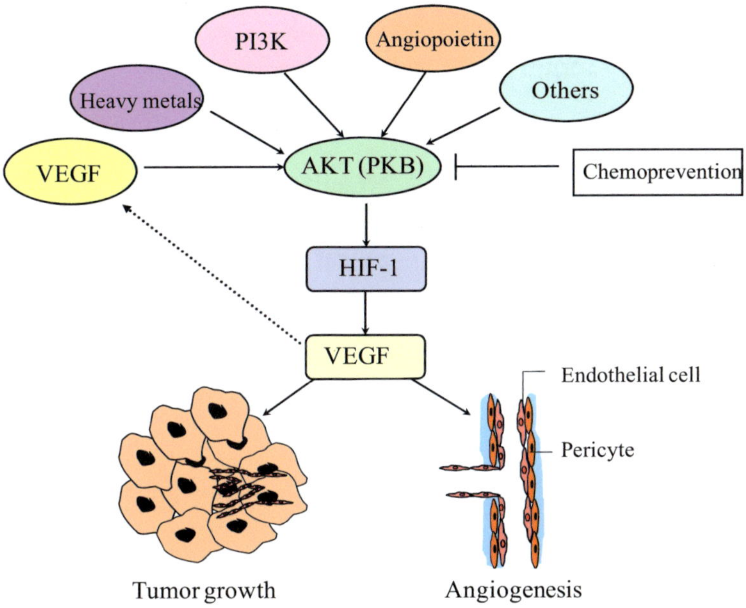

Figure 2: The outline of AKT signaling in regulating tumor growth and angiogenesis. AKT is activated by several upstream inducers such as VEGF, angiopoietins, PI3K, and heavy metals. AKT activation induces tumor growth and angiogenesis through the expression of HIF-1 and VEGF. AKT and VEGF may form an autocrine loop for regulating the cellular functions. Some natural compounds used for chemoprevention inhibit AKT signaling pathway for inhibiting tumor growth and angiogenesis.

AKT upstream molecules such as Ras, PI3K, and PTEN are commonly detected in many human cancers. The development of AKT inhibitors would also offer an advantage by targeting a central signaling molecule for transmitting these upstream signals. Since AKT has three different isoforms with some structure and function difference, it is possible to develop isoform-specific AKT inhibitors that could inhibit AKT membrane localization and function regulated by its PH domain in the cells. In addition, mammalian target of rapamycin (mTOR) is one of AKT downstream targets. The ongoing preclinical and clinical study indicates that mTOR inhibitors, rapamycin analogs CCI-779 and RAD001 are effective for inhibiting tumor growth. This ongoing development further supports the perspective targeting of AKT for cancer treatment. However, AKT signaling is also required for normal cell survival and proliferation, the selective targeting of AKT downstream targets for regulating angiogenesis would be an ideal choice to achieve the specific inhibition of human tumor development and growth without affecting normal tissues and organs. Therefore, it would be important to study the mechanism of AKT in regulating angiogenesis and to identify AKT downstream targets that are specifically required for inducing angiogenesis.

ACKNOWLEDGEMENTS

This work was supported in part by the National Key Basic Research Program of China (2011CB504003), by National Natural Science Foundation of China (81071642 and 30871296), and by National Cancer Institute, NIH (R01CA109460).

CONFLICT OF INTEREST

The author(s) confirm that this chapter content has no conflict of interest.

DISCLOSURE

The chapter submitted for the eBook Series entitled **"Advances in Cancer Drug Targets, Volume 1"** is an update of our article in **Current Cancer Drug Targets, Volume 8, Issue 1, 2008,** with additional text and references.

ABBREVIATIONS

PI3K = phosphatidylinositol 3-kinase

VEGF = vascular endothelial growth factor

VEGFR = vascular endothelial growth factor receptor

PKB = protein kinase B

PTKs = protein tyrosine kinases

NOS = nitric oxide synthase

NF-κB = nuclear factor-kappaB

PTEN = phosphatase and tensin homolog deleted on chromosome ten

FGF = fibroblast growth factors

EGF = epidermal growth factor

HGF = hepatocyte growth factor

IGF = insulin-like growth factor

CAM = chicken chorioallantoic membrane

Tie = tyrosine kinase with immunoglobulin (Ig) and EGF homology domains

Ang = angiopoietin

siRNA = small interference RNA

eNOS = endothelial nitric oxide synthase

TSP = thrombospondins

EPC = endothelial progenitor cell

HIF-1 = hypoxia-inducable factor-1

iNOS = inducible nitric oxide synthase

PHDs = prolyl hydroxylases

ODD = oxygen-dependent degradation

VHL = von Hipple-Lindau

DMBA = 7,12-dimethylbenz(a)anthracene

TPA = 2-O-tetradecanoylphorbol-13-acetate

mTOR = mammalian target of rapamycin

REFERENCES

[1] Datta SR, Brunet A, Greenberg ME: Cellular survival: a play in three Akts. *Genes Dev.* 1999, 13:2905-2927.

[2] Duronio V, Scheid MP, Ettinger S: Downstream signalling events regulated by phosphatidylinositol 3-kinase activity. *Cell Signal.* 1998, 10:233-239.

[3] Chan TO, Rittenhouse SE, Tsichlis PN: AKT/PKB and other D3 phosphoinositide-regulated kinases: kinase activation by phosphoinositide-dependent phosphorylation. *Annu. Rev. Biochem.* 1999, 68:965-1014.

[4] Kandel ES, Hay N: The regulation and activities of the multifunctional serine/threonine kinase Akt/PKB. *Exp. Cell Res.* 1999, 253:210-229.

[5] Jiang BH, Zheng JZ, Aoki M, Vogt PK: Phosphatidylinositol 3-kinase signaling mediates angiogenesis and expression of vascular endothelial growth factor in endothelial cells. *Proc. Natl. Acad. Sci. U. S. A* 2000, 97:1749-1753.

[6] Franke TF, Hornik CP, Segev L, Shostak GA, Sugimoto C: PI3K/Akt and apoptosis: size matters. *Oncogene* 2003, 22:8983-8998.

[7] Alessi DR, Cohen P: Mechanism of activation and function of protein kinase B. *Curr. Opin. Genet. Dev.* 1998, 8:55-62.

[8] Carpenter CL, Duckworth BC, Auger KR, Cohen B, Schaffhausen BS, Cantley LC: Purification and characterization of phosphoinositide 3-kinase from rat liver. *J. Biol. Chem.* 1990, 265:19704-19711.

[9] Chen HC, Guan JL: Association of focal adhesion kinase with its potential substrate phosphatidylinositol 3-kinase. *Proc. Natl. Acad. Sci. U. S. A* 1994, 91:10148-10152.

[10] Izuhara K, Feldman RA, Greer P, Harada N: Interleukin-4 induces association of the c-fes proto-oncogene product with phosphatidylinositol-3 kinase. *Blood* 1996, 88:3910-3918.

[11] Karnitz LM, Sutor SL, Abraham RT: The Src-family kinase, Fyn, regulates the activation of phosphatidylinositol 3-kinase in an interleukin 2-responsive T cell line. *J. Exp. Med.* 1994, 179:1799-1808.

[12] Cheng JQ, Godwin AK, Bellacosa A, Taguchi T, Franke TF, Hamilton TC, Tsichlis PN, Testa JR: AKT2, a putative oncogene encoding a member of a subfamily of protein-serine/threonine kinases, is amplified in human ovarian carcinomas. *Proc. Natl. Acad. Sci. U. S. A* 1992, 89:9267-9271.

[13] Cheng JQ, Ruggeri B, Klein WM, Sonoda G, Altomare DA, Watson DK, Testa JR: Amplification of AKT2 in human pancreatic cells and inhibition of AKT2 expression and tumorigenicity by antisense RNA. *Proc. Natl. Acad. Sci. U. S. A* 1996, 93:3636-3641.

[14] Staal SP: Molecular cloning of the akt oncogene and its human homologues AKT1 and AKT2: amplification of AKT1 in a primary human gastric adenocarcinoma. *Proc. Natl. Acad. Sci. U. S. A* 1987, 84:5034-5037.

[15] Dimmeler S, Fleming I, Fisslthaler B, Hermann C, Busse R, Zeiher AM: Activation of nitric oxide synthase in endothelial cells by Akt-dependent phosphorylation. *Nature* 1999, 399:601-605.

[16] Fulton D, Gratton JP, McCabe TJ, Fontana J, Fujio Y, Walsh K, Franke TF, Papapetropoulos A, Sessa WC: Regulation of endothelium-derived nitric oxide production by the protein kinase Akt. *Nature* 1999, 399:597-601.

[17] Romashkova JA, Makarov SS: NF-kappaB is a target of AKT in anti-apoptotic PDGF signalling. *Nature* 1999, 401:86-90.

[18] Ozes ON, Mayo LD, Gustin JA, Pfeffer SR, Pfeffer LM, Donner DB: NF-kappaB activation by tumour necrosis factor requires the Akt serine-threonine kinase. *Nature* 1999, 401:82-85.

[19] Kane LP, Shapiro VS, Stokoe D, Weiss A: Induction of NF-kappaB by the Akt/PKB kinase. *Curr. Biol.* 1999, 9:601-604.

[20] del Peso L, Gonzalez-Garcia M, Page C, Herrera R, Nunez G: Interleukin-3-induced phosphorylation of BAD through the protein kinase Akt. *Science* 1997, 278:687-689.

[21] Cheatham B, Vlahos CJ, Cheatham L, Wang L, Blenis J, Kahn CR: Phosphatidylinositol 3-kinase activation is required for insulin stimulation of pp70 S6 kinase, DNA synthesis, and glucose transporter translocation. *Mol. Cell Biol.* 1994, 14:4902-4911.

[22] Monfar M, Lemon KP, Grammer TC, Cheatham L, Chung J, Vlahos CJ, Blenis J: Activation of pp70/85 S6 kinases in interleukin-2-responsive lymphoid cells is mediated by phosphatidylinositol 3-kinase and inhibited by cyclic AMP. *Mol. Cell Biol.* 1995, 15:326-337.

[23] Cross DA, Alessi DR, Cohen P, Andjelkovich M, Hemmings BA: Inhibition of glycogen synthase kinase-3 by insulin mediated by protein kinase B. *Nature* 1995, 378:785-789.

[24] Klippel A, Reinhard C, Kavanaugh WM, Apell G, Escobedo MA, Williams LT: Membrane localization of phosphatidylinositol 3-kinase is sufficient to activate multiple signal-transducing kinase pathways. *Mol. Cell Biol.* 1996, 16:4117-4127.

[25] Cantley LC, Neel BG: New insights into tumor suppression: PTEN suppresses tumor formation by restraining the phosphoinositide 3-kinase/AKT pathway. *Proc. Natl. Acad. Sci. U. S. A* 1999, 96:4240-4245.

[26] Carmeliet P, Lampugnani MG, Moons L, Breviario F, Compernolle V, Bono F, Balconi G, Spagnuolo R, Oostuyse B, Dewerchin M, Zanetti A, Angellilo A, Mattot V, Nuyens D, Lutgens E, Clotman F, de Ruiter MC, Gittenberger-de Groot A, Poelmann R, Lupu F, Herbert JM, Collen D, Dejana E: Targeted deficiency or cytosolic truncation of the VE-cadherin gene in mice impairs VEGF-mediated endothelial survival and angiogenesis. *Cell* 1999, 98:147-157.

[27] Ong SH, Hadari YR, Gotoh N, Guy GR, Schlessinger J, Lax I: Stimulation of phosphatidylinositol 3-kinase by fibroblast growth factor receptors is mediated by coordinated recruitment of multiple docking proteins. *Proc. Natl. Acad. Sci. U. S. A* 2001, 98:6074-6079.

[28] Zubilewicz A, Hecquet C, Jeanny JC, Soubrane G, Courtois Y, Mascarelli F: Two distinct signalling pathways are involved in FGF2-stimulated proliferation of choriocapillary endothelial cells: a comparative study with VEGF. *Oncogene* 2001, 20:1403-1413.

[29] Burgering BM, Coffer PJ: Protein kinase B (c-Akt) in phosphatidylinositol-3-OH kinase signal transduction. *Nature* 1995, 376:599-602.

[30] Zhong H, Chiles K, Feldser D, Laughner E, Hanrahan C, Georgescu MM, Simons JW, Semenza GL: Modulation of hypoxia-inducible factor 1alpha expression by the epidermal growth factor/phosphatidylinositol 3-kinase/PTEN/AKT/FRAP pathway in human prostate

cancer cells: implications for tumor angiogenesis and therapeutics. *Cancer Res.* 2000, 60:1541-1545.

[31] Dong G, Chen Z, Li ZY, Yeh NT, Bancroft CC, Van Waes C: Hepatocyte growth factor/scatter factor-induced activation of MEK and PI3K signal pathways contributes to expression of proangiogenic cytokines interleukin-8 and vascular endothelial growth factor in head and neck squamous cell carcinoma. *Cancer Res.* 2001, 61:5911-5918.

[32] Khwaja A, Lehmann K, Marte BM, Downward J: Phosphoinositide 3-kinase induces scattering and tubulogenesis in epithelial cells through a novel pathway. *J. Biol. Chem.* 1998, 273:18793-18801.

[33] Kulik G, Klippel A, Weber MJ: Antiapoptotic signalling by the insulin-like growth factor I receptor, phosphatidylinositol 3-kinase, and Akt. *Mol. Cell Biol.* 1997, 17:1595-1606.

[34] Oh JS, Kucab JE, Bushel PR, Martin K, Bennett L, Collins J, DiAugustine RP, Barrett JC, Afshari CA, Dunn SE: Insulin-like growth factor-1 inscribes a gene expression profile for angiogenic factors and cancer progression in breast epithelial cells. *Neoplasia.* 2002, 4:204-217.

[35] Papapetropoulos A, Fulton D, Mahboubi K, Kalb RG, O'Connor DS, Li F, Altieri DC, Sessa WC: Angiopoietin-1 inhibits endothelial cell apoptosis *via* the Akt/survivin pathway. *J. Biol. Chem.* 2000, 275:9102-9105.

[36] Hennessy BT, Smith DL, Ram PT, Lu Y, Mills GB: Exploiting the PI3K/AKT pathway for cancer drug discovery. *Nat. Rev. Drug Discov.* 2005, 4:988-1004.

[37] Shayesteh L, Lu Y, Kuo WL, Baldocchi R, Godfrey T, Collins C, Pinkel D, Powell B, Mills GB, Gray JW: PIK3CA is implicated as an oncogene in ovarian cancer. *Nat. Genet.* 1999, 21:99-102.

[38] Kang S, Bader AG, Zhao L, Vogt PK: Mutated PI 3-kinases: cancer targets on a silver platter. *Cell Cycle* 2005, 4:578-581.

[39] Knobbe CB, Reifenberger G: Genetic alterations and aberrant expression of genes related to the phosphatidyl-inositol-3'-kinase/protein kinase B (Akt) signal transduction pathway in glioblastomas. *Brain Pathol.* 2003, 13:507-518.

[40] Bellacosa A, de Feo D, Godwin AK, Bell DW, Cheng JQ, Altomare DA, Wan M, Dubeau L, Scambia G, Masciullo V, Ferrandina G, Benedetti PP, Mancuso S, Neri G, Testa JR: Molecular alterations of the AKT2 oncogene in ovarian and breast carcinomas. *Int. J. Cancer* 1995, 64:280-285.

[41] Nakatani K, Thompson DA, Barthel A, Sakaue H, Liu W, Weigel RJ, Roth RA: Up-regulation of Akt3 in estrogen receptor-deficient breast cancers and androgen-independent prostate cancer lines. *J. Biol. Chem.* 1999, 274:21528-21532.

[42] Liu LZ, Zhou XD, Qian G, Shi X, Fang J, Jiang BH: AKT1 amplification regulates cisplatin resistance in human lung cancer cells through the mammalian target of rapamycin/p70S6K1 pathway. *Cancer Res.* 2007, 67:6325-6332.

[43] Jain RK, Schlenger K, Hockel M, Yuan F: Quantitative angiogenesis assays: progress and problems. *Nat. Med.* 1997, 3:1203-1208.

[44] Risau W: Mechanisms of angiogenesis. *Nature* 1997, 386:671-674.

[45] Folkman J: Angiogenesis. *Annu. Rev. Med.* 2006, 57:1-18.

[46] Carmeliet P, Jain RK: Angiogenesis in cancer and other diseases. *Nature* 2000, 407:249-257.

[47] Ferrara N: Molecular and biological properties of vascular endothelial growth factor. *J. Mol. Med.* 1999, 77:527-543.

[48] Gale NW, Yancopoulos GD: Growth factors acting *via* endothelial cell-specific receptor tyrosine kinases: VEGFs, angiopoietins, and ephrins in vascular development. *Genes Dev.* 1999, 13:1055-1066.

[49] Yancopoulos GD, Klagsbrun M, Folkman J: Vasculogenesis, angiogenesis, and growth factors: ephrins enter the fray at the border. *Cell* 1998, 93:661-664.
[50] Folkman J: Seminars in Medicine of the Beth Israel Hospital, Boston. Clinical applications of research on angiogenesis. *N. Engl. J. Med.* 1995, 333:1757-1763.
[51] Fidler IJ: Angiogenesis and cancer metastasis. *Cancer J.* 2000, 6 Suppl 2:S134-S141.
[52] Gupta K, Zhang J: Angiogenesis: a curse or cure? *Postgrad. Med. J.* 2005, 81:236-242.
[53] Rosen EM, Lamszus K, Laterra J, Polverini PJ, Rubin JS, Goldberg ID: HGF/SF in angiogenesis. *Ciba Found. Symp.* 1997, 212:215-226.
[54] Folkman J: Endogenous angiogenesis inhibitors. *APMIS* 2004, 112:496-507.
[55] Azam F, Mehta S, Harris AL: Mechanisms of resistance to antiangiogenesis therapy. *Eur. J. Cancer* 2010, 46:1323-1332.
[56] Loges S, Mazzone M, Hohensinner P, Carmeliet P: Silencing or fueling metastasis with VEGF inhibitors: antiangiogenesis revisited. *Cancer Cell* 2009, 15:167-170.
[57] Shojaei F: Anti-angiogenesis therapy in cancer: Current challenges and future perspectives. *Cancer Lett.* 2012, 320:130-137.
[58] Grothey A, Galanis E: Targeting angiogenesis: progress with anti-VEGF treatment with large molecules. *Nat. Rev. Clin. Oncol.* 2009, 6:507-518.
[59] Mackey JR, Kerbel RS, Gelmon KA, McLeod DM, Chia SK, Rayson D, Verma S, Collins LL, Paterson AH, Robidoux A, Pritchard KI: Controlling angiogenesis in breast cancer: A systematic review of anti-angiogenic trials. *Cancer Treat. Rev.* 2012.
[60] Ullrich A, Schlessinger J: Signal transduction by receptors with tyrosine kinase activity. *Cell* 1990, 61:203-212.
[61] Folkman J: Angiogenesis in cancer, vascular, rheumatoid and other disease. *Nat. Med.* 1995, 1:27-31.
[62] Fong GH, Rossant J, Gertsenstein M, Breitman ML: Role of the Flt-1 receptor tyrosine kinase in regulating the assembly of vascular endothelium. *Nature* 1995, 376:66-70.
[63] Plate KH, Breier G, Weich HA, Risau W: Vascular endothelial growth factor is a potential tumour angiogenesis factor in human gliomas *in vivo*. *Nature* 1992, 359:845-848.
[64] Shalaby F, Rossant J, Yamaguchi TP, Gertsenstein M, Wu XF, Breitman ML, Schuh AC: Failure of blood-island formation and vasculogenesis in Flk-1-deficient mice. *Nature* 1995, 376:62-66.
[65] Gerber HP, McMurtrey A, Kowalski J, Yan M, Keyt BA, Dixit V, Ferrara N: Vascular endothelial growth factor regulates endothelial cell survival through the phosphatidylinositol 3'-kinase/Akt signal transduction pathway. Requirement for Flk-1/KDR activation. *J. Biol. Chem.* 1998, 273:30336-30343.
[66] Ilan N, Mahooti S, Madri JA: Distinct signal transduction pathways are utilized during the tube formation and survival phases of *in vitro* angiogenesis. *J. Cell Sci.* 1998, 111 (Pt 24):3621-3631.
[67] Fujio Y, Walsh K: Akt mediates cytoprotection of endothelial cells by vascular endothelial growth factor in an anchorage-dependent manner. *J. Biol. Chem.* 1999, 274:16349-16354.
[68] Dumont DJ, Gradwohl G, Fong GH, Puri MC, Gertsenstein M, Auerbach A, Breitman ML: Dominant-negative and targeted null mutations in the endothelial receptor tyrosine kinase, tek, reveal a critical role in vasculogenesis of the embryo. *Genes Dev.* 1994, 8:1897-1909.
[69] Sato TN, Tozawa Y, Deutsch U, Wolburg-Buchholz K, Fujiwara Y, Gendron-Maguire M, Gridley T, Wolburg H, Risau W, Qin Y: Distinct roles of the receptor tyrosine kinases Tie-1 and Tie-2 in blood vessel formation. *Nature* 1995, 376:70-74.

[70] Hayes AJ, Huang WQ, Mallah J, Yang D, Lippman ME, Li LY: Angiopoietin-1 and its receptor Tie-2 participate in the regulation of capillary-like tubule formation and survival of endothelial cells. *Microvasc. Res.* 1999, 58:224-237.

[71] Lin P, Polverini P, Dewhirst M, Shan S, Rao PS, Peters K: Inhibition of tumor angiogenesis using a soluble receptor establishes a role for Tie2 in pathologic vascular growth. *J. Clin. Invest* 1997, 100:2072-2078.

[72] Vikkula M, Boon LM, Carraway KL, III, Calvert JT, Diamonti AJ, Goumnerov B, Pasyk KA, Marchuk DA, Warman ML, Cantley LC, Mulliken JB, Olsen BR: Vascular dysmorphogenesis caused by an activating mutation in the receptor tyrosine kinase TIE2. *Cell* 1996, 87:1181-1190.

[73] Davis S, Aldrich TH, Jones PF, Acheson A, Compton DL, Jain V, Ryan TE, Bruno J, Radziejewski C, Maisonpierre PC, Yancopoulos GD: Isolation of angiopoietin-1, a ligand for the TIE2 receptor, by secretion-trap expression cloning. *Cell* 1996, 87:1161-1169.

[74] Maisonpierre PC, Suri C, Jones PF, Bartunkova S, Wiegand SJ, Radziejewski C, Compton D, McClain J, Aldrich TH, Papadopoulos N, Daly TJ, Davis S, Sato TN, Yancopoulos GD: Angiopoietin-2, a natural antagonist for Tie2 that disrupts *in vivo* angiogenesis. *Science* 1997, 277:55-60.

[75] Valenzuela DM, Griffiths JA, Rojas J, Aldrich TH, Jones PF, Zhou H, McClain J, Copeland NG, Gilbert DJ, Jenkins NA, Huang T, Papadopoulos N, Maisonpierre PC, Davis S, Yancopoulos GD: Angiopoietins 3 and 4: diverging gene counterparts in mice and humans. *Proc. Natl. Acad. Sci. U. S. A* 1999, 96:1904-1909.

[76] Tsigkos S, Koutsilieris M, Papapetropoulos A: Angiopoietins in angiogenesis and beyond. *Expert. Opin. Investig. Drugs* 2003, 12:933-941.

[77] Kim I, Kim HG, So JN, Kim JH, Kwak HJ, Koh GY: Angiopoietin-1 regulates endothelial cell survival through the phosphatidylinositol 3'-Kinase/Akt signal transduction pathway. *Circ. Res.* 2000, 86:24-29.

[78] Kim I, Kim HG, Moon SO, Chae SW, So JN, Koh KN, Ahn BC, Koh GY: Angiopoietin-1 induces endothelial cell sprouting through the activation of focal adhesion kinase and plasmin secretion. *Circ. Res.* 2000, 86:952-959.

[79] Fujikawa K, de AS, I, Jain SK, Presman E, Christensen RA, Varticovski L: Role of PI 3-kinase in angiopoietin-1-mediated migration and attachment-dependent survival of endothelial cells. *Exp. Cell Res.* 1999, 253:663-672.

[80] Kim I, Kim JH, Moon SO, Kwak HJ, Kim NG, Koh GY: Angiopoietin-2 at high concentration can enhance endothelial cell survival through the phosphatidylinositol 3'-kinase/Akt signal transduction pathway. *Oncogene* 2000, 19:4549-4552.

[81] Tsigkos S, Zhou Z, Kotanidou A, Fulton D, Zakynthinos S, Roussos C, Papapetropoulos A: Regulation of Ang2 release by PTEN/PI3-kinase/Akt in lung microvascular endothelial cells. *J. Cell Physiol* 2006, 209:239.

[82] Lee HJ, Cho CH, Hwang SJ, Choi HH, Kim KT, Ahn SY, Kim JH, Oh JL, Lee GM, Koh GY: Biological characterization of angiopoietin-3 and angiopoietin-4. *FASEB J.* 2004, 18:1200-1208.

[83] Olsen MW, Ley CD, Junker N, Hansen AJ, Lund EL, Kristjansen PE: Angiopoietin-4 inhibits angiogenesis and reduces interstitial fluid pressure. *Neoplasia.* 2006, 8:364-372.

[84] Lai EC: Micro RNAs are complementary to 3' UTR sequence motifs that mediate negative post-transcriptional regulation. *Nat. Genet.* 2002, 30:363-364.

[85] Lee RC, Ambros V: An extensive class of small RNAs in Caenorhabditis elegans. *Science* 2001, 294:862-864.

[86] Ambros V: microRNAs: tiny regulators with great potential. *Cell* 2001, 107:823-826.

[87] Xu N, Papagiannakopoulos T, Pan G, Thomson JA, Kosik KS: MicroRNA-145 regulates OCT4, SOX2, and KLF4 and represses pluripotency in human embryonic stem cells. *Cell* 2009, 137:647-658.

[88] le Sage C, Nagel R, Egan DA, Schrier M, Mesman E, Mangiola A, Anile C, Maira G, Mercatelli N, Ciafre SA, Farace MG, Agami R: Regulation of the p27(Kip1) tumor suppressor by miR-221 and miR-222 promotes cancer cell proliferation. *EMBO J.* 2007, 26:3699-3708.

[89] Yoo AS, Staahl BT, Chen L, Crabtree GR: MicroRNA-mediated switching of chromatin-remodelling complexes in neural development. *Nature* 2009, 460:642-646.

[90] Calin GA, Sevignani C, Dumitru CD, Hyslop T, Noch E, Yendamuri S, Shimizu M, Rattan S, Bullrich F, Negrini M, Croce CM: Human microRNA genes are frequently located at fragile sites and genomic regions involved in cancers. *Proc. Natl. Acad. Sci. U. S. A* 2004, 101:2999-3004.

[91] Zhang H, Li Y, Lai M: The microRNA network and tumor metastasis. *Oncogene* 2010, 29:937-948.

[92] Wang X, Zhang X, Ren XP, Chen J, Liu H, Yang J, Medvedovic M, Hu Z, Fan GC: MicroRNA-494 targeting both proapoptotic and antiapoptotic proteins protects against ischemia/reperfusion-induced cardiac injury. *Circulation* 2010, 122:1308-1318.

[93] Fu X, Tian J, Zhang L, Chen Y, Hao Q: Involvement of microRNA-93, a new regulator of PTEN/Akt signaling pathway, in regulation of chemotherapeutic drug cisplatin chemosensitivity in ovarian cancer cells. *FEBS Lett.* 2012, 586:1279-1286.

[94] Bar N, Dikstein R: miR-22 forms a regulatory loop in PTEN/AKT pathway and modulates signaling kinetics. *PLoS. One.* 2010, 5:e10859.

[95] Kong G, Zhang J, Zhang S, Shan C, Ye L, Zhang X: Upregulated microRNA-29a by hepatitis B virus X protein enhances hepatoma cell migration by targeting PTEN in cell culture model. *PLoS. One.* 2011, 6:e19518.

[96] Wang C, Bian Z, Wei D, Zhang JG: miR-29b regulates migration of human breast cancer cells. *Mol. Cell Biochem.* 2011, 352:197-207.

[97] Garofalo M, Di Leva G, Romano G, Nuovo G, Suh SS, Ngankeu A, Taccioli C, Pichiorri F, Alder H, Secchiero P, Gasparini P, Gonelli A, Costinean S, Acunzo M, Condorelli G, Croce CM: miR-221&222 regulate TRAIL resistance and enhance tumorigenicity through PTEN and TIMP3 downregulation. *Cancer Cell* 2009, 16:498-509.

[98] Shi W, Gerster K, Alajez NM, Tsang J, Waldron L, Pintilie M, Hui AB, Sykes J, P'ng C, Miller N, McCready D, Fyles A, Liu FF: MicroRNA-301 mediates proliferation and invasion in human breast cancer. *Cancer Res.* 2011, 71:2926-2937.

[99] Yang H, Kong W, He L, Zhao JJ, O'Donnell JD, Wang J, Wenham RM, Coppola D, Kruk PA, Nicosia SV, Cheng JQ: MicroRNA expression profiling in human ovarian cancer: miR-214 induces cell survival and cisplatin resistance by targeting PTEN. *Cancer Res.* 2008, 68:425-433.

[100] Small EM, O'Rourke JR, Moresi V, Sutherland LB, McAnally J, Gerard RD, Richardson JA, Olson EN: Regulation of PI3-kinase/Akt signaling by muscle-enriched microRNA-486. *Proc. Natl. Acad. Sci. U. S. A* 2010, 107:4218-4223.

[101] Greene SB, Gunaratne PH, Hammond SM, Rosen JM: A putative role for microRNA-205 in mammary epithelial cell progenitors. *J. Cell Sci.* 2010, 123:606-618.

[102] Zhang L, Deng T, Li X, Liu H, Zhou H, Ma J, Wu M, Zhou M, Shen S, Li X, Niu Z, Zhang W, Shi L, Xiang B, Lu J, Wang L, Li D, Tang H, Li G: microRNA-141 is involved in a nasopharyngeal carcinoma-related genes network. *Carcinogenesis* 2010, 31:559-566.

[103] Kato M, Putta S, Wang M, Yuan H, Lanting L, Nair I, Gunn A, Nakagawa Y, Shimano H, Todorov I, Rossi JJ, Natarajan R: TGF-beta activates Akt kinase through a microRNA-dependent amplifying circuit targeting PTEN. *Nat. Cell Biol.* 2009, 11:881-889.

[104] Meng F, Henson R, Wehbe-Janek H, Ghoshal K, Jacob ST, Patel T: MicroRNA-21 regulates expression of the PTEN tumor suppressor gene in human hepatocellular cancer. *Gastroenterology* 2007, 133:647-658.

[105] Fang YX, Xue JL, Shen Q, Chen J, Tian L: miR-7 inhibits tumor growth and metastasis by targeting the PI3K/AKT pathway in hepatocellular carcinoma. *Hepatology* 2012.

[106] Zhu N, Zhang D, Xie H, Zhou Z, Chen H, Hu T, Bai Y, Shen Y, Yuan W, Jing Q, Qin Y: Endothelial-specific intron-derived miR-126 is down-regulated in human breast cancer and targets both VEGFA and PIK3R2. *Mol. Cell Biochem.* 2011, 351:157-164.

[107] Lin RJ, Lin YC, Yu AL: miR-149* induces apoptosis by inhibiting Akt1 and E2F1 in human cancer cells. *Mol. Carcinog.* 2010, 49:719-727.

[108] Watanabe A, Tagawa H, Yamashita J, Teshima K, Nara M, Iwamoto K, Kume M, Kameoka Y, Takahashi N, Nakagawa T, Shimizu N, Sawada K: The role of microRNA-150 as a tumor suppressor in malignant lymphoma. *Leukemia* 2011, 25:1324-1334.

[109] Foley NH, Bray IM, Tivnan A, Bryan K, Murphy DM, Buckley PG, Ryan J, O'Meara A, O'Sullivan M, Stallings RL: MicroRNA-184 inhibits neuroblastoma cell survival through targeting the serine/threonine kinase AKT2. *Mol. Cancer* 2010, 9:83.

[110] Iliopoulos D, Polytarchou C, Hatziapostolou M, Kottakis F, Maroulakou IG, Struhl K, Tsichlis PN: MicroRNAs differentially regulated by Akt isoforms control EMT and stem cell renewal in cancer cells. *Sci. Signal.* 2009, 2:ra62.

[111] Bronisz A, Godlewski J, Wallace JA, Merchant AS, Nowicki MO, Mathsyaraja H, Srinivasan R, Trimboli AJ, Martin CK, Li F, Yu L, Fernandez SA, Pecot T, Rosol TJ, Cory S, Hallett M, Park M, Piper MG, Marsh CB, Yee LD, Jimenez RE, Nuovo G, Lawler SE, Chiocca EA, Leone G, Ostrowski MC: Reprogramming of the tumour microenvironment by stromal PTEN-regulated miR-320. *Nat. Cell Biol.* 2012, 14:159-167.

[112] Rao E, Jiang C, Ji M, Huang X, Iqbal J, Lenz G, Wright G, Staudt LM, Zhao Y, McKeithan TW, Chan WC, Fu K: The miRNA-17 approximately 92 cluster mediates chemoresistance and enhances tumor growth in mantle cell lymphoma *via* PI3K/AKT pathway activation. *Leukemia* 2011.

[113] Sachdeva M, Wu H, Ru P, Hwang L, Trieu V, Mo YY: MicroRNA-101-mediated Akt activation and estrogen-independent growth. *Oncogene* 2011, 30:822-831.

[114] Uesugi A, Kozaki K, Tsuruta T, Furuta M, Morita K, Imoto I, Omura K, Inazawa J: The tumor suppressive microRNA miR-218 targets the mTOR component Rictor and inhibits AKT phosphorylation in oral cancer. *Cancer Res.* 2011, 71:5765-5778.

[115] Li D, Liu X, Lin L, Hou J, Li N, Wang C, Wang P, Zhang Q, Zhang P, Zhou W, Wang Z, Ding G, Zhuang SM, Zheng L, Tao W, Cao X: MicroRNA-99a inhibits hepatocellular carcinoma growth and correlates with prognosis of patients with hepatocellular carcinoma. *J. Biol. Chem.* 2011, 286:36677-36685.

[116] Liu P, Wilson MJ: miR-520c and miR-373 upregulate MMP9 expression by targeting mTOR and SIRT1, and activate the Ras/Raf/MEK/Erk signaling pathway and NF-kappaB factor in human fibrosarcoma cells. *J. Cell Physiol* 2012, 227:867-876.

[117] Grundmann S, Hans FP, Kinniry S, Heinke J, Helbing T, Bluhm F, Sluijter JP, Hoefer I, Pasterkamp G, Bode C, Moser M: MicroRNA-100 regulates neovascularization by suppression of mammalian target of rapamycin in endothelial and vascular smooth muscle cells. *Circulation* 2011, 123:999-1009.

[118] Sun D, Lee YS, Malhotra A, Kim HK, Matecic M, Evans C, Jensen RV, Moskaluk CA, Dutta A: miR-99 family of MicroRNAs suppresses the expression of prostate-specific antigen and prostate cancer cell proliferation. *Cancer Res.* 2011, 71:1313-1324.

[119] Fornari F, Milazzo M, Chieco P, Negrini M, Calin GA, Grazi GL, Pollutri D, Croce CM, Bolondi L, Gramantieri L: MiR-199a-3p regulates mTOR and c-Met to influence the doxorubicin sensitivity of human hepatocarcinoma cells. *Cancer Res.* 2010, 70:5184-5193.

[120] Xu Q, Liu LZ, Qian X, Chen Q, Jiang Y, Li D, Lai L, Jiang BH: MiR-145 directly targets p70S6K1 in cancer cells to inhibit tumor growth and angiogenesis. *Nucleic Acids Res.* 2012, 40:761-774.

[121] Shi ZM, Wang J, Yan Z, You YP, Li CY, Qian X, Yin Y, Zhao P, Wang YY, Wang XF, Li MN, Liu LZ, Liu N, Jiang BH: MiR-128 inhibits tumor growth and angiogenesis by targeting p70S6K1. *PLoS. One.* 2012, 7:e32709.

[122] Osaki M, Oshimura M, Ito H: PI3K-Akt pathway: its functions and alterations in human cancer. *Apoptosis.* 2004, 9:667-676.

[123] Xia C, Meng Q, Cao Z, Shi X, Jiang BH: Regulation of angiogenesis and tumor growth by p110 alpha and AKT1 *via* VEGF expression. *J. Cell Physiol* 2006, 209:56-66.

[124] Zhao YW, Jin L, Li ZM, Zhao CJ, Wei YQ, Yang HS: Enhanced antitumor efficacy by blocking activation of the phosphatidylinositol 3-kinase/Akt pathway during anti-angiogenesis therapy. *Cancer Sci.* 2011, 102:1469-1475.

[125] Su JD, Mayo LD, Donner DB, Durden DL: PTEN and phosphatidylinositol 3'-kinase inhibitors up-regulate p53 and block tumor-induced angiogenesis: evidence for an effect on the tumor and endothelial compartment. *Cancer Res.* 2003, 63:3585-3592.

[126] Liu LZ, Fang J, Zhou Q, Hu X, Shi X, Jiang BH: Apigenin inhibits expression of vascular endothelial growth factor and angiogenesis in human lung cancer cells: implication of chemoprevention of lung cancer. *Mol. Pharmacol.* 2005, 68:635-643.

[127] Min JK, Han KY, Kim EC, Kim YM, Lee SW, Kim OH, Kim KW, Gho YS, Kwon YG: Capsaicin inhibits *in vitro* and *in vivo* angiogenesis. *Cancer Res.* 2004, 64:644-651.

[128] Petrangolini G, Pratesi G, De Cesare M, Supino R, Pisano C, Marcellini M, Giordano V, Laccabue D, Lanzi C, Zunino F: Antiangiogenic effects of the novel camptothecin ST1481 (gimatecan) in human tumor xenografts. *Mol. Cancer Res.* 2003, 1:863-870.

[129] Zhong XS, Zheng JZ, Reed E, Jiang BH: SU5416 inhibited VEGF and HIF-1alpha expression through the PI3K/AKT/p70S6K1 signaling pathway. *Biochem. Biophys. Res. Commun.* 2004, 324:471-480.

[130] Zhu XF, Xie BF, Zhou JM, Feng GK, Liu ZC, Wei XY, Zhang FX, Liu MF, Zeng YX: Blockade of vascular endothelial growth factor receptor signal pathway and antitumor activity of ON-III (2',4'-dihydroxy-6'-methoxy-3',5'-dimethylchalcone), a component from Chinese herbal medicine. *Mol. Pharmacol.* 2005, 67:1444-1450.

[131] Xia C, Meng Q, Liu LZ, Rojanasakul Y, Wang XR, Jiang BH: Reactive oxygen species regulate angiogenesis and tumor growth through vascular endothelial growth factor. *Cancer Res.* 2007, 67:10823-10830.

[132] Jo M, Nishikawa T, Nakajima T, Okada Y, Yamaguchi K, Mitsuyoshi H, Yasui K, Minami M, Iwai M, Kagawa K, Itoh Y, Yoshikawa T: Oxidative stress is closely associated with tumor angiogenesis of hepatocellular carcinoma. *J. Gastroenterol.* 2011, 46:809-821.

[133] Ushio-Fukai M, Alexander RW: Reactive oxygen species as mediators of angiogenesis signaling: role of NAD(P)H oxidase. *Mol. Cell Biochem.* 2004, 264:85-97.

[134] Coso S, Harrison I, Harrison CB, Vinh A, Sobey CG, Drummond GR, Williams ED, Selemidis S: NADPH oxidases as regulators of tumor angiogenesis: current and emerging concepts. *Antioxid. Redox. Signal.* 2012, 16:1229-1247.

[135] Gupta SC, Hevia D, Patchva S, Park B, Koh W, Aggarwal BB: Upsides and downsides of reactive oxygen species for cancer: the roles of reactive oxygen species in tumorigenesis, prevention, and therapy. *Antioxid. Redox. Signal.* 2012, 16:1295-1322.

[136] Sun JF, Phung T, Shiojima I, Felske T, Upalakalin JN, Feng D, Kornaga T, Dor T, Dvorak AM, Walsh K, Benjamin LE: Microvascular patterning is controlled by fine-tuning the Akt signal. *Proc. Natl. Acad. Sci. U. S. A* 2005, 102:128-133.

[137] Coffer PJ, Jin J, Woodgett JR: Protein kinase B (c-Akt): a multifunctional mediator of phosphatidylinositol 3-kinase activation. *Biochem. J.* 1998, 335 (Pt 1):1-13.

[138] Chen WS, Xu PZ, Gottlob K, Chen ML, Sokol K, Shiyanova T, Roninson I, Weng W, Suzuki R, Tobe K, Kadowaki T, Hay N: Growth retardation and increased apoptosis in mice with homozygous disruption of the Akt1 gene. *Genes Dev.* 2001, 15:2203-2208.

[139] Cho H, Thorvaldsen JL, Chu Q, Feng F, Birnbaum MJ: *Akt1*/PKBalpha is required for normal growth but dispensable for maintenance of glucose homeostasis in mice. *J. Biol. Chem.* 2001, 276:38349-38352.

[140] Yang ZZ, Tschopp O, Hemmings-Mieszczak M, Feng J, Brodbeck D, Perentes E, Hemmings BA: Protein kinase B alpha/Akt1 regulates placental development and fetal growth. *J. Biol. Chem.* 2003, 278:32124-32131.

[141] Chen J, Somanath PR, Razorenova O, Chen WS, Hay N, Bornstein P, Byzova TV: Akt1 regulates pathological angiogenesis, vascular maturation and permeability *in vivo*. *Nat. Med.* 2005, 11:1188-1196.

[142] Ackah E, Yu J, Zoellner S, Iwakiri Y, Skurk C, Shibata R, Ouchi N, Easton RM, Galasso G, Birnbaum MJ, Walsh K, Sessa WC: Akt1/protein kinase Balpha is critical for ischemic and VEGF-mediated angiogenesis. *J. Clin. Invest* 2005, 115:2119-2127.

[143] Cho H, Mu J, Kim JK, Thorvaldsen JL, Chu Q, Crenshaw EB, III, Kaestner KH, Bartolomei MS, Shulman GI, Birnbaum MJ: Insulin resistance and a diabetes mellitus-like syndrome in mice lacking the protein kinase Akt2 (PKB beta). *Science* 2001, 292:1728-1731.

[144] Easton RM, Cho H, Roovers K, Shineman DW, Mizrahi M, Forman MS, Lee VM, Szabolcs M, de Jong R, Oltersdorf T, Ludwig T, Efstratiadis A, Birnbaum MJ: Role for Akt3/protein kinase Bgamma in attainment of normal brain size. *Mol. Cell Biol.* 2005, 25:1869-1878.

[145] Brown LF, Berse B, Jackman RW, Tognazzi K, Manseau EJ, Senger DR, Dvorak HF: Expression of vascular permeability factor (vascular endothelial growth factor) and its receptors in adenocarcinomas of the gastrointestinal tract. *Cancer Res.* 1993, 53:4727-4735.

[146] Byrne AM, Bouchier-Hayes DJ, Harmey JH: Angiogenic and cell survival functions of vascular endothelial growth factor (VEGF). *J. Cell Mol. Med.* 2005, 9:777-794.

[147] Mazure NM, Chen EY, Laderoute KR, Giaccia AJ: Induction of vascular endothelial growth factor by hypoxia is modulated by a phosphatidylinositol 3-kinase/Akt signaling pathway in Ha-ras-transformed cells through a hypoxia inducible factor-1 transcriptional element. *Blood* 1997, 90:3322-3331.

[148] Cao Z, Fang J, Xia C, Shi X, Jiang BH: trans-3,4,5'-Trihydroxystibene inhibits hypoxia-inducible factor 1alpha and vascular endothelial growth factor expression in human ovarian cancer cells. *Clin. Cancer Res.* 2004, 10:5253-5263.

[149] Fang J, Xia C, Cao Z, Zheng JZ, Reed E, Jiang BH: Apigenin inhibits VEGF and HIF-1 expression *via* PI3K/AKT/p70S6K1 and HDM2/p53 pathways. *FASEB J.* 2005, 19:342-353.

[150] Skinner HD, Zheng JZ, Fang J, Agani F, Jiang BH: Vascular endothelial growth factor transcriptional activation is mediated by hypoxia-inducible factor 1alpha, HDM2, and p70S6K1 in response to phosphatidylinositol 3-kinase/AKT signaling. *J. Biol. Chem.* 2004, 279:45643-45651.

[151] Huang C, Li J, Song L, Zhang D, Tong Q, Ding M, Bowman L, Aziz R, Stoner GD: Black raspberry extracts inhibit benzo(a)pyrene diol-epoxide-induced activator protein 1 activation and VEGF transcription by targeting the phosphotidylinositol 3-kinase/Akt pathway. *Cancer Res.* 2006, 66:581-587.

[152] Mirshahi P, Toprak SK, Faussat AM, Dubrulle S, Marie JP, Soria C, Soria J, Mirshahi M: Malignant hematopoietic cells induce an increased expression of VEGFR-1 and VEGFR-3 on bone marrow endothelial cells *via* AKT and mTOR signalling pathways. *Biochem. Biophys. Res. Commun.* 2006, 349:1003-1010.

[153] Larrivee B, Lane DR, Pollet I, Olive PL, Humphries RK, Karsan A: Vascular endothelial growth factor receptor-2 induces survival of hematopoietic progenitor cells. *J. Biol. Chem.* 2003, 278:22006-22013.

[154] Jiang BH, Rue E, Wang GL, Roe R, Semenza GL: Dimerization, DNA binding, and transactivation properties of hypoxia-inducible factor 1. *J. Biol. Chem.* 1996, 271:17771-17778.

[155] Wang GL, Jiang BH, Rue EA, Semenza GL: Hypoxia-inducible factor 1 is a basic-helix-loop-helix-PAS heterodimer regulated by cellular O2 tension. *Proc. Natl. Acad. Sci. U. S. A* 1995, 92:5510-5514.

[156] Dang CV, Semenza GL: Oncogenic alterations of metabolism. *Trends Biochem. Sci.* 1999, 24:68-72.

[157] Semenza GL: HIF-1 and tumor progression: pathophysiology and therapeutics. *Trends Mol. Med.* 2002, 8:S62-S67.

[158] Jiang BH, Agani F, Passaniti A, Semenza GL: V-SRC induces expression of hypoxia-inducible factor 1 (HIF-1) and transcription of genes encoding vascular endothelial growth factor and enolase 1: involvement of HIF-1 in tumor progression. *Cancer Res.* 1997, 57:5328-5335.

[159] Maxwell PH, Dachs GU, Gleadle JM, Nicholls LG, Harris AL, Stratford IJ, Hankinson O, Pugh CW, Ratcliffe PJ: Hypoxia-inducible factor-1 modulates gene expression in solid tumors and influences both angiogenesis and tumor growth. *Proc. Natl. Acad. Sci. U. S. A* 1997, 94:8104-8109.

[160] Ryan HE, Lo J, Johnson RS: HIF-1 alpha is required for solid tumor formation and embryonic vascularization. *EMBO J.* 1998, 17:3005-3015.

[161] Iyer NV, Kotch LE, Agani F, Leung SW, Laughner E, Wenger RH, Gassmann M, Gearhart JD, Lawler AM, Yu AY, Semenza GL: Cellular and developmental control of O2 homeostasis by hypoxia-inducible factor 1 alpha. *Genes Dev.* 1998, 12:149-162.

[162] Bruick RK, McKnight SL: A conserved family of prolyl-4-hydroxylases that modify HIF. *Science* 2001, 294:1337-1340.

[163] Epstein AC, Gleadle JM, McNeill LA, Hewitson KS, O'Rourke J, Mole DR, Mukherji M, Metzen E, Wilson MI, Dhanda A, Tian YM, Masson N, Hamilton DL, Jaakkola P, Barstead R, Hodgkin J, Maxwell PH, Pugh CW, Schofield CJ, Ratcliffe PJ: C. elegans EGL-9 and mammalian homologs define a family of dioxygenases that regulate HIF by prolyl hydroxylation. *Cell* 2001, 107:43-54.

[164] Yu F, White SB, Zhao Q, Lee FS: HIF-1alpha binding to VHL is regulated by stimulus-sensitive proline hydroxylation. *Proc. Natl. Acad. Sci. U. S. A* 2001, 98:9630-9635.

[165] Hirota K, Semenza GL: Regulation of hypoxia-inducible factor 1 by prolyl and asparaginyl hydroxylases. *Biochem. Biophys. Res. Commun.* 2005, 338:610-616.

[166] Zundel W, Schindler C, Haas-Kogan D, Koong A, Kaper F, Chen E, Gottschalk AR, Ryan HE, Johnson RS, Jefferson AB, Stokoe D, Giaccia AJ: Loss of PTEN facilitates HIF-1-mediated gene expression. *Genes Dev.* 2000, 14:391-396.

[167] Jiang BH, Jiang G, Zheng JZ, Lu Z, Hunter T, Vogt PK: Phosphatidylinositol 3-kinase signaling controls levels of hypoxia-inducible factor 1. *Cell Growth Differ.* 2001, 12:363-369.

[168] Mayo LD, Donner DB: A phosphatidylinositol 3-kinase/Akt pathway promotes translocation of Mdm2 from the cytoplasm to the nucleus. *Proc. Natl. Acad. Sci. U. S. A* 2001, 98:11598-11603.

[169] Bardos JI, Chau NM, Ashcroft M: Growth factor-mediated induction of HDM2 positively regulates hypoxia-inducible factor 1alpha expression. *Mol. Cell Biol.* 2004, 24:2905-2914.

[170] Montesano R, Pepper MS, Belin D, Vassalli JD, Orci L: Induction of angiogenesis *in vitro* by vanadate, an inhibitor of phosphotyrosine phosphatases. *J. Cell Physiol* 1988, 134:460-466.

[171] Soucy NV, Ihnat MA, Kamat CD, Hess L, Post MJ, Klei LR, Clark C, Barchowsky A: Arsenic stimulates angiogenesis and tumorigenesis *in vivo*. *Toxicol. Sci.* 2003, 76:271-279.

[172] Gao N, Ding M, Zheng JZ, Zhang Z, Leonard SS, Liu KJ, Shi X, Jiang BH: Vanadate-induced expression of hypoxia-inducible factor 1 alpha and vascular endothelial growth factor through phosphatidylinositol 3-kinase/Akt pathway and reactive oxygen species. *J. Biol. Chem.* 2002, 277:31963-31971.

[173] Skinner HD, Zhong XS, Gao N, Shi X, Jiang BH: Arsenite induces p70S6K1 activation and HIF-1alpha expression in prostate cancer cells. *Mol. Cell Biochem.* 2004, 255:19-23.

[174] Lee M, Hwang JT, Yun H, Kim EJ, Kim MJ, Kim SS, Ha J: Critical roles of AMP-activated protein kinase in the carcinogenic metal-induced expression of VEGF and HIF-1 proteins in DU145 prostate carcinoma. *Biochem. Pharmacol.* 2006, 72:91-103.

[175] Hwang JT, Lee M, Jung SN, Lee HJ, Kang I, Kim SS, Ha J: AMP-activated protein kinase activity is required for vanadate-induced hypoxia-inducible factor 1alpha expression in DU145 cells. *Carcinogenesis* 2004, 25:2497-2507.

[176] Chen CJ, Wang CJ: Ecological correlation between arsenic level in well water and age-adjusted mortality from malignant neoplasms. *Cancer Res.* 1990, 50:5470-5474.

[177] Chiou HY, Hsueh YM, Liaw KF, Horng SF, Chiang MH, Pu YS, Lin JS, Huang CH, Chen CJ: Incidence of internal cancers and ingested inorganic arsenic: a seven-year follow-up study in Taiwan. *Cancer Res.* 1995, 55:1296-1300.

[178] Chen CJ, Chen CW, Wu MM, Kuo TL: Cancer potential in liver, lung, bladder and kidney due to ingested inorganic arsenic in drinking water. *Br. J. Cancer* 1992, 66:888-892.

[179] Gao N, Shen L, Zhang Z, Leonard SS, He H, Zhang XG, Shi X, Jiang BH: Arsenite induces HIF-1alpha and VEGF through PI3K, Akt and reactive oxygen species in DU145 human prostate carcinoma cells. *Mol. Cell Biochem.* 2004, 255:33-45.

[180] Duyndam MC, Hulscher TM, Fontijn D, Pinedo HM, Boven E: Induction of vascular endothelial growth factor expression and hypoxia-inducible factor 1alpha protein by the oxidative stressor arsenite. *J. Biol. Chem.* 2001, 276:48066-48076.
[181] Liu LZ, Jiang Y, Carpenter RL, Jing Y, Peiper SC, Jiang BH: Role and mechanism of arsenic in regulating angiogenesis. *PLoS. One.* 2011, 6:e20858.
[182] Jing Y, Liu LZ, Jiang Y, Zhu Y, Guo NL, Barnett J, Rojanasakul Y, Agani F, Jiang BH: Cadmium increases HIF-1 and VEGF expression through ROS, ERK, and AKT signaling pathways and induces malignant transformation of human bronchial epithelial cells. *Toxicol. Sci.* 2012, 125:10-19.
[183] Wen G, Hong M, Calaf GM, Roy D, Partridge MA, Li B, Hei TK: Phosphoproteomic profiling of arsenite-treated human small airway epithelial cells. *Oncol. Rep.* 2010, 23:405-412.
[184] Stueckle TA, Lu Y, Davis ME, Wang L, Jiang BH, Holaskova I, Schafer R, Barnett JB, Rojanasakul Y: Chronic occupational exposure to arsenic induces carcinogenic gene signaling networks and neoplastic transformation in human lung epithelial cells. *Toxicol. Appl. Pharmacol.* 2012.
[185] Costa M: Molecular mechanisms of nickel carcinogenesis. *Annu. Rev. Pharmacol. Toxicol.* 1991, 31:321-337.
[186] Li J, Davidson G, Huang Y, Jiang BH, Shi X, Costa M, Huang C: Nickel compounds act through phosphatidylinositol-3-kinase/Akt-dependent, p70(S6k)-independent pathway to induce hypoxia inducible factor transactivation and Cap43 expression in mouse epidermal Cl41 cells. *Cancer Res.* 2004, 64:94-101.
[187] Fotsis T, Pepper MS, Aktas E, Breit S, Rasku S, Adlercreutz H, Wahala K, Montesano R, Schweigerer L: Flavonoids, dietary-derived inhibitors of cell proliferation and *in vitro* angiogenesis. *Cancer Res.* 1997, 57:2916-2921.
[188] Wei H, Tye L, Bresnick E, Birt DF: Inhibitory effect of apigenin, a plant flavonoid, on epidermal ornithine decarboxylase and skin tumor promotion in mice. *Cancer Res.* 1990, 50:499-502.
[189] Fang J, Zhou Q, Liu LZ, Xia C, Hu X, Shi X, Jiang BH: Apigenin inhibits tumor angiogenesis through decreasing HIF-1{alpha} and VEGF expression. *Carcinogenesis* 2006.
[190] Bagli E, Stefaniotou M, Morbidelli L, Ziche M, Psillas K, Murphy C, Fotsis T: Luteolin inhibits vascular endothelial growth factor-induced angiogenesis; inhibition of endothelial cell survival and proliferation by targeting phosphatidylinositol 3'-kinase activity. *Cancer Res.* 2004, 64:7936-7946.
[191] Fang J, Zhou Q, Shi XL, Jiang BH: Luteolin inhibits insulin-like growth factor 1 receptor signaling in prostate cancer cells. *Carcinogenesis* 2006.
[192] Hwang DM, Kundu JK, Shin JW, Lee HJ, Surh YJ: cis-9,trans-11-Conjugated linoleic acid down-regulates phorbol ester-induced NF-{kappa}B activation and subsequent COX-2 expression in hairless mouse skin by targeting I{kappa}B kinase and PI3K-Akt. *Carcinogenesis* 2006.
[193] Palozza P, Sheriff A, Serini S, Boninsegna A, Maggiano N, Ranelletti FO, Calviello G, Cittadini A: Lycopene induces apoptosis in immortalized fibroblasts exposed to tobacco smoke condensate through arresting cell cycle and down-regulating cyclin D1, pAKT and pBad. *Apoptosis.* 2005, 10:1445-1456.

[194] Akimoto T, Nonaka T, Ishikawa H, Sakurai H, Saitoh JI, Takahashi T, Mitsuhashi N: Genistein, a tyrosine kinase inhibitor, enhanced radiosensitivity in human esophageal cancer cell lines *in vitro*: possible involvement of inhibition of survival signal transduction pathways. *Int. J. Radiat. Oncol. Biol. Phys.* 2001, 50:195-201.

Advances in Cancer Drug Targets, Vol. 1, 2013, 51-119

CHAPTER 3

Inhibitors of Cyclin Dependent Kinases: Useful Targets for Cancer Treatment (An Update)

P. Sapra Sharma* and R. Sharma

Department of Chemistry, C.S.S.S. (P.G.) College, Machhra, Meerut, Uttar Pradesh, India

Abstract: Cyclin-dependent kinases (CDKs) are serine/threonine protein kinases, which regulate multiple pathways such as the cell division cycle, apoptosis, transcription, and neuronal functions. Their sequential activation ensures the correct timing and ordering of events required for cell cycle progression. Uncontrolled proliferation is a hallmark of cancer cells. Over the past two decades, it has become increasingly clear that in many human cancers, hyperactivity of CDKs is one of the mechanisms underlying the physiological hyper-proliferation. Therefore, inhibition of CDKs, through the insertion of small molecules into its ATP binding pocket has emerged as a potential therapy method for cancers. For these reasons an intensive search for pharmacological inhibitors of these protein kinases has been carried out during the last decade. Consequently, a number of small molecules with CDK inhibitory properties have been developed. Many of these have been evaluated as potent inhibitors and some are currently in clinical-trials for various types of cancer. This review reports various CDK inhibitors, natural as well as small molecules, along with their reported activities for various CDKs. It will highlight the potential for the development of novel anti-cancer molecules.

Keywords: Cyclin dependent kinase, CKIs, small molecule inhibitors, anticancer agents, cell cycle, apoptosis.

INTRODUCTION

The worldwide epidemic of cancer has been stimulating the search for new concept and targets for the treatment of this incurable disease. Most traditional therapies [1] aim to exploit the proliferative machinery, for example DNA replication or chromosome segregation. As such, they demonstrate only partial selectivity for tumor cells compared with normal proliferating tissues such as the gut and bone marrow. Although efforts to refine and incrementally improve

***Address correspondence to P. Sapra Sharma:** Department of Chemistry, C.S.S.S. (P. G.) College, Machhra, Meerut, Uttar Pradesh, India; E-mail: poojasapra.sharma@gmail.com

Atta-ur-Rahman (Ed)

existing classes of anticancer agents continue, the recent shift of emphasis is towards novel mechanistic targets that have emerged as a direct consequence of the intense study of the underlying genetic changes associated with the cancerous state.

Recently, pharmaceutical attention has been focused on the proteins driving cellular proliferation, transformation, differentiation, and metastasis [2]. Approximately 518 different protein kinases are encoded in the human genome [3]. Among them a key class of cell cycle proteins, the Cyclin Dependent Kinases (CDKs), are a group of serine/threonine kinases involved in the regulation of the cell cycle, neuronal functions, transcription and apoptosis [4]. Their activity is highly regulated at several levels by multiple mechanisms, including association with cyclin regulatory subunit (CDK binding protein). The oscillating concentration of the cyclin during the cell cycle is the basis for the stage-dependent activity of the CDKs. Different CDK/cyclin pairs are active during each phase of the cell cycle [5]. To date at least 13 CDKs and more than 25 different cyclin families [6] have been described. Individual family members have a limited ability to assort a heterodimeric complex.

It is now recognized that in various human tumors, hyperactivity and deregulation of CDKs (mutation, deletion, and overexpression) are the primary causes for the uncontrolled proliferation [7]. This led to the initiation of ATP-competitive low molecular weight CDK inhibitor and their evaluation as anticancer agents [7-9]. The significance of these potential drug targets is clearly evidenced by the high incidence of alteration in the genes that code for these proteins in tumors. Targeting of protein kinase is a relatively recent activity for medicinal chemists. The design principles gleaned from these efforts have emerged as novel therapeutic that are more specific, efficacious, lesser toxic than their predecessors and target a wide range of protein kinase with broad therapeutic potential. A number of natural product-derived as well as synthetic kinase inhibitors have been discovered and characterized [10]. Presently more than a dozen kinase inhibitors have been approved for clinical use and about 150 are undergoing clinical trials [11].

There are many challenges in the rational development of specific inhibitors for protein kinases due to the similarity of the mechanism of different protein kinases and structure of their catalytic domains [12]. To achieve success, two main issues must be explored: First the selectivity among the kinases for efficacious and safe control of cell cycle. The clinical efficacy of these inhibitors critically depends not only on their potency, that is their ability to bind to CDKs, more stable than ATP (**1**), but also on their selectivity for the specific CDK over other highly homologous members of the CDK family and also other protein kinases. Non - selective inhibition carries the risk of undesired and potentially toxic side effect [13]. Thus along with potency, selectivity is crucial issue in inhibitor design [14,15]. Second as evidenced from those compounds with nanomolar potency for the CDK enzymes, two hydrogen bonds between the substrate and the CDK in the ATP pocket are preferred. As there have been no compounds disclosed with picomolar potency, it remains a possibility that an additional binding interaction will be key in achieving better potency and selectivity [16].

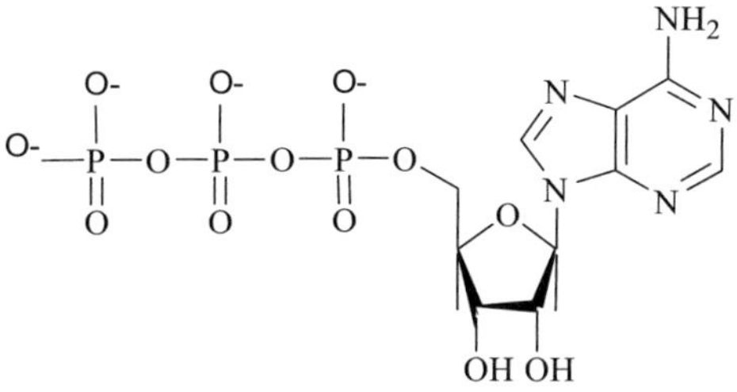

(1)

This review highlights small molecule inhibitors of CDKs (natural as well as synthetic) as potential drug molecules for cancer treatment. It also provides a brief insight into CDK inhibitory proteins (CKIs).

CDK INHIBITORS

The CDK inhibitors can be visualized as belonging to the following categories:

CDK Inhibitory Proteins or CKIs

Small Molecule Inhibitors

These are an additional regulatory subunit for the CDKs, a protein that binds to the CDK/cyclin complex and inhibits its activity. These proteins are termed CDK inhibitory proteins (CKIs). INK4 {(p16(Ink4a), p15(Ink4b), p18(Ink4c) and p19(Ink4d)} and Cip1/Waf1/Kip1-2 family {(p21(Cip1/Waf1), p27(Kip1), p57(Kip2)} are two families of CKIs targeting CDK4, CDK6 and CDK2, respectively [17,18]. Both of these families are shown in the context of proliferation regulators and as contributors to the apoptotic machinery [19]. Most known CKIs are involved in putting a brake on the cell cycle: some play a role in response to extra cellular signals, whereas other appear to function in intrinsic steps of the cell cycle [20,21].

Cip/Kip Family

The p21 protein was identified by its ability to bind to CDK2/cyclin complexes and functions as a CKI to inhibit their activity. p21 is a universal inhibitor of CDKs, as it inhibits the activity of each member of the CDK/cyclin family [22]. Emerging evidence now suggests additional functions for p21 in diverse cellular processes including a role as a modulator of apoptosis. Several mechanisms are postulated by which p21 interferes with the apoptotic machinery that encompass either CDK-independent events such as transcriptional regulation and direct binding to pro-apoptotic gene products in the cytoplasm [23].

Crystal structure of p27 bound to CDK2/cyclin A complex indicates that p27 associates with both CDK and cyclin subunits. The binding of p27 to CDK2/cyclin A complexes seems to be a two step event, where p27 first binds with cyclin followed by CDK binding [24]. Similarly biochemical studies of p27 complexes suggest that p27/p21-cyclin complexes are formed more readily than p27/p21-CDK complexes [25]. The association of p27 to CDK2/cyclin A complex cause conformational changes in the catalytic cleft of CDK2 that inactivate the kinase by hindering of ATP binding and blocking of the CAK (CDK-activating kinase) phosphorylation site. In accordance to the structural data studied, it is indicated that one molecule of p21 or p27 bound to CDK2/cyclin A complex is enough to inhibit the kinase activity [26].

INK4 Family

INK4 proteins are a group of ankyrin repeat-containing proteins, which specifically bind to CDK4 and CDK6 [27,28].

p16 specifically inhibit CDK4/cyclin kinase activity *in vitro*. Over expression of p16 leads to G1 arrest in various cell lines and suppresses cellular transformation, whereas overexpression of p16 in cell lacking functional pRb did not arrest cells in G1 [29]. In the crystal structure of the p16–CDK6 complex, p16 binds to one side of the catalytic cleft of CDK6 opposite to the cyclin–binding site. The concave surface of p16 contacts the N lobe of CDK6.

p15 and p16 are close homologue of each other especially in the exon two area [30]. The increased p15 levels associated with CDK4 and CDK6 inhibit their activity [31] and their overexpression prevents cellular growth. The coding sequence for p15 was not found to be altered in tumor cell lines examined in contrast to p16 sequence and therefore p15 was first thought to be a pseudogene.

p18 is a homologue of the important tumor suppressor p16. The global conformation of the twenty-four rationally designed mutants was characterized by NMR, while the function was assayed by inhibition of CDK4. Most of these mutants have unperturbed global structures [32], thus the changes in their inhibitory abilities can be attributed to the mutated residues. Some residues at loop 1 and 2 but not 3, are important for the inhibitory function of p18 similar to p16. Two residues at the first helix-turn-helix motif and two at the third are important for inhibition. Most importantly, the extra loop of p18 appears to contribute to the function of p18. p18 interacts with the preassembled CDK4/cyclin D2 complex in a similar way as predicted from the crystal structure of p16- CDK6 and p19-CDK6 binary complex.

p19 is another INK4 protein which inhibit CDK6 activity. Although the global folds and contacts of the two binary complexes, p16-CDK6 and p19-CDK6 are very similar, they differ in some specific interaction as well as in the surface area of the binding interface. Some of these differences are due to the surface residues in the two proteins that have contrasting charges. For example, Arg-24 of p16 corresponds to Asp-20 in p19. In the p16-CDK6 complex Arg-24 of p16 interacts with Asp-104 and Thr-106 of CDK6, while in the p19-CDK6 complex Asp-20 interacts with Arg-168 of CDK6. Differences in specific interaction arise where there is sequence identity between p16 and p19. For example Glu-27 of p16 forms a salt bridge with Arg-168 of CDK6 whereas Gln-22 of p19 interacts with Arg-168 of CDK6 [33].

Small Molecules as CDK Inhibitors

Of even greater importance to the successful development of small molecule kinase inhibitor is the understanding of the primary interactions of endogenous inhibitor to their substrates.

The kinase substrate ATP was co-crystallized with CDK2 [34]. The key interactions in the ATP pocket include hydrogen bonds between Leu-83 to N1, Glu-81 to N(6)H2, and Asp-86 to O(2)H, in addition to the phosphate chain interaction with the pocket at Lys-33, Asn-132, Asp-145, Lys-129, Thr-14, and Wat-558. This type of structural information has led to the employment of three main approaches to the inhibition of CDKs, which include ATP-competitive inhibitors, noncompetitive inhibitors that bind in the region of natural peptide inhibitors and molecules incorporating both of these approaches. The majority of published reports on CDK inhibitors utilize a small molecule approach to develop ATP-competitive inhibitors [16]. Frequently, first generation approaches to inhibitors rely on similarities to known inhibitor of analogous substrates. This type of approach has been modestly successful for kinase inhibitors. Indeed, for many kinases, small molecule ATP-competitive inhibitor approaches are being tested in clinical studies.

Staurosporine and Analogues

Staurosporine (**2**), a natural product that belongs to a family of microbial alkaloids was isolated from *Streptomyces staurosporeus* [35]. Compound (**2**) showed significant CDK inhibition IC_{50} (CDK2/cyclin A = 0.007 μM, [36] CDK4/cyclin D = 3-10 μM) [37]. At present, several (**2**) cognates are in advanced clinical trials as anticancer agents, with the potential to join the other protein kinase inhibitors now approved for clinical use [38].

The 7-hydroxystaurosporine analogue UCN-01 (**3**) [39] isolated from the culture broth of *Streptomyces* sp., is selective but non-specific inhibitor of kinases with good activity against PKC and CDKs (IC_{50} PKC = 0.0068 μM, CDK1 = 0.031 μM, and CDK2 = 0.03 μM). Compound (**3**) is currently in clinical trials to evaluate the compound's tolerability and pharmacokinetics (PK) [40, 41]. Five human cancer cell lines (MKN 45, HT-29, WiDr, PAN-3-JCK, and CRL 1420) were used to evaluate the antitumor spectrum of (**3**), which suppressed the growth of these digestive cancer cell lines. The determinant of sensitivity to (**3**) lies in the balance of CDK2 kinase activity and p21 protein induction [42].

The furanosylated indolocarbazole, K252a (**4**) is known to inhibit proliferation, stimulate apoptosis and induce cell cycle arrest of cancer cells [43]. 3-(4,5-Dimethylthiazol-2-yl)-2,5-diphenyltetrazolium bromide (MTT) assays showed that the ovarian cancer cell line SK-OV-3 was sensitive to the growth inhibitory effect of (**4**). Cell cycle analysis indicated that their exposure to (**4**) decreased the proportion of cells in the S-phase and increased the proportion of cells in the G(0)/G(1) phase of the cell cycle [44]. In response to the challenging chemistry of this series synthesis of (**2**), (**3**) and the furanyl analogue (**4**) have been reported [45-47].

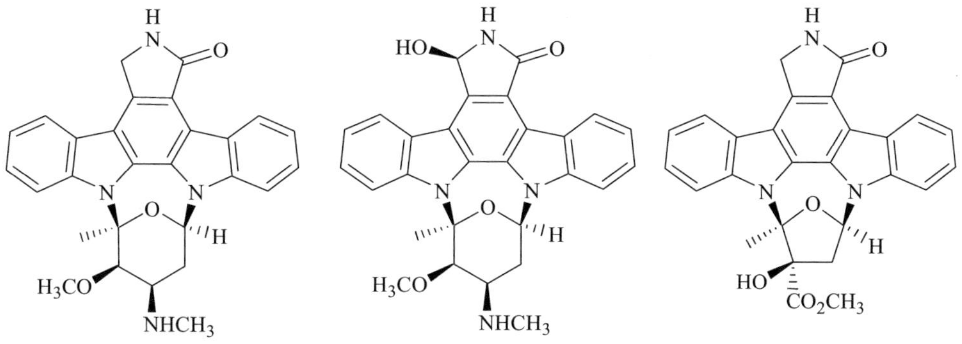

(**2**) (**3**) (**4**)

Flavonoid Derivatives

Quercetin (**5**) an ubiquitous bioactive plant flavonoid, has been shown to inhibit the proliferation of cancer cells over a range of concentration from 0.01-10 μM [48]. Due to its anti-oxidant, anti-tumor, and anti-inflammatory activity, (**5**) has been studied extensively as a chemoprevention agent in several cancer models. Since most of these studies used higher doses of (**5**) than clinically achievable, a study to determine the effectiveness of physiologically relevant doses was carried out. A low dose of (**5**) exerted cancer cell-specific inhibition of proliferation and this inhibition resulted from cell cycle arrest at the G(1) phase. Compound (**5**) induced p21 CDK inhibitor with a concomitant decrease of phosphorylation of pRb, which inhibits the G(1)/S cell cycle progression by trapping transcription factor E2F1 [49].

Alvocidib (Flavopiridol, NSC-649890, L86-8275) (**6**) is a semi-synthetic flavone analog of the alkaloid, rohitukine, a compound from an Indian tree, *Dysoxylum binectariferum*. It has been shown to inhibit CDKs, causing cell cycle arrest and growth inhibition [50]. This flavone is the most advanced CDK inhibitor, currently in Phase I clinical trials for solid tumors [51]. The compound (**6**) is a non-selective kinase inhibitor showing *in vitro* activity with IC_{50} (CDK4/cyclin D = 0.4 μM, CDK2/cyclin A = 0.1 μM, CAK = 0.3 μM [52] and CDK1/cyclin B = 0.4 μM [53]) and with very slight activity for Epidermal Growth Factor (EGF) receptor tyrosine kinase (IC_{50} = 21 μM) and Protein Kinase A (PKA) (IC_{50} = 122 μM) [54]. The compound (**6**) has also shown promising results in combination therapy, enhancing the activity of Bortezomib in human trials [55]. The design and synthesis of a small library of 8-amidoflavone, 8-sulfonamidoflavone, 8-amido-7-hydroxyflavone, and heterocyclic analogues of flavopiridol is reported. The potential activity of these compounds as kinase inhibitors was evaluated by cytotoxicity studies in MCF-7 and ID-8 cancer cell lines and inhibition of CDK2/cyclin A enzyme activity *in vitro*. The antiproliferative and CDK2/Cyclin A inhibitory activity of these analogues was significantly lower than the activity of (**6**) [56].

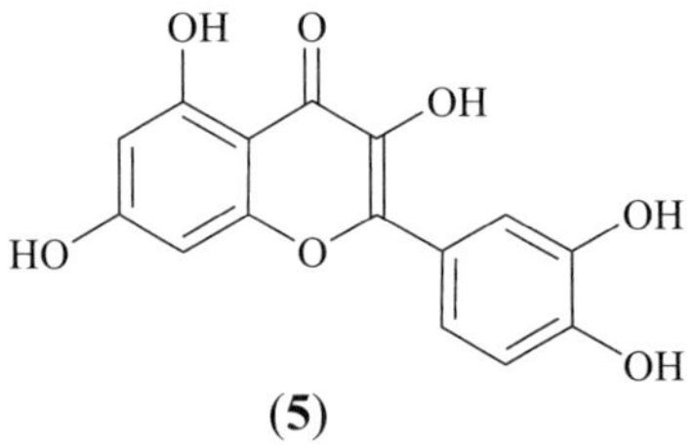

(5)

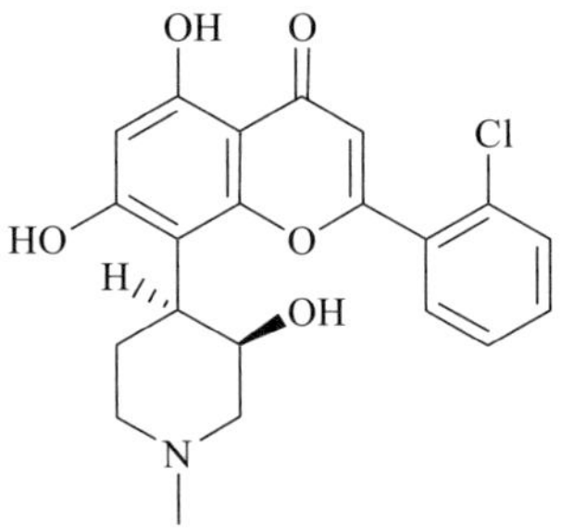

(6)

Wogonin (**7d**) has been shown to induce apoptosis in different cancer cells and to suppress growth of human cancer xenografts *in vivo*. The (**7d**)-containing herb *Scutellaria baicalensis* has successfully been used for curing various diseases in traditional Chinese medicine. A recent study demonstrated for the first time that (**7d**) and structurally related natural flavones, for example, apigenin (**7a**), chrysin (**7b**) and luteolin (**7c**), are inhibitors of CDK9 and block phosphorylation of the carboxy-terminal domain of RNA polymerase II at Ser2. Pull-down and *in silico* docking studies demonstrate that (**7d**) directly binds to CDK9, presumably to the ATP-binding pocket. In contrast, (**7d**) does not inhibit CDK2, CDK4 and CDK6 at doses that inhibit CDK9 activity [57].

P276-00 (**8**) shows 40-fold selectivity toward CDK4/cyclin D1, compared with CDK2/cyclin E. The specificity toward 14 other related and unrelated kinases was also determined [58]. Compound (**8**) was found to be more selective with IC_{50}s <100 nM for CDK4, CDK1, and CDK9, as compared with other CDKs, and less selective for non-CDK kinases. Compound (**8**) showed potent antiproliferative effects against various human cancer cell lines, with an IC_{50} ranging from 300-800 nM and was further compared for its antiproliferative activity against cancer and normal fibroblast cell lines. Compound (**8**) was found to be highly selective for cancer cells as compared with normal fibroblast cells [59].

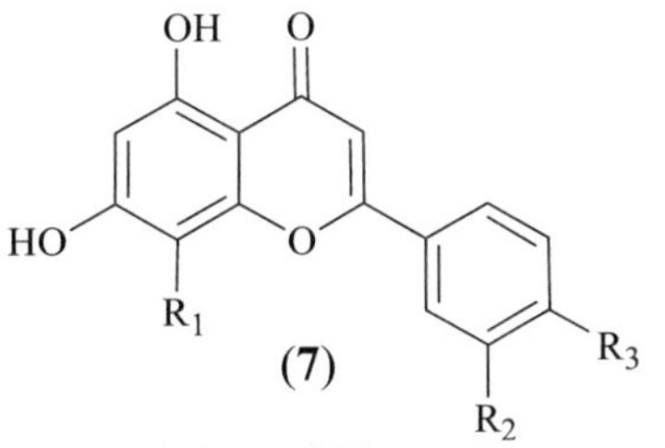

a. R_1, R_2= H; R_3 = OH
b. R_1, R_2, R_3 = H
c. R_1 = H; R_2, R_3 = OH
d. R_1 = OCH_3; R_2, R_3 = H

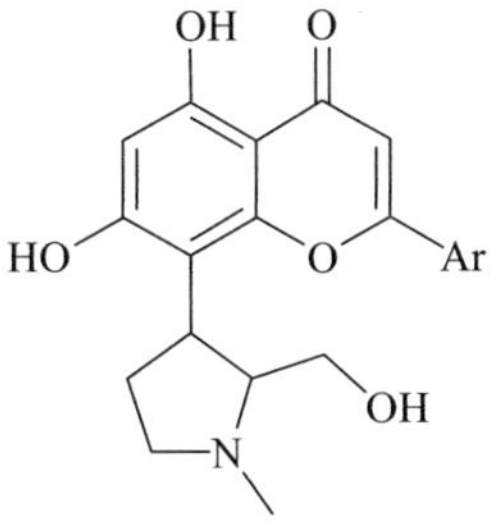

(**8**)

A metabolite of Daidzein (**9a**), 6,7,4'-Trihydroxyisoflavone (6,7,4'-THIF, **9b**) suppressed anchorage-dependent and -independent growth of HCT-116 and DLD1 human colon cancer cells more effectively than (**9a**). In addition, (**9b**) induced cell cycle arrest at the S and G2/M phases in HCT-116 human colon cancer cells. Western blot analysis revealed that (**9b**) effectively suppressed the expression of CDK2, but had no effect on other S- or G2/M-phase regulatory proteins such as cyclin A, cyclin B1 or CDK1 [60].

Fisetin (3,7,3',4'-Tetrahydroxyflavone) (**10**) is a natural flavonol present in edible vegetables, fruits, and wine, reported to exert anticarcinogenic effects. Compound (**10**) is a relatively small flavonol inhibitor with a hydroxyl group in the 3-position of the benzopyran ring. This distinguishes it from several other flavone inhibitors whose inhibitory activity on CDK6/cyclin V was determined. The 4-keto group and the 3-hydroxy group of (**10**) are hydrogen bonded with the backbone in the hinge region between the N-terminal and C-terminal kinase domain, as has been observed for many CDK inhibitors. Compound (**10**) inhibits CDK6 with an IC_{50} = 0.85 μM [61].

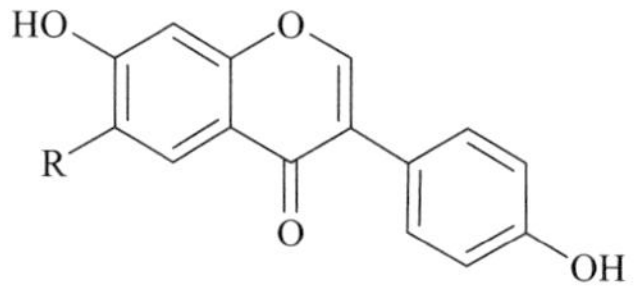

(**9**)

a. R = H
b. R = OH

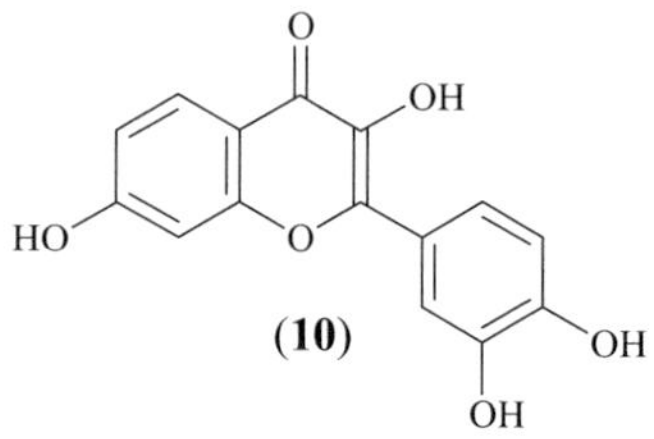

(**10**)

A novel series of 3-hydroxychromones (**11**) were prepared and found to be CDK inhibitors. Isothiazolidine 1,1-dioxide analogues (**12**) of (**11**) showed potent CDK1 and CDK2 inhibitory activities and inhibited proliferation of EJ, HCT-116, SW620, and MDAMB468 cancer cells [62]. The CDK2 inhibitory values for (**11a,b**) as IC_{50} = 4 μM, 5 μM and (**12a,b**) IC_{50} = 0.087 μM, 0.075 μM respectively are reported.

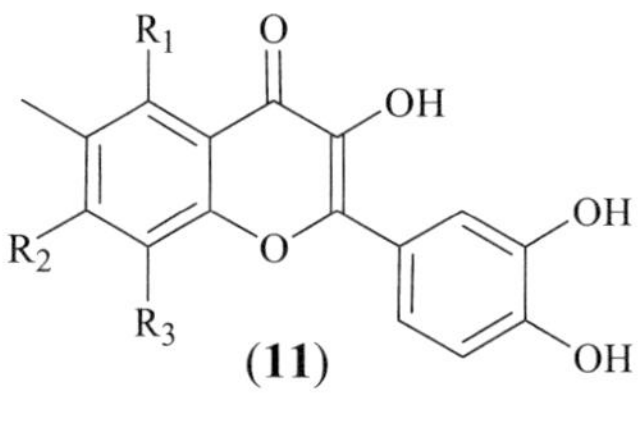

(**11**)

a. $R_1 = R_2 = R_3 = H$
b. $R_1 = R_3 = H$; $R_2 = OH$

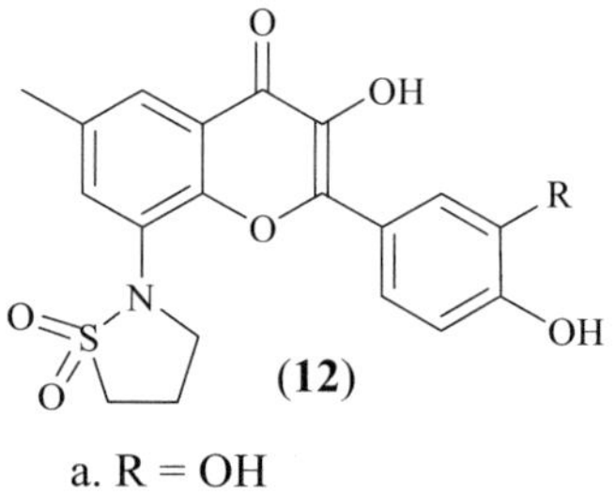

(**12**)

a. R = OH
b. R = Br

Purine Derivatives

The purines ring system is used in a number of CDK inhibitors, such as Olomoucine (**13**) which was identified as an active lead compound through the screening of substituted purines with modest potency {IC_{50} (CDK1/cyclin B = 7 μM, CDK2/cyclin A = 7 μM, CDK2/cyclin E = 7 μM and CDK5/p35 = 3 μM)} [63], whereas it has an antitumor potency with IC_{50} = 56 μM for HCT-116 cancer cells [64]. The effects of (**13**) in gamma-irradiation mediated cell growth inhibition and apoptosis were studied in the Raji cell line (Burkitt's lymphoma). The combination of (**13**) with irradiation caused an increased G2 arrest, decreased cell survival and DNA synthesis in the non-apoptotic fraction of the Raji cells [65].

Olomoucine II {6-[(2-hydroxybenzyl)amino]-2-[[1-(hydroxymethyl)propyl]amino]-9-isopropylpurine} (**14**) displays 10 times higher inhibitory activity than Roscovitine (**15**), a potent and specific CDK1 inhibitor. Compound (**14**) *in vitro* cytotoxic activity exceeds Purvalanol A (**19a**), a potent CDK inhibitor, as it kills the CEM cells with IC_{50} = 3.0 μM. Compound (**14**) shows IC_{50} of 0.02 μM against CDK1/cyclin B [66]. Apart from the main cell cycle-regulating kinase CDK1 and CDK2, (**14**) also exerts specificity for CDK7 and CDK9, with important functions in the regulation of RNA transcription [67].

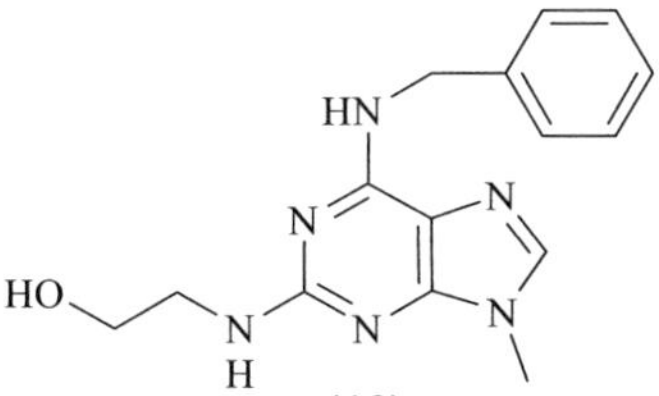

(**13**)

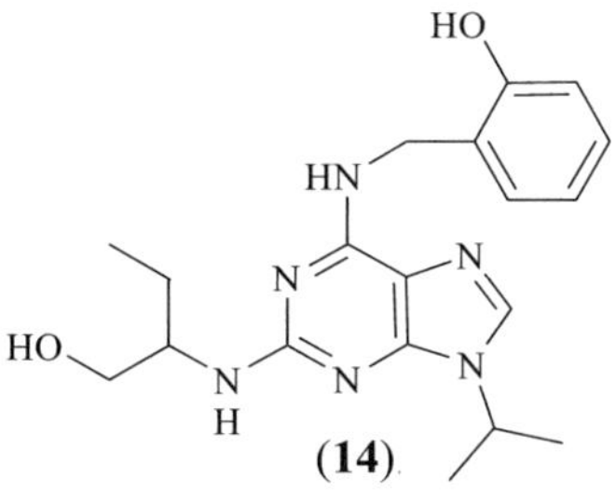

(**14**)

Compound (**15**) is a second-generation purine derivative in which the 2- and 9-substituents are bulky as compared to (**13**). This compound shows a 10-fold improved potency for CDK1/cyclin B (IC_{50} = 0.7 μM), CDK2/cyclin E (IC_{50} = 0.7 μM) and CDK5/p35 (IC_{50} = 0.16 μM) while maintaining selectivity with respect to a number of other kinases [68]. The R-isomer of (**15**) displays higher CDK1 and CDK5 inhibitory activity than the S-isomer. R-Roscovitine (Seliciclib or CYC202) (**16**) gave active concentration in the tumor, modulation of pharmacodynamic markers, and inhibition of tumor growth with IC_{50} = 15 μM for HCT-116 cell lines [64]. Compound (**16**) completely inhibits CDK5/p25 in the concentration range of 10 to 50 μM [69]. Being more orally available (**16**) is currently in Phase II clinical trials for Non-Small Cell Lung (NSCL) cancer and nasopharyngeal cancers and Phase I trials for glomerulonephritis. Preclinical investigations of the role of roscovitine in the treatment of neurodegenerative disorders such as Alzheimer's disease, viral infections, protozoal infections and inflammatory diseases are ongoing [70]. Compound (**15**) can reduce cell proliferation and survival of hormone therapy-resistant breast cancer cells supporting an emerging concept that inhibition of CDK2 activity has the potential to abrogate growth of hormonal therapy-resistant cells [71].

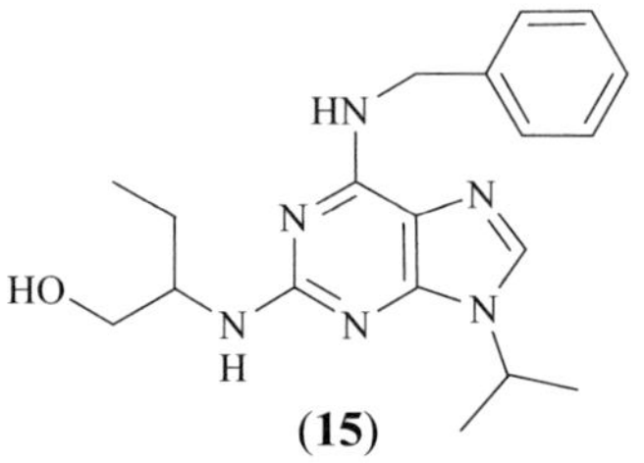

(15)

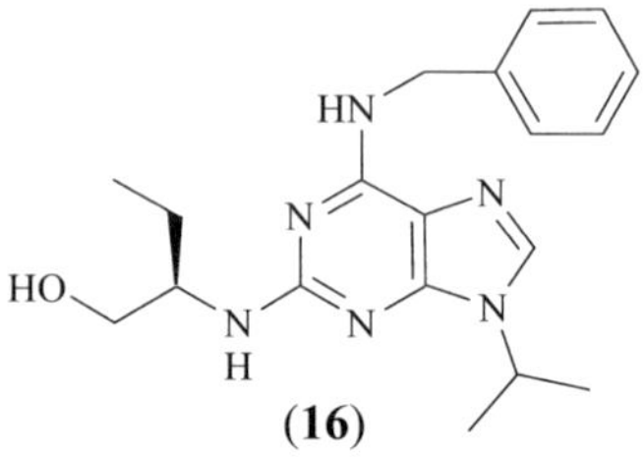

(16)

Recently, it has been shown that **(15)** exerts potent antiangiogenic effects. These findings introduce CDK5 as novel target for antiangiogenic therapy, and CDK5 inhibitors as an attractive therapeutic approach. A study reported the antiangiogenic profile of 15 derivatives of **(15)** *in vitro* and *in vivo* and provided structure activity relationships of the **(15)** analogs [72]. This study provides first information on how to modify **(15)** to develop CDK inhibitors with increased antiangiogenic activity and suggests the application of existing and the development of new CDK inhibitors to inhibit both, cancer cell proliferation and angiogenesis.

Hepatocellular carcinoma (HCC) is frequently associated with abnormalities in cell cycle regulation, leading to increased activity of CDKs due to the loss, or low expression of, CDK inhibitors. Ibulocydine [**17b**, an isobutyrate prodrug of the specific CDK inhibitor, BMK-Y101 **(17a)**] due to its high activity against CDK7/cyclin H/Mat1 and CDK9/cyclin T is a candidate anti-cancer drug for HCC. Compound **(17b)** inhibited the growth of HCC cells more effectively than other CDK inhibitors, including **(13)** and **(15)** [73].

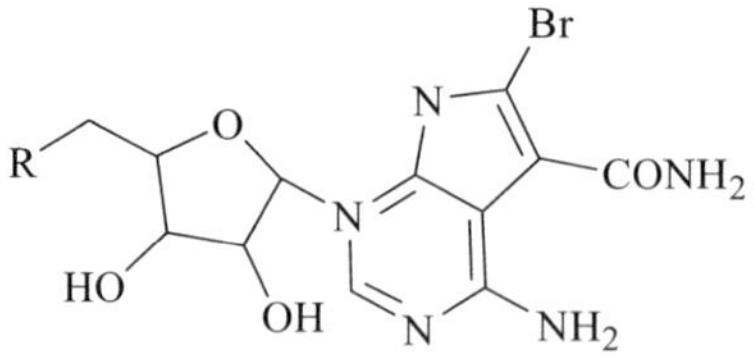

(17)

a. R = OH
b. R = $(CH_3)_2CHCOO$

Bohemine (**18**), a purine based analogue of (**13**) substituted with a 6-benzylamine and a 2-amino alcohol has been reported to have weak inhibitory effect on CDKs [74]. The cellular and molecular pharmacology of the new class of anticancer drugs, in which the CDK inhibitor (**18**) and its analogues are coordinated to Pt(II) to form cisplatin derivatives, was investigated. The results revealed the unique anticancer profile of a cisplatin-derived platinum(II) dichlorido complex involving N^7-coordinated bohemine. Although the IC_{50} values were ~6-fold higher for coordinated complexes than for cisplatin in cisplatin-sensitive tumor cells, the tumor cells in which complex was also active are those which acquired resistance to cisplatin [75].

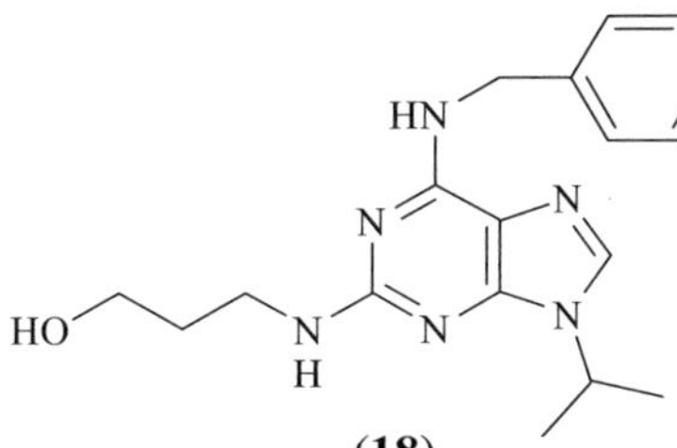

(18)

In an attempt to enhance the competitive binding of purines to CDKs, elements of diversity were introduced at the 2-, 6- and 9- position, which yielded the Purvalanol A,B (**19a,b**). These compounds show selectivity with respect to CDK4/cyclin D1, Extracellular Signal-Regulated Kinase (ERK), PKC and RAF in addition to other kinases. Purvalanol B (**19b**) was shown to be active for CDK2/cyclin E (IC_{50} = 0.009 μM), CDK5/p35 (IC_{50} = 0.006 μM) and CDK2/cyclin A (IC_{50} = 0.006 μM) [76]. Purvalanol A (**19a**) is one of the most potent compounds in this group, but its pharmacological profile may be inferior to that for (**15**). Compound (**19a**) effectively suppressed the growth of human colon cancer HT29 and SW480 cells, in which Src family kinases and CDKs both are activated. These findings demonstrated that the coordinated inhibition of cell cycle progression and tyrosine kinase signaling by the multi-selective (**19a**) is effective in suppressing cancer progression associated with c-Src up-regulation [77].

Medulloblastoma is the most prevalent of childhood brain malignancies, constituting 25% of childhood brain tumors. VMY-1-103 (**20**, a novel dansylated analog of **19b**) inhibited cell cycle progression and proliferation in prostate and breast cancer cells more effectively than (**19b**). Compound (**20**) significantly decreased the proportion of cells in S phase and increased the proportion of cells in G(2)/M. It increased the sub G(1) fraction of apoptotic cells, induced PARP and caspase-3 cleavage and increased the levels of the Death Receptors DR4 and DR5, Bax and Bad while decreasing the number of viable cells, all supporting apoptosis as a mechanism of cell death. p21(CIP1/WAF1) levels were greatly suppressed. (**20**) was unique in its ability to severely disrupt the mitotic spindle apparatus significantly delaying metaphase and disrupting mitosis. This data suggest that (**20**) possesses unique antiproliferative capabilities and that this compound may form the basis of a new candidate drug to treat medulloblastoma [78].

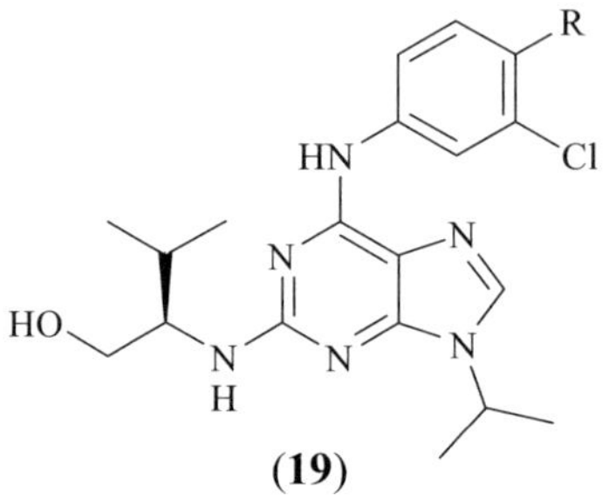

(**19**)

a. R = H
b. R = COOH

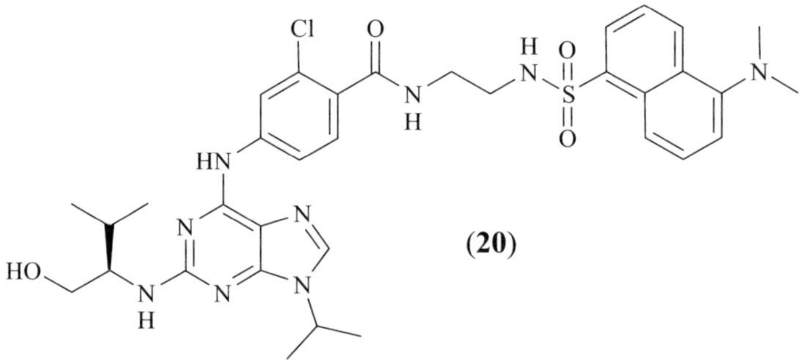

(**20**)

Recently, a novel series of purines with greater solubility, lower metabolic clearance, and enhanced potency *versus* CDKs is reported. These compounds exhibit novel selectivity profiles *versus* CDK isoforms. Compound αSβR-21 (**21**) inhibited CDK2/cyclin E with IC_{50} = 30 nM, CDK7-cyclin H (IC_{50} = 1.3 μM), and CDK9-cyclinT (IC_{50} = 0.11 μM); stopped proliferation of HCT116 colon cancer cells *in vitro* with GI_{50} = 0.7 μM; and showed antitumour activity when dosed *p.o.* at 50 mg/kg to mice bearing HCT-116 solid human tumour xenografts [79].

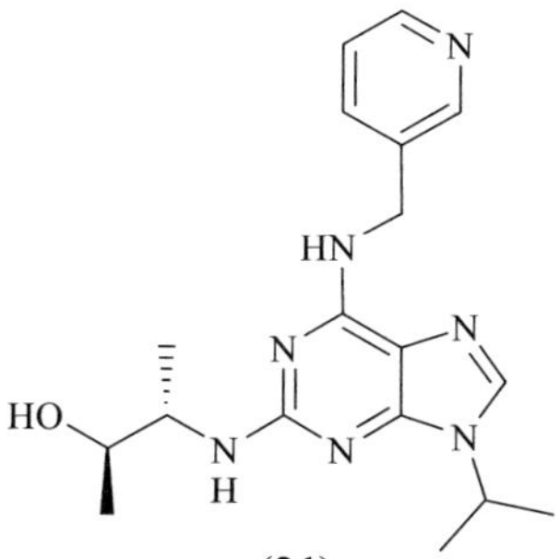

(21)

A series of 2-arylsubstituted purine derivatives has been synthesized by Suzuki Pd^0 coupling reactions. Moderate *in vitro* inhibitory activity against CDK5 and CDK1 was observed but were found to be inactive against Glycogen Synthase Kinase (GSK3) [80].

A family of O-alkylguanine-based CDK inhibitors was reported which lack the seemingly crucial secondary amine substituent at C-6. From the crystal structure of the initial lead compound NU2058 (**22a**) with CDK2 (IC_{50} = 12 μM) it was determined that (**22a**) binds in the ATP site in yet another orientation. Phenyl substituted NU6094 (**22b**) has CDK2 IC_{50} value of 1 μM [81, 82].

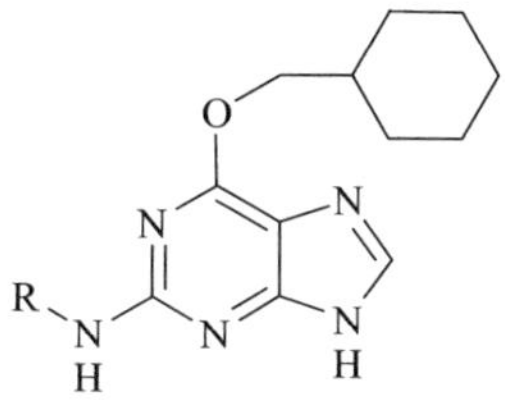

(22)

a. R = H
b. R = Phenyl

CDKs and Casein Kinases 1 (CK1) are involved in the two key molecular features of Alzheimer's disease, production of amyloid-beta peptides (extracellular plaques) and hyper-phosphorylation of Tau (intracellular neurofibrillary tangles). A series of 2,6,9-trisubstituted purines, structurally related to the (**15**) has been synthesized. They mainly differ by the substituent on the C-6 position. These compounds were screened for kinase inhibitory activities and antiproliferative effects. Several biaryl derivatives displayed potent inhibition of both CDKs and CK1 [83].

C-6 Biarylmethylamino purine derivatives of (**15**) inhibited CDKs and demonstrated potent antiproliferative activity. Replacement of the aryl rings of the C-6 biarylmethylamino group with heterobiaryl rings has provided compounds with significantly improved activity [84, 85].

A set of 38 6-benzylaminopurine (BAP) derivatives were prepared by the condensation of 6-chloropurine with corresponding substituted benzylamines. These were later assaysed in cytokinin and CDK2 inhibition bioassays. Several of the tested compounds showed stronger inhibitory activity and cytotoxicity than BAP. There was also a significant positive correlation of the inhibitory effects on human and plant CDKs with cell proliferation of cancer and cytokinin-dependent tobacco cells, respectively. This suggests that at least a part of the antiproliferative effect of the new cytokinins was due to the inhibition of CDK activity [86].

A novel series of 8-Azapurines (1,2,3-triazolo[4,5-d]pyrimidines) is reported as new inhibitors of CDKs. The introduced N at position 8 of the purine ring generally lowered CDK2 inhibitory activity of new 8-azapurines in comparison to the model trisubstituted purines, whereas the antiproliferative potential of some derivatives remained very high, reflecting their ability to activate p53 tumor suppressor [87].

Optimized N-6 anilino/benzylamino inhibitors discovered for the most part through screening of large libraries of 2,6,9-trisubstituted purines are reported [88-90]. Zinc(II) complexes with potent inhibitors of CDK derived from 6-benzylaminopurine [91] are synthesized and their activities are reported.

Indole Derivatives

Oxindoles (**23**) are reported as potent CDK2 inhibitors. Two closely related classes of oxindole based compounds, 1H-indole-2,3-dione-3-phenylhydrazone (**23a**) and 3-(anilinomethylene)-1,3-dihydro-2H-indole-2-ones (**23b**) were shown to potently inhibit CDK2 [92]. Compound in this series inhibited CDK2 with a potency ~10 fold greater than that for CDK1. 5-Oxazolyl derivative of compound (**23a**) has IC_{50} value for CDK1 as 0.01 μM and for CDK2 0.0023 μM, and for (**23b**) the values are 0.017 μM and 0.0025 μM, respectively. A hydrogen bond between inhibitor and the backbone NH of Asp-86 near the opening of the ATP binding cleft of CDK2 was of particular interest and appeared to play a significant role in affinity.

With the purpose of designing new chemical entities with better inhibitory potencies against CDK2 and CDK1, the 3D-QSAR CoMFA studies has been carried out on oxindole derivatives as inhibitors of these kinases was reported [93].

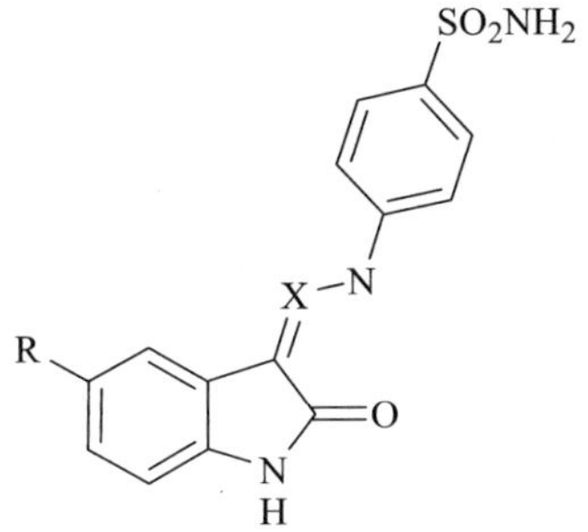

(23)

a. X = N; R = H, Br, Cl, oxazolyl
b. X = CH; R = H, Cl, oxazolyl

A novel series of oxindole-type inhibitors of CDK2 that have heteroatom substituted alkynyl moieties at their C-4 position is reported. These novel 4-alkynyl-substituted inhibitors have superior potency relative to their parent compound in free enzyme and in cell based assays. The crystal structure of CDK2 in complex with one of these analogues was determined and gives insight to their increased potency [94].

Indolinone scaffold has provided a large number of tyrosine kinase inhibitor (TKIs). In search for better potent inhibitor, (E)-Ethyl 3,5-dimethyl-4-[(indolin-2-one-3-ylidene)methyl]-1H-pyrrole-2-carboxylate (B5, **24**) was one of the novel pyrrole-substituted indolinones synthesized with the initial aim of developing selective EGFR inhibitor. However, (**24**) exhibited weak inhibitory potency against a variety of PTKs including EGFR, but potent kinase inhibition against several members of CDK family [95].

Indigoids (**25**), a class of bis-indole derivatives represents a promising protein kinase inhibitor scaffold. Oxidation of indole by cytochrome P450 has been shown to generate species (indoxyl, isatin) that couple to yield indigo and indirubin. Incubation study of 27 substituted indole derivatives with *Escherichia coli*-expressed human P450 2A6 mutants isolated from a randomized library were screened for inhibition of human CDK1, CDK5 and GSK3. The extracts from cultures incubated with 5- and 5'-methoxyindole (**25a,b**) with IC_{50} (CDK1/cyclin B = 2.1, 1.5 μM, CDK5/p25 = 1.2, 1.2 μM, respectively) were the most inhibitory [96].

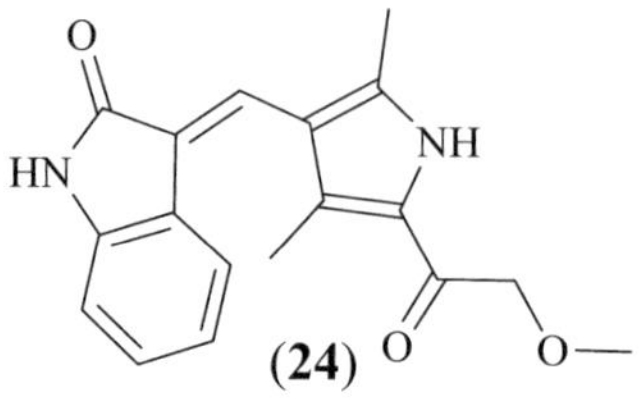

(24)

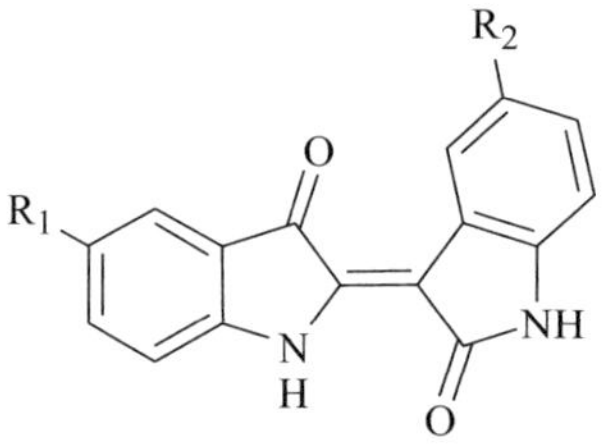

(25)

a. R_1 = H; R_2 = OCH_3
b. R_1 = OCH_3; R_2 = H

6-Substituted indolocarbazoles (**26a** and **26b**) represent a new class of CDK4/cyclin D1 inhibitors, which are structural homologue of (**2**). These compounds are potent, selective and ATP-competitive CDK4/cyclin D1 inhibitors and are capable of inhibiting cell growth in the human tumor cell lines, HCT-116 and NCI H460. Compound (**26a,b**) had the most potent CDK4/cyclin D1 enzyme inhibitory activity with IC_{50} values of 0.076 and 0.042 μM respectively [97].

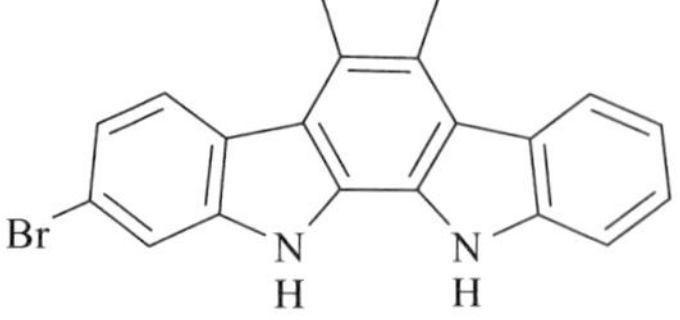

(26a)

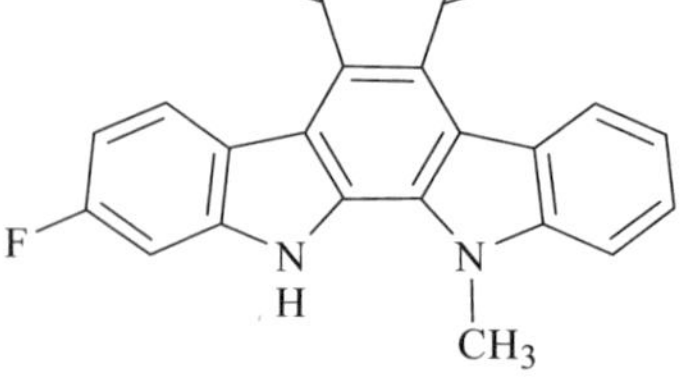

(26b)

High Throughput Screening (HTS) of the Lilly compound collection against the CDK4/cyclin D1 enzyme complex yielded an indolocarbazole, SB-210878 (**27**) which is a Checkpoint Kinase 1 (ChK1) and PKC inhibitor and has an IC_{50} of 0.54 μM against CDK4/cyclin D1 [98]. Subsequent testing of other indolocarbazoles indicated that the naturally occurring Arcyriaflavin A (**28**) also showed moderate inhibitory activity against CDK4/cyclin D1 [97].

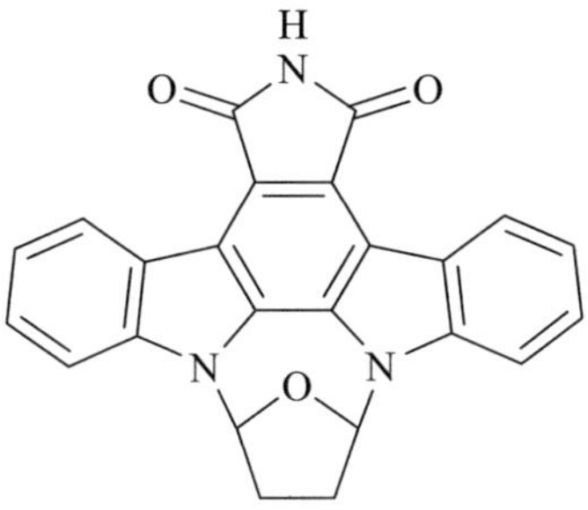

(**27**)

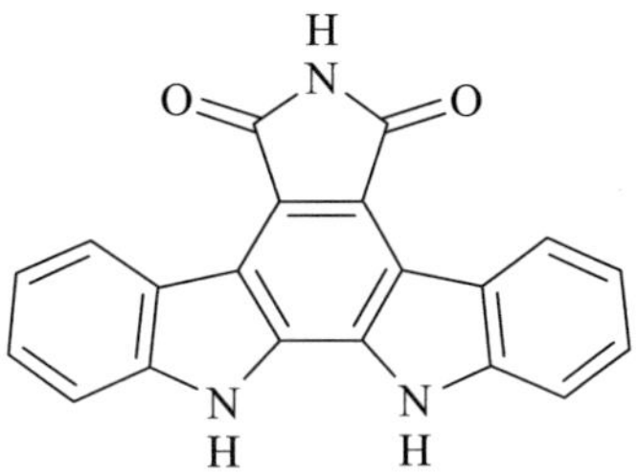

(**28**)

A series of (**26**) and their precursors were synthesized in order to compare their activity as CDK4/cyclin D inhibitors. Both enzymatic and antiproliferative assays have shown that the structurally more constrained (**26**) are consistently more active (8-42 fold) in head-to-head comparison with their counterparts [98].

Cyclin-D1binds to CDK-4/6 to form a holoenzyme that phosphorylates the Rb protein to promote cell cycle progression from G1 to S phase. Therefore, targeting CDK4/6 may be a good strategy for chemotherapy of cancer. To test this hypothesis, MCF7, MB231, MCF15, T47D and GI101Ap human breast cancer cells were analyzed for the efficacy of NPCD (**29**, Naphtho [2, 1-a] pyrrolo [3, 4-c] carbazole-5, 7 (6H, 12H)-dione) with MTT and clonogenic assays, with FACS and staining for ethidium bromide and acridine orange for cell death and cell cycle profile. Western blot, reverse transcription and PCR were used for studies of gene expression, and co-immunoprecipitation for protein-complex formation. MTT assay showed that (**29**) caused growth arrest and apoptosis of MCF7, MDA-MB231, T47D, MCF15 and GI101Ap cells with an IC_{50} ranging between 3 to 8 μM given as a single dose. The growth arrest persisted for many days after cessation of the treatment, as shown in a clonogenic assay [99].

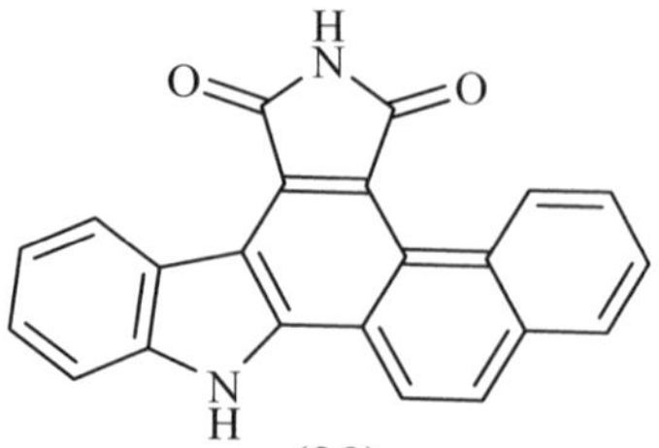

(29)

The chemistry and biology of indolocarbazole products is reviewed [100].

Pyridine Derivatives

Ciclopirox olamine (**30**, CPX, 6-cyclohexyl-1-hydroxy-4-methylpyridin-2(1H)-one) is a synthetic antifungal agent clinically used to treat mycoses of the skin and nails. In a study (**30**) inhibited tumor growth in human breast cancer MDA-MB-231 xenografts. Further, compound (**30**) inhibited cell proliferation and induced apoptosis in human rhabdomyosarcoma (Rh30), breast carcinoma (MDA-MB231) and colon adenocarcinoma (HT-29) cells in a concentration-dependent manner. By cell cycle analysis, (**30**) induced accumulation of cells in G(1)/G(0) phase of the cell cycle. Concurrently, (**30**) downregulated cellular protein expression of cyclins (A, B1, D1 and E), CDK2, CDK4 and upregulated expression of the CDK inhibitor p21(Cip1), leading to hypophosphorylation of retinoblastoma protein [101].

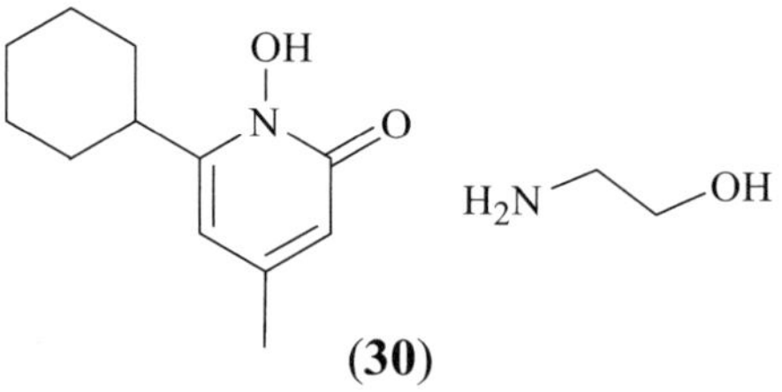

(30)

SCH 727965 (**31**, (S)-3-(((3-ethyl-5-(2-(2-hydroxyethyl)piperidin-1-yl)pyrazolo[1,5-a]pyrimidin-7-yl)amino)methyl)pyridine 1-oxide) was selected as a clinical candidate using a functional screen *in vivo* that integrated both efficacy and safety parameters (IC_{50} CDK2, CDK5, CDK1, and CDK9 = of 0.001, 0.001, 0.003, and 0.004 μM, respectively) [102]. The therapeutic efficacy of (**31**) on human pancreatic cancer cells was tested using *in vitro* and *in vivo* model systems where (**31**) significantly reduced *in vitro* cell growth, motility and colony formation in soft agar of MIAPaCa-2 and Pa20C cells. These phenotypic changes were accompanied by marked reduction of phosphorylation of Retinoblastoma (Rb) suggesting that (**31**) alone or in combination is a highly promising novel experimental therapeutic strategy against pancreatic cancer [103].

A novel series of 3-[(2-indolyl)]-5-phenyl-3,5-pyridine, 3-[(2-indolyl)]-5-phenyl-2,4-pyridine and 3-[(2-indolyl)]-5-phenyl-2,6-pyrazine derivatives are reported as potential CDK inhibitors. The synthesis included Stille or Suzuki type reactions, which were carried out on the 3,5-dibromopyridine, 2,4-dichloropyridine and 2,6-dichloro-1-4-pyrazine moieties. Cell effects of the V-shaped family were in the micromolar range. Kinase assays were conducted and showed that compound (**32**) inhibited CDK5 with an inhibitory concentration of 160 nM with a moderate selectivity over GSK3 [104].

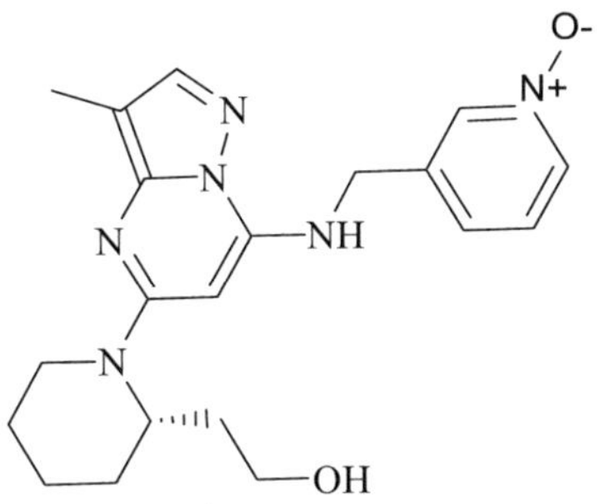

(**31**)

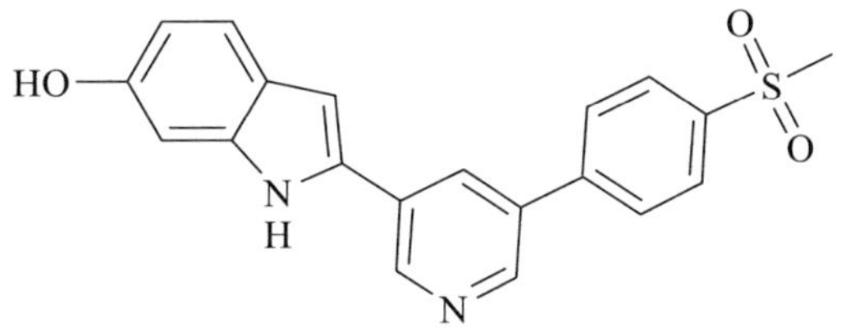

(**32**)

A new series of 3,5-disubstituted pyrazolo[3,4-b]pyridine showed potency and selectivity towards CDKs and inhibited *in vitro* cellular proliferation in cultured human tumor cells. Selected compounds were evaluated in an *in vivo* tumor xenograft model. The synthesis and biological evaluation of these pyrazolo[3,4-b]pyridines and related compounds are reported [105].

3-(1H-Benzimidazol-2-yl)-5-isoquinolin-4-yl-pyrazolo[1,2-*b*]pyridine (**33**) has been reported as a potent CDK1 inhibitor (IC_{50} = 0.023 μM). Compound (**33**) inhibited the proliferation of HeLa cervical adenocarcinoma, A375 malignant melanoma and HCT-116 colon carcinoma cells with IC_{50} values of 1.7, 0.87 and 0.55 μM respectively. Compound (**33**) also inhibited Vascular Endothelial Growth Factor Receptor (VEGFR-2) kinase with an IC_{50} value of 1.46 μM revealing approximately 60-fold selectivity in favour of CDK1 inhibition [106].

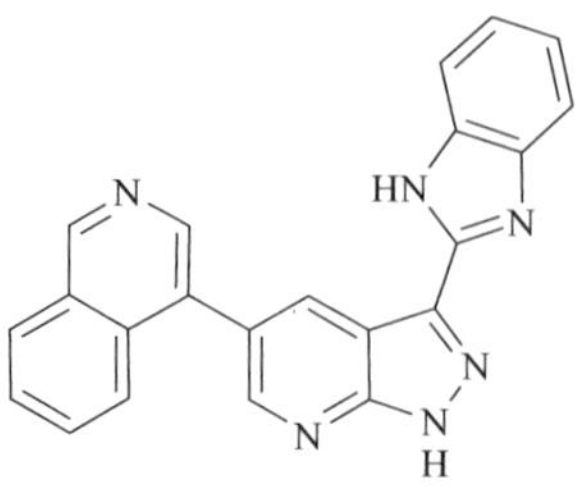

(33)

In vitro studies revealed that AZ703 (**34**), a novel imidazopyridine derivative is a selective inhibitor of CDK1 and CDK2. Compound (**34**) displays a mode of action consistent with the induction of G1, S, and G2-M phase arrest. (**34**) also showed potent anti-proliferative activity across a wide range of tumor cell lines [107]. The inhibitory activities of (**34**) are IC_{50} (CDK2/cyclin E = 0.004 μM, CDK2/cyclin A = 0.003 μM, CDK1/cyclin B = 0.006 μM, CDK4/cyclin D = 3.058 μM, CDK7/cyclin H = 1.510 μM).

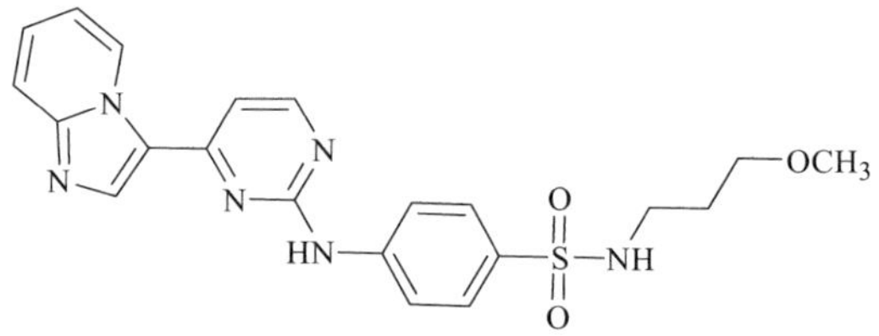

(34)

A series of 6-substituted 2-(N-trifluoroacetylamino)imidazopyridines have been synthesized and their bioactivities were evaluated. Compounds **35a-c** were the most active compounds with modest cytotoxic activity against six human cancer cell lines U251, PC-3, K-562, HCT-15, MCF7 and SK-LU-1. The cell cycle analysis showed that compounds induce a G2/M phase cell cycle arrest on SK-LU-1 cell line where inhibition of CDK1 and CDK2 may be implicated [108].

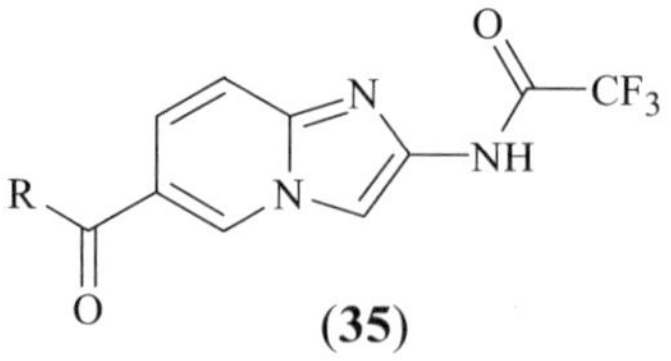

(35)

a. R = 3-Fluoro-4-methylphenyl
b. R = 2-Fluoro-5-methylphenyl
c. R = 1-Methyl-1H-indole-3-yl

Pyrimidines Derivatives

The phenylpyrimidine, CGP-60474 (**36**) was found to be a potent inhibitor of both CDK1 (IC_{50} = 0.017 μM) and CDK2 (IC_{50} = 0.05-0.08 μM) [109], while displaying weaker submicromolar to low micromolar activity for PKCα, ERK-1 and CDK4. Other growth-related protein kinase were unaffected by exposure to (**36**) including JNK, p38 and other PKC sub type.

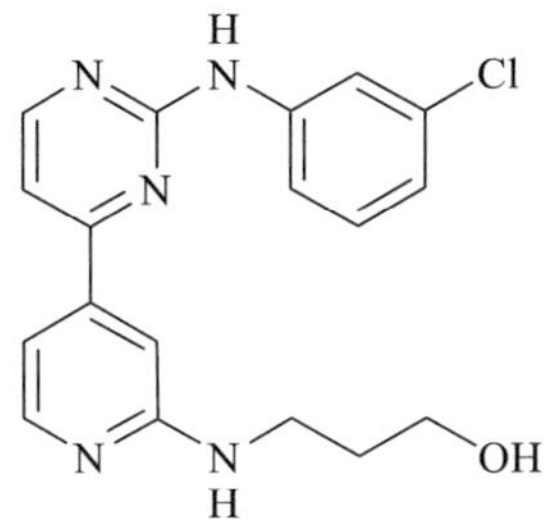

(**36**)

2-Aminopyrido[2,3-*d*]pyrimidine (**37**) derivatives are potent inhibitors of CDK4 and synthesis of its derivatives *via* a three-component reaction under microwave irradiation without catalyst is reported [110].

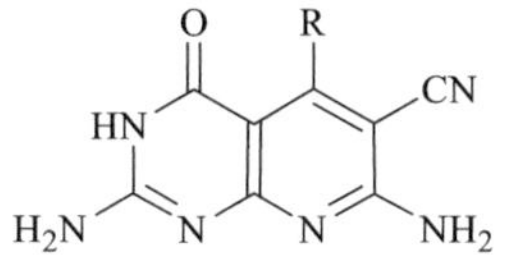

(**37**)

R = C_6H_5, 4-$NO_2C_6H_4$, 4-FC_6H_4, CH_3CH_2

The pyrido[2,3-*d*]pyrimidin-7-one template (**38**) had been identified as a privileged structure for the inhibition of ATP-dependent kinase and good potency against CDKs had been reported for representative examples [111]. The introduction of the methyl substituent at the C-5 position of (**38**) confered excellent selectivity for CDK4 *versus* other CDKs and representative tyrosine kinases. A structure activity relationship for derivative of (**38**) and inhibition of CDK4 was studied, and the interesting results associated with modification at the C-5 (**39a**) and C-6 (**39b**) position of this template are given in the Tables **1** and **2**, respectively. Remarkable levels of selectivity for CDKs *versus* other kinases had been achieved by appropriate substitution at these two positions [112].

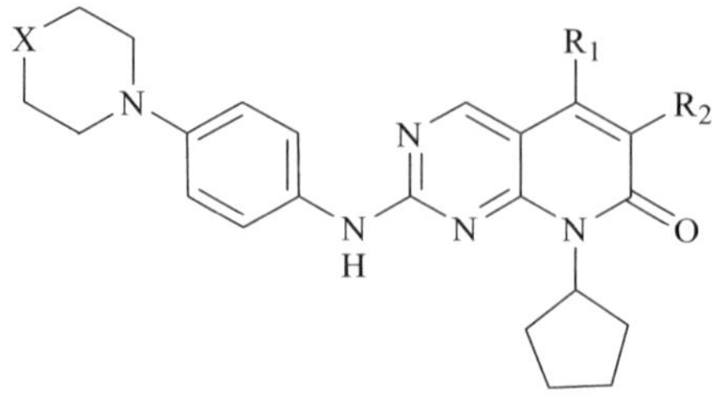

(38)

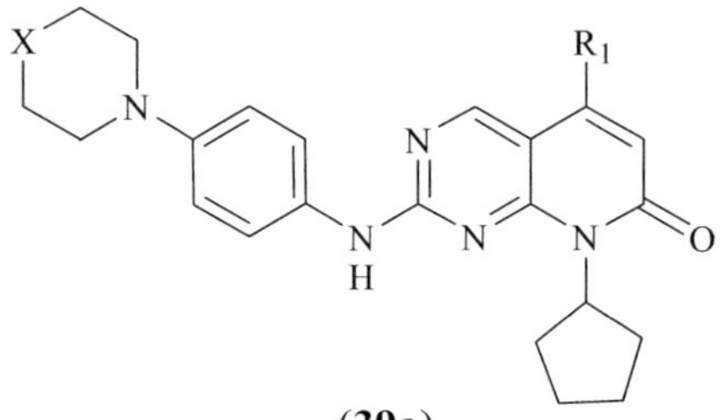

(39a)

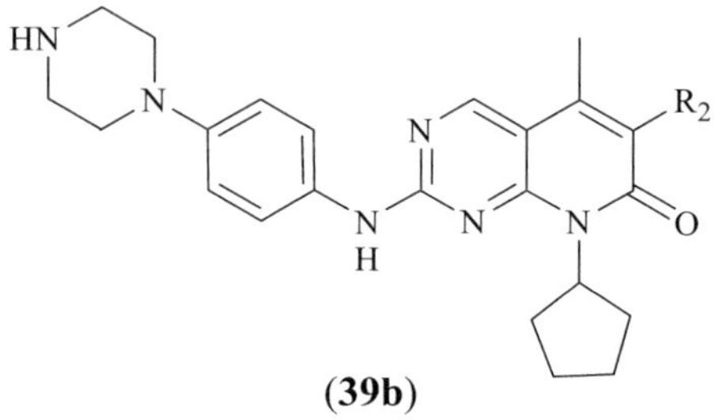

(39b)

Table 1: Effect of the C-5 substitution on Compound (**39a**). The values are IC_{50} in μM.

	R_1	X	CDK4/D	CDK1/B	CDK2/A	CDK2/E
i	H	O	0.01	0.275	0.028	0.085
ii	H	CH_2	0.01	0.57	0.66	0.246
iii	Me	O	0.116	1.12	>5	>5

Table 2: Effect of the C-6 substitution on Compound (**39b**). The values are IC_{50} in μM.

	R_2	CDK4/D	CDK1/B	CDK2/A	CDK2/E
i	Et	0.025	4.119	1.538	1.65
ii	F	0.03	>5	>5	>5
iii	Cl	0.016	>5	1.625	1.5
iv	Br	0.005	2.615	0.439	0.95
v	I	0.005	1.865	0.443	0.365
vi	COMe	0.002	-	0.23	-

Further, the introduction of a 2-aminopyridyl substituent at the C-2 position of (**39b**) substantially biases the selectivity of these compounds towards selective inhibition of CDK4/cyclin D1 *versus* other serine/threonine and tyrosine kinases. One of the derivative of the series, PD 0332991 (**40**) is a potent inhibitor of CDK4/cyclin D1 with IC_{50} value of 0.011 μM, for CDK2/cyclin A $IC_{50} > 5$ μM, and for MDA-MB435 $IC_{50} = 0.160$ μM [113]. Compound (**40**) displays good pharmocokinetic properties in rats (CL = 37.5 ± 1.7 mL/min/Kg, 56% oral bioavailability) and a high level of selectivity for CDK4/cyclin D1 *versus* over 36 other kinases. On the basis of its selectivity profile and pharmacokinetic profile, compound (**40**) was identified as a drug candidate for the treatment of cancer and is presently under Phase I clinical trials for advanced cancers [114].

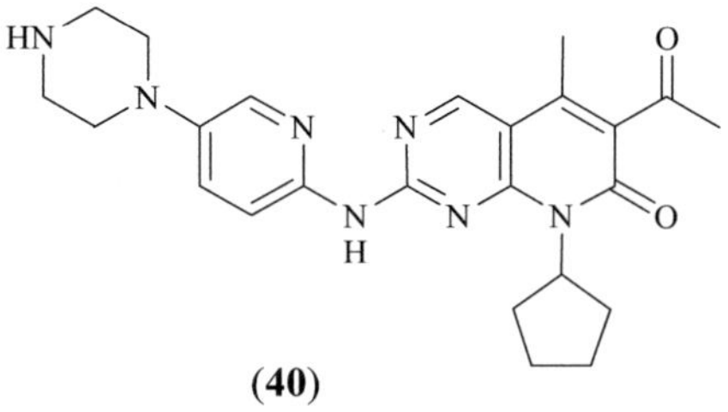

(**40**)

Using a HTS strategy, a series of 1-aryl-4,5-dihydro-1H-pyrazolo[3,4-*d*]pyrimidin-4-ones (**41a**) were identified that inhibit the CDK4/cyclin D1 complex-mediated phosphorylation of a protein substrate with IC_{50}s in the low micromolar range. The inhibitor molecule binds as ATP and other reported inhibitors, in the deep cleft between the N-terminal and C-terminal domains. This series appears to be selective for CDKs over several other protein kinases. The best CKD4/cyclin D1 inhibitors in this series are 50-330 times more potent than the screening hit and are characterized by having a relatively acidic hydrogen bond donor in the meta-position of the pyrazolopyrimidineR_6benzyl. The best antiproliferative activity is seen in those compounds having anilide group at the para position of the pyrazolopyrimidineR_6benzyl group (**41b**) (IC_{50} CDK4/cyclin D1 = 1.3 μM, CDK2/cyclin E = 0.009 μM) [115].

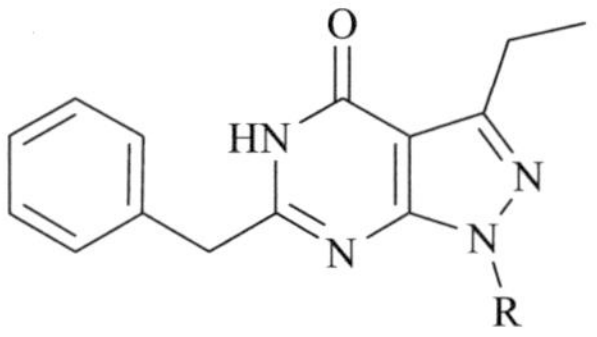

(**41a**)

R = benzyl, 2,3;2,4;2,6-dichlorophenyl, 2,4,6-trichlorophenyl

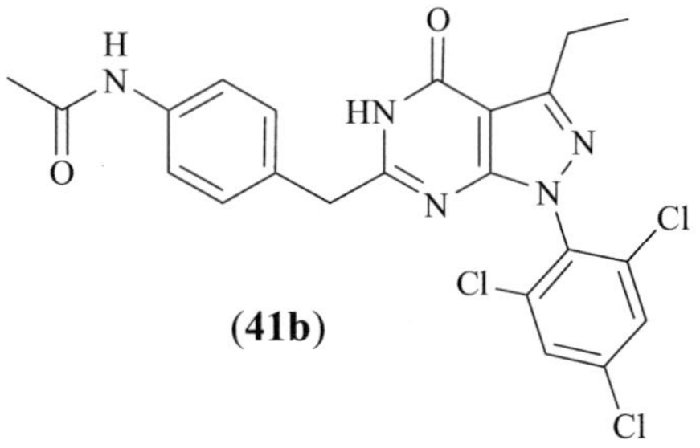

(**41b**)

A series of 2,5,7-trisubstituted pyrimido[4,5-d]pyrimidine CDK2 inhibitors is designed and synthesized. 6-Amino-2-thiouracil is reacted with an aldehyde and thiourea to prepare the pyrimido[4,5-d]-pyrimidines. Alkylation and amination of the latter ones give different amino derivatives. These compounds show potent and selective CDK inhibitory activities and inhibit *in vitro* cellular proliferation in cultured human tumor cells. Compound (**42**) has an IC_{50} of 0.05 μM making it more active than compound (**15**) [116].

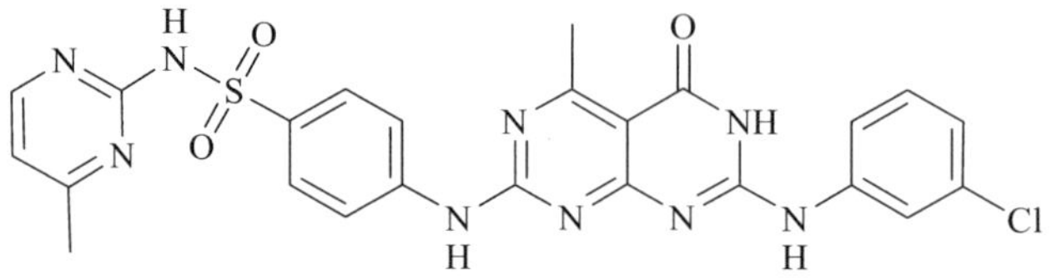

(**42**)

The synthetic chemistry, structure guided design approach, and SAR led to the discovery of 2-anilino-4-(thiazol-5-yl)pyrimidines**,** as ATP-antagonistic CDK2 inhibitors, many with very low nanomolar K_i's against CDK2 [117]. The most potent CDK2 inhibitor of this class is compound (**43**), where the presence of the primary NH_2 group leads to increased electrostatic interactions with the chains of Asp-145 and Asn-132. The side chain of Asn-132 is found to adopt two alternative conformations, only one of which interacts with the NH_2 group. The significantly tighter binding of (**43**) may also be explained by additional interaction involving the nitro substituent. The potency was highest against CDK2 but other CDKs, particularly CDK9, were also inhibited at somewhat reduced potency. Unlike other small-molecule ATP-antagonist CDK inhibitors, compound (**43**) did not have a significant effect on the catalytic activity of the structurally related ERK-2 kinase. On the other hand, GSK3 was inhibited with sub-micromolar potency. There was also a large increase in cell death after treatment of HeLa cells with (**43**) (IC_{50} = 0.5 μM) [117].

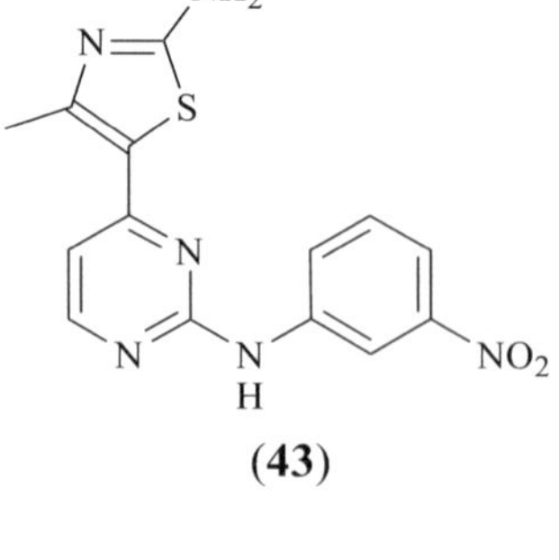

(**43**)

TG02/SB1317 [(16E)-14-methyl-20-oxa-5,7,14,26-tetraazatetracyclo[19.3.1.1(2,6).1 (8,12)]heptacosa-1(25),2(26),3,5,8(27),9,11,16,21,23-decaene), **44**] is a novel pyrimidine-based multi-kinase inhibitor that inhibits CDKs 1, 2, 7 and 9 together with Janus kinase 2 (JAK2) and Fms-like tyrosine kinase receptor-3 (FLT3) [118]. Compound (**44**) is anti-proliferative in a broad range of tumor cell lines, inducing G1 cell cycle arrest and apoptosis. Primary cultures of progenitor cells derived from acute myeloid leukemia (AML) and polycythemia vera patients are very sensitive to (**44**) [119].

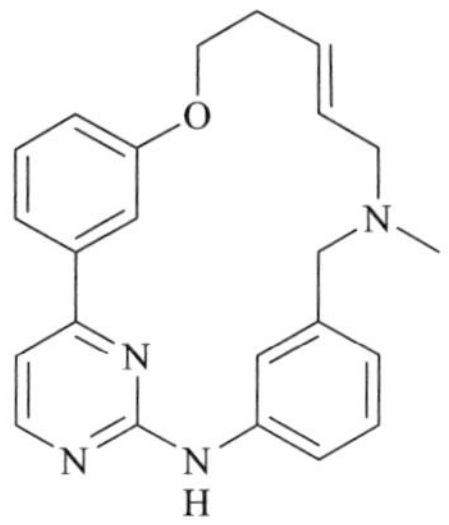

(44)

The main difficulty in the development of ATP antagonist kinase inhibitors is target specificity, since the ATP-binding motif is present in many proteins. Employing a screening cascade of cellular phenotypic assays based on mitotic index and nuclear p53 protein accumulation permitted to classify compounds into transcriptional, cell cycle, and mitotic inhibitor groups. This strategy identified compounds from a kinase inhibitor library that block the cyclin-dependent kinases responsible for regulating transcription, *i.e.*, CDK7 and especially CDK9. A structural selectivity rationale was used to optimize potency and biopharmaceutical properties and led to the development of a transcriptional inhibitor, 3,4-dimethyl-5-[2-(4-piperazin-1-yl-phenylamino)-pyrimidin-4-yl]-3H-thiazol-2-one (**45**), with anticancer activity in animal models [120].

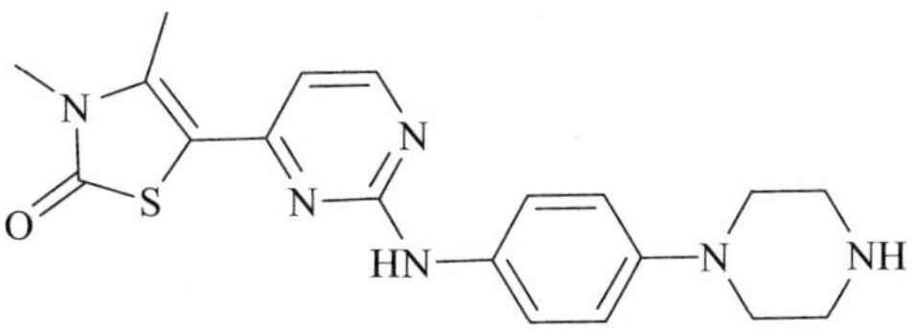

(45)

Pyrazolo[1,5-a]pyrimidine based compound, BS-194 [**46**, (2S,3S)-3-(7-Benzylamino-3-isopropyl-pyrazolo[1.5-a]pyrimdin-5-ylamino)-butane-1,2,4-triol)], is a selective and potent CDK inhibitor, which inhibits CDK2, CDK1, CDK5, CDK7 and CDK9 (IC_{50} = 0.003, 0.03, 0.03, 0.25 and 0.09 μM, respectively). Cell-based studies showed inhibition of the phosphorylation of CDK substrates, Rb and the RNA polymerase II C-terminal domain, down-regulation of cyclins A, E, and D1, and cell cycle block in the S and G2/M phases [121].

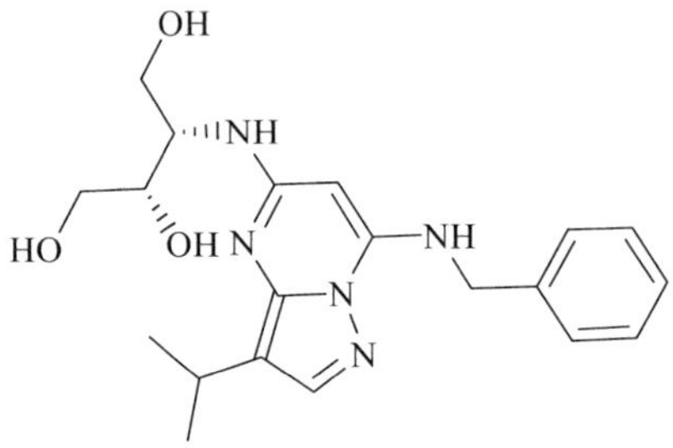

(**46**)

A novel series of 2-amino-4-(7-azaindol-3-yl)pyrimidines was reported as CDK1 inhibitors. A number of analogues showed good potency for CDK1 and exhibited cellular antiproliferative activity. Most potent 4-substituted derivatives (**47a,b**) have CDK1 activity of IC_{50} = 0.001 μM and 0.0006 μM, respectively [122].

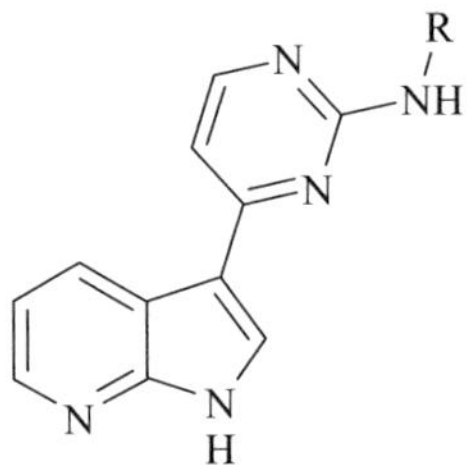

(**47**)

a. R = 4-[Piperidin-1-yl-$(CH_2)_2$]-2-CH_3-phenyl
b. R = 4-[Pyrrolidin-1-yl-$(CH_2)_2$]-2-CH_3-phenyl

Triazolo[1,5-*a*]pyrimidines are identified as novel and potent inhibitors of CDK2, with selectivity over GSK3β. One of its member, compound (**48**) has CDK2 IC_{50} of 0.12 μM and a GSK3β IC_{50} of 20 μM, with selectivity over GSK3β of 167-fold [123].

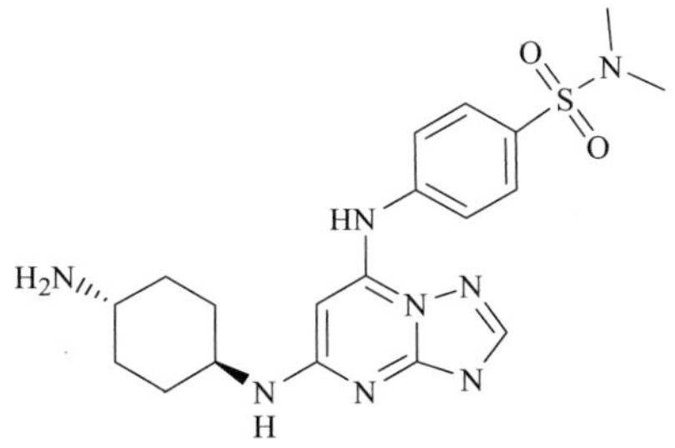

(48)

7-Benzylamino-5(R)-[2-(hydroxymethyl)propyl]amino-3-isopropyl-1(2)H-pyrazolo[4,3-d]pyrimidine (**49**) was prepared as a bioisostere of the well-known CDK inhibitor (**15**). An X-ray crystal structure of compound (**49**) bound to CDK2 has been determined, revealing a binding mode similar to that of (**15**). Protein kinase selectivity profile of (**49**) and its biological effects (cell cycle arrest, dephosphorylation of the retinoblastoma protein, accumulation of the tumor suppressor protein p53, induction of apoptosis, inhibition of homologous recombination) are consistent with CDK inhibition as a primary mode of action. Importantly, as the anticancer activities of the pyrazolo[4,3-d]pyrimidine (**49**) exceed those of its bioisostere (**15**), it may be preferable for cancer therapy [124].

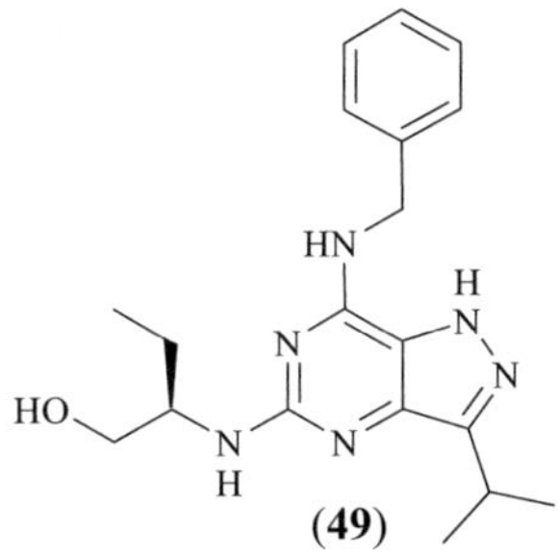

(49)

5-substituted O^4-alkylpyrimidines are developed as potent CDK2 inhibitory drug leads. Variation of the 5-substituent in the 2,6-diaminopyrimidine series confirmed the 5-nitroso substituent as optimal, and showed that 5-formyl and 5-acetyl substituents were also tolerated at this position. A series of O^4-alkyl-N^2-aryl-5-substituted-6-aminopyrimidines revealed interesting SAR. In the 5-nitroso series, the optimum O^4-alkyl substituents were cyclohexylmethyl or sec-butyl, combined with a 2-sulfanilyl group. By contrast, in the N^2-arylsulfonamido-5-formyl series, the cyclohexylmethyl compound showed relatively poor activity compared with the sec-butyl derivative (**50**, (R)-4-(4-amino-6-sec-butoxy-5-formylpyrimidin-2-ylamino)benzenesulfonamide; CDK2 IC_{50} = 0.8 nM). Similarly, in the N^2-arylsulfonamido-5-(hydroxyiminomethyl) series the O^4-sec-butyl substituent conferred greater potency than the cyclohexylmethyl (**51**, (rac)-4-(4-amino-6-sec-butoxy-5-(hydroxyiminomethyl)pyrimidin-2-ylamino)benzenesulfonamide; CDK2 IC_{50} = 7.4 nM). The 5-formyl derivatives show selectivity for CDK2 over other CDK family members, and are growth inhibitory in tumour cells (*e.g.* **50**, GI_{50} = 0.57 μM) [125].

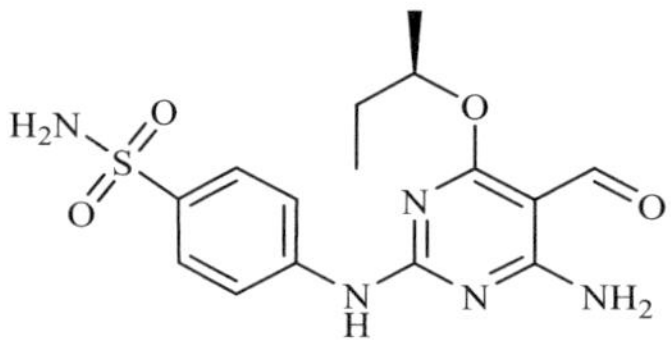

(50)

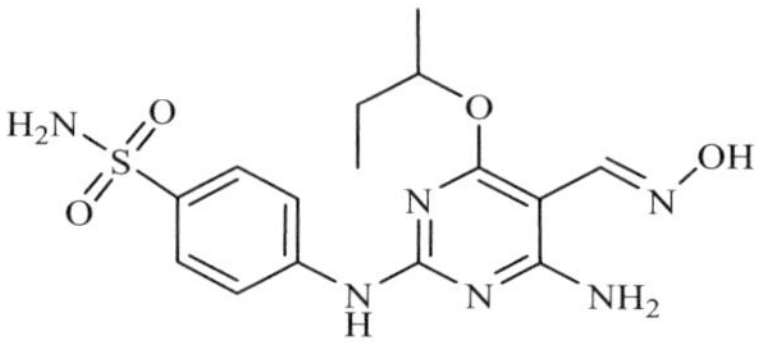

(51)

A pyrazolo[1,5-a]pyrimidine-derived compound, BS-181 (**52**, N^6-(6-Amino-hexyl)-N^7-benzyl-3-isopropyl-pyrolo[1,5-a]pyrimidine-5,7-diamine), inhibited CAK activity with an IC_{50} of 21 nM. Testing of other CDKs as well as another 69 kinases showed that (**52**) only inhibited CDK2 at concentrations lower than 1 μM, with CDK2 being inhibited 35-fold less potently (IC_{50} = 880 nM) than CDK7. In MCF-7 cells, (**52**) inhibited the phosphorylation of CDK7 substrates, promoted cell cycle arrest and apoptosis to inhibit the growth of cancer cell lines, and showed antitumor effects *in vivo*. The drug was stable *in vivo* with a plasma elimination half-life in mice of 405 minutes after i.p. administration of 10 mg/kg. The same dose of drug inhibited the growth of MCF-7 human xenografts in nude mice. Compound (**52**) provides the first example of a potent and selective CDK7 inhibitor with potential as an anticancer agent [126].

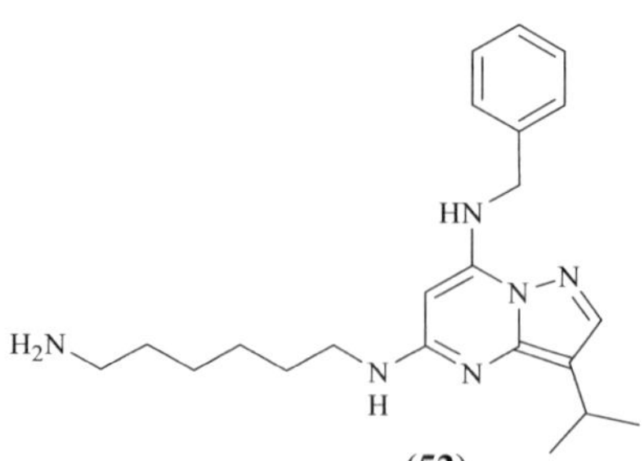

(52)

AZD5438 (**53**, 4-(1-isopropyl-2-methylimidazol-5-yl)-2-(4-methylsulphonylanilino) pyrimidine) a potent inhibitor of CDK 1, 2, and 9 (IC_{50} = 0.016, 0.006, and 0.02 μM, respectively). *In vitro*, (**53**) showed significant antiproliferative activity in human tumor cell lines (IC_{50} range, 0.2-1.7 μM), causing inhibition of the phosphorylation of cdk substrates pRb, nucleolin, protein phosphatase 1a, and RNA polymerase II COOH-terminal domain and blocking cell cycling at G(2)-M, S, and G(1) phases. *In vivo*, when orally administered at either 50 mg/kg twice daily or 75 mg/kg once daily, (**53**) inhibited human tumor xenograft growth (maximum percentage tumor growth inhibition, range, 38-153; $P < 0.05$). *In vivo*, (**53**) also reduced the proportion of actively cycling cells [127]. Three Phase I studies assessed the clinical safety, tolerability, PK and pharmacodynamics (PD) of (**53**) when administered in different dosing schedules. Compound (**53**) was generally well tolerated in a weekly dosing schedule, but not in continuous schedules. The clinical development programme for (**53**) was discontinued owing to tolerability and exposure data from these studies [128].

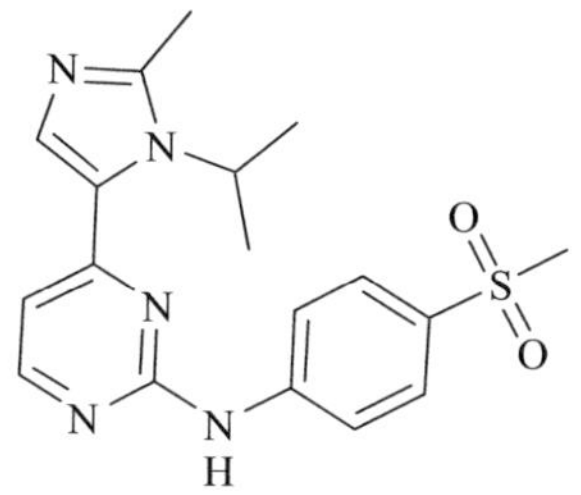

(53)

A similar molecule AZD5597 (**54**, [4-[[5-Fluoro-4-[2-methyl-1-(1-methylethyl)-1H-imidazol-5-yl]-2-pyrimidinyl]amino]phenyl][(3S)-3-(methylamino)-1-pyrrolidinyl]methanone) too shows excellent potency against CDK1,2 (IC_{50} = 0.011, 0.002 μM, respectively) [129].

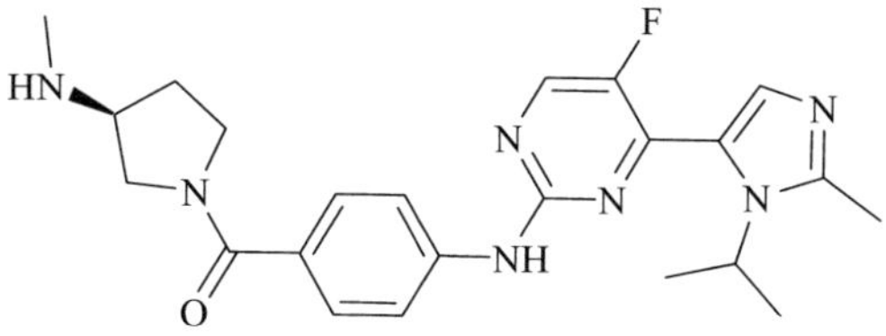

(54)

Xylocydine (**55**) selectively down-regulates the activity of CDK1 and CDK2, accompanied by significant cell growth inhibition in HCC cells. (**55**) also strongly inhibited the activity of CDK7 and CDK9, *in vitro* as well as in cell cultures that is temporally associated with apoptotic cell death in xylocydine-induced HCC cells. This is associated with inhibition of phosphorylation of RNA polymerase II at serine residues 5 and 2, which are targets of CDK7 and CDK9, respectively [130]. A series of (**55**) analogues bearing an aryl and hetaryl group in position 6 were prepared and their biological activities were assessed by *in vitro* CDK1/Cyclin B1 and CDK2/Cyclin A2 kinase assay [131].

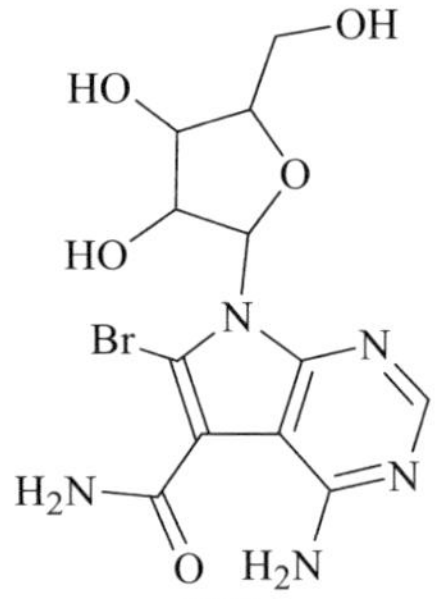

(55)

The development of a novel series of imidazole pyrimidine amides as CDK inhibitors is reported. The series was found to have much improved CDK2 inhibition and potent *in vitro* anti-proliferative effects against cancer cell lines. Control of overall lipophilicity was important to achieve good *in vitro* potency along with acceptable physiochemical properties and margins against inhibition of both CYP isoforms and the hERG potassium ion channel. A compound (**56**) with an attractive overall balance of properties (IC_{50} CDK1, 2, 4 = 0.06, <0.001, 0.05 μM) was profiled *in vivo* and possessed suitable physiochemical and pharmacokinetic profiles for oral dosing [132].

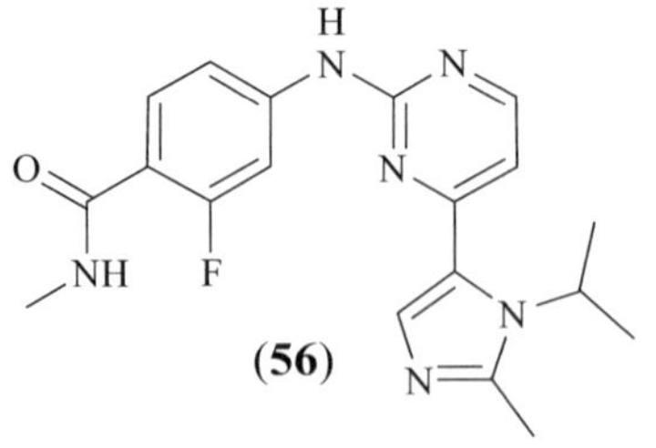

(56)

A potent and selective ATP-competitive inhibitor R547 {[4-Amino-2-(1-methanesulfonylpiperidin-4-ylamino)pyrimidin-5-yl](2,3-difluoro-6-methoxyphenyl)methanone} (**57**) showed significant *in vivo* antitumor activity [133]. In cell-free assays, compound (**57**) effectively inhibited CDK1/cyclin B, CDK2/cyclin E, and CDK4/cyclin D1 (K_i = 0.001-0.003 μM) and was inactive (K_i > 5 μM) against a panel of >120 unrelated kinases. In *in vitro* assays, compound (**57**) effectively inhibited the proliferation of human tumor cell lines HCT-116 (IC_{50} = 0.08 μM). The growth-inhibitory activity of (**57**) is characterized by a cell cycle block at G1 and G2 phases and induction of apoptosis. Due to superior drug like profile the compound (**57**) is currently being evaluated in Phase I clinical trials for the treatment of cancer [134].

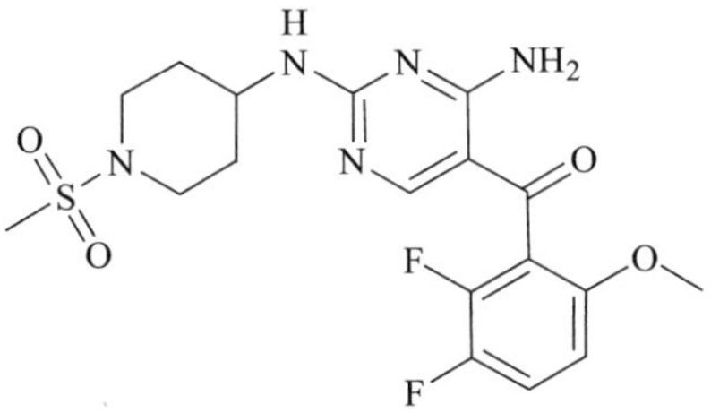

(**57**)

Pyrimidine derivatives like thiopyrimidines [135], macrocyclic aminopyrimidines [136], imidazole pyrimidine amides [137], pyrido[2,3-d]pyrimidin-7-ones [138], 4-(pyrazol-4-yl)-pyrimidines [139] are reported as CDK inhibitiors using a combination of experimental and computational methodology.

Indirubin Derivatives

Indirubin (**58**), an isomer of indigo, is reported as an inhibitor of CDKs (IC_{50} CDK1/cyclin B = 10 μM, CDK5/p25 = 10 μM) and GSK3 (IC_{50} = 1 μM) as well as an agonist of the aryl hydrocarbon receptor (AhR). Compound (**58**) is the active ingredient of a Ganggui Lohui Wan, a traditional Chinese medicinal recipe used against Chronic Myelogenous Leukemia (CML) [140]. Compound (**58**) and a few indirubin derivatives have been reported to inhibit CDKs by competing in the ATP-binding sites with high selectivity among several kinase families [141, 142]. The anti-proliferative effect of (**58**) on the human cancer cells was reported to have resulted from inhibiting the genes or proteins of regulating cell cycle progression, arresting G2/M phase of the cell cycle [143].

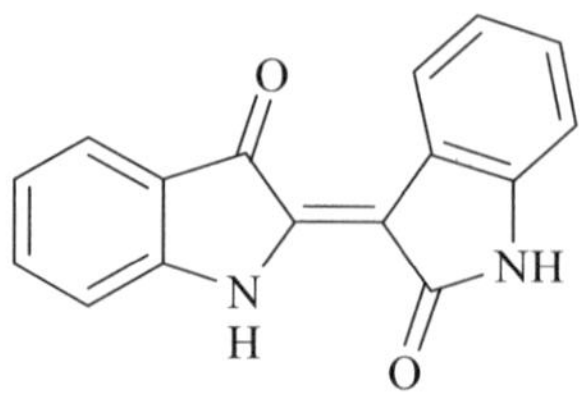

(58)

E226 (Indirubin-5-sulphonate) (**59**) is a potential anti-tumour agent and a potent inhibitor of CDK2 with IC_{50} value 0.035 μM. The binding of compound (**59**) has been studied by kinetic and crystallographic methods [144].

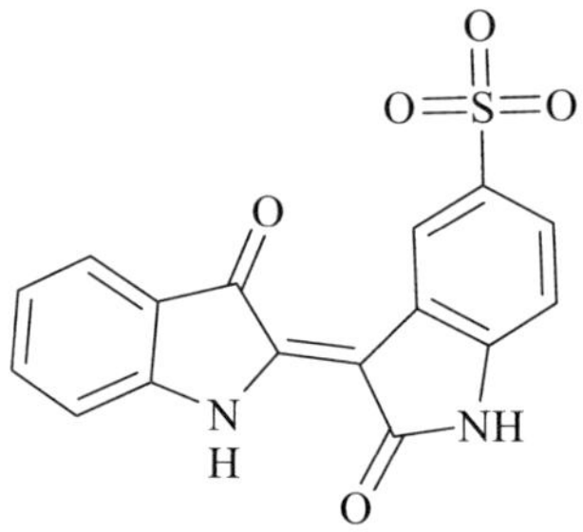

(59)

A cell permeable derivative Indirubin-3'-monoxime (**60**), is a selective and potent inhibitor of CDKs. Compound (**60**) shows inhibition activity with IC_{50} values for CDK1/cyclin B = 0.18 μM, CDK5/p25 = 0.10 μM and for GSK3 = 0.022 μM, respectively [145]. Compound (**60**) and derivatives are evaluated as anti-solid tumor agents, using their anti-proliferative activity in monolayers, as well as in multicellular spheroids (MCS) cultures of human colorectal cancer cells, DLD-1 and HT-29. The MCS model is an *in vitro* solid tumor model that is increasingly used for the evaluation of anti-solid tumor activity. 5-Nitro-indirubin-3'-oxime and 5'-Bromo-5-nitro-indirubin-3'-oxime compared to 5-Trimethylacetamido-indirubin-3'-oxime and 5-Diphenylacetamido-indirubin-3'-oxime showed greater anti-proliferative effects in monolayers, but lower anti-proliferative effects in MCS. These compounds are worth further investigation with respect to their anti-solid tumor activity and their mechanism of action in various solid tumor models [146].

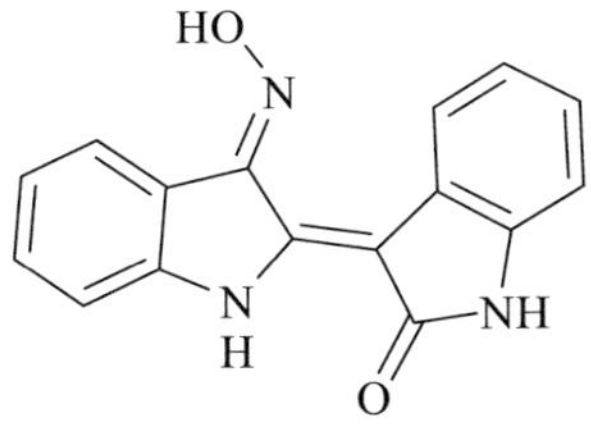

(60)

Simulation studies detected the displacement of a water molecule in the active site of CDK/indirubin-3'-oxime system. This resulted in a more conserved binding pattern than the water-excluded structure. Hence, it was suggested that in the design of new (**58**) like inhibitors, it is important to include the water molecule in the analysis [147].

A new series of indirubin-3'-oxime derivatives with combined substitutions at the 5 and 5' positions is synthesized showing nanomolar potency against CDK2 kinase [148].

7-Bromoindirubin-3'-oxime (7BIO) (**61**) has only a marginal inhibitory activity towards CDKs and GSK3 in contrast to its 5-, and 6-bromo isomers. Unexpectedly, (**61**) triggers a rapid cell death process distinct from apoptosis. Compound (**61**) induces the appearance of large pycnotic nuclei, without classical features of apoptosis such as chromatin condensation and nuclear fragmentation. Thus, in contrast to previously described indirubins, (**61**) triggers the activation of non-apoptotic cell death, possibly through necroptosis or autophagy. Although their molecular targets remain to be identified, 7-substituted indirubins may constitute a new class of potential antitumor compounds that would retain their activity in cells refractory to apoptosis [149].

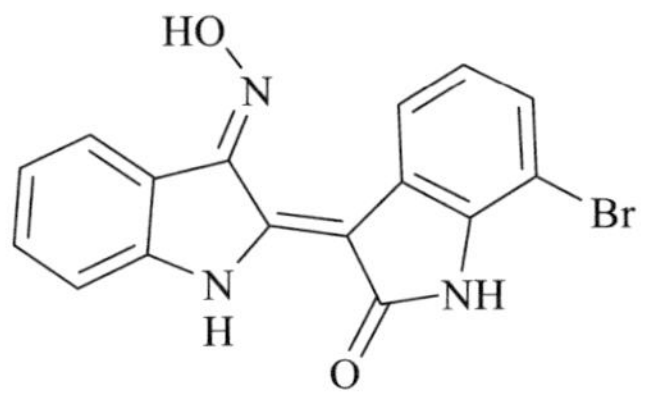

(61)

Numerous indirubin analogues (**62**) have been synthesized to optimize this promising kinase inhibitor scaffold [150]. Inhibitory activity for indirubin derivatives against a panel of kinases is given in Table **3**.

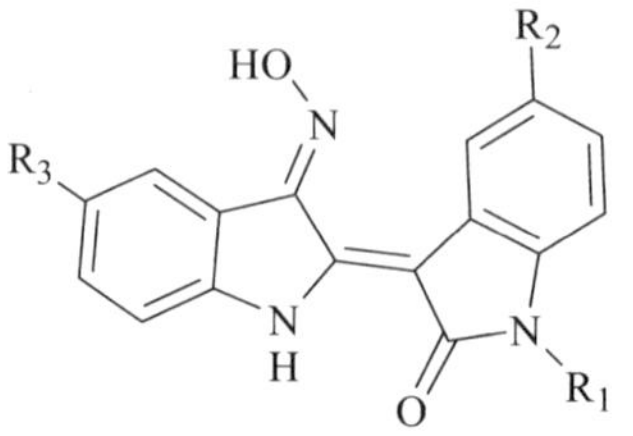

(62)

Table 3: Inhibitory activities for indirubin analogues (**62**). The values are IC_{50} in μM.

	R_1	R_2	R_3	CDK1	CDK5	GSK3
a	H	NO_2	H	0.019	0.006	0.0021
b	Me	NO_2	H	2.2	1.4	0.53
c	H	NO_2	Br	0.16	0.05	0.055
d	Me	NO_2	Br	8	3.3	9.3

Pyrazole Derivatives

Among several classes of potential CDK2/cyclin A inhibitors emerging from internal HTS efforts, 3-aminopyrazoles are getting attention because of low molecular weight of the scaffold and amenability for rapid class expansion. QSAR study was performed using Electrotopological State Atom (ETSA) index, Refractotopological State Atom (RTSA) index, indicator parameters and atomic charges to consider quantitatively the effect of the structural variation on the antitumor activity of 3-aminopyrazole [151]. X-ray crystallographic data of early compound in this series PNU292137 [(N-5-cyclopropyl-1H-pyrazol-3-yl)-2-(2-napthyl)acetamide] (**63**) was reported. Compound (**63**) showed nanomolar inhibiton of CDK2/cyclin A with IC_{50} = 0.037 μM. (**63**) was assessed for its selectivity against a panel of 33 kinases. Among the members of the CDK family that were tested, it was found to inhibit CDK2/cyclin E, CDK5/p25 and less potently CDK1/cyclin B but displayed selectivity for CDK4/cyclin D1. It had a 60 fold higher IC_{50} for GSK3β while IC_{50} values for all other enzymes in the panel were higher than 10 μM. Compound (**63**) and (**16**) are shown superimposed in the ATP binding pocket of CDK2/cyclin A [152].

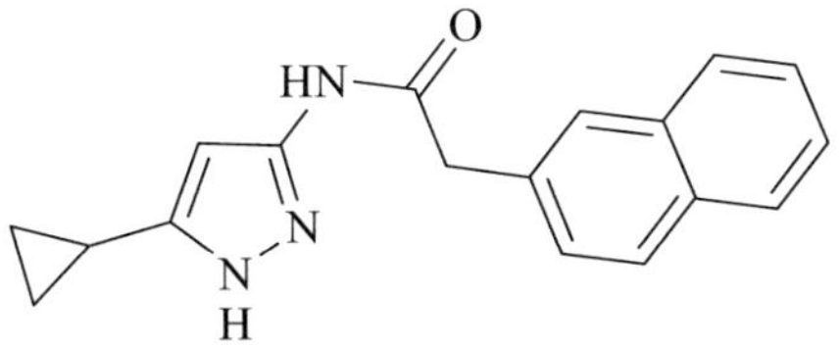

(63)

By introducing a methyl group in the S-configuration on the benzylic position of (**63**) and by changing the naphthyl moiety into a 4-lactam-1-yl phenyl group a new CDK inhibitor was prepared with improved physicochemical properties, notably solubility and plasma protein binding. This lead optimization process brought to the discovery of PHA-533533 [(2S)-N-(5-cyclopropyl-1H-pyrazol-3-yl)-2-[4-(2-oxo-1-pyrrolidinyl)phenyl]propanamide] (**64**) [153], a compound with a balanced activity *versus* drug like profile. This compound inhibited CDK2/cyclin A with K_i of 0.031 μM and IC_{50} of 0.037 μM, counteracting tumor cell proliferation of different cell lines with an IC_{50} in the sub-micromolar range. The synthesis and activity of the major metabolite of (**63**) was reported [154].

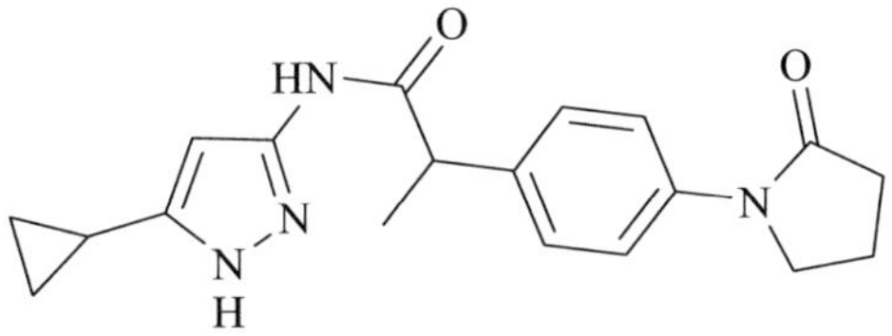

(64)

Improvement of inhibitory potency against multiple CDKs, antiproliferative activity against cancer cell lines and optimization of the physico-chemical properties led to the identification of highly potent compounds. like PHA-793887 (**56**, 3-Methyl-N-[1,4,5,6-tetrahydro-6,6-dimethyl-5-[(1-methyl-4-piperidinyl)carbonyl]pyrrolo[3,4-c]pyrazol-3-yl] butanamide) (IC_{50} CDK1, CKD2/E, CDK2/A = 0.45, 0.090, 0.060 μM, respectively) that showed good efficacy in the human ovarian A2780, colon HCT-116 and pancreatic BX-PC3 carcinoma xenograft models and was well tolerated upon daily treatments by i.v. administration. It was identified as a drug candidate for clinical evaluation in patients with solid tumors [155]. Compound (**56**) induced severe, dose-related hepatic toxicity, which was not predicted by pre-clinical models and currently precludes its further clinical development [156].

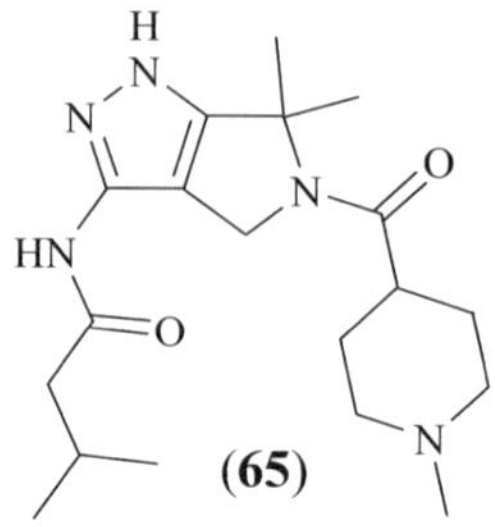

(65)

AT7519 (**66**, N-(4-Piperidinyl)-4-(2,6-dichlorobenzoylamino)-1H-pyrazole-3-carboxamide) is an inhibitor of multiple CDKs (IC_{50} CDK2 = 0.047 μM) [157]. Based on potent antitumor activity in preclinical models, a first-in-human clinical trial in refractory solid tumors investigated its safety, tolerability, PK and PD [158].

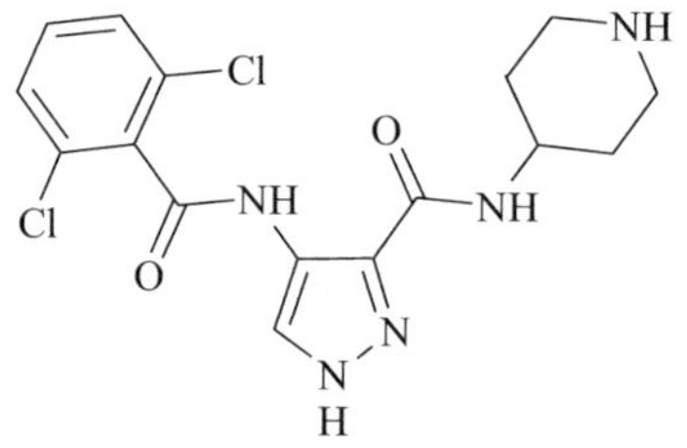

(66)

Indeno[1,2-*c*]pyrazol-4-ones are novel series of indenopyrazoles based CDK inhibitors. Molecular modeling studies indicate that these molecules create a similar hydrogen bond donating/accepting network as found in many other known small molecule CDK inhibitors [159]. With the objective of designing new chemical entities having enhanced inhibitory potencies against CDK2 and CDK4, the 3D-QSAR CoMFA studies carried out on indenopyrazole derivatives as inhibitors of kinases are reported [160].

Thiazole Derivatives

Compound A (**67**, {[5-(2-Cyclohexyloxy-6-methylpyrimidin-4-yl)-thiazol-2-yl]-[5-(4-methyl-piperazin-1-ylmethyl)-pyrazin-2-yl]-amine} has potent CDK4 and CCK6 inhibitory activity (IC_{50} = 9.2 and 7.8 nM, respectively). (**67**) is more than 57-fold selective against CDKs involved in cell cycle regulation (1, 2, 7) and CDKs with functions in other than cell cycle regulation (5, 7, 9) [161].

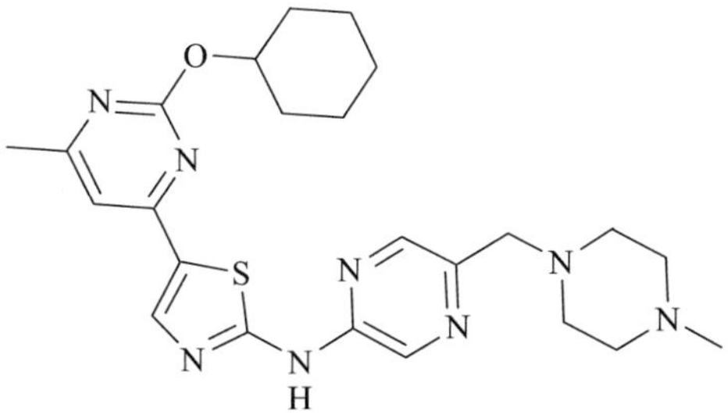

(67)

The 3D-QSAR CoMFA study was carried out on 47 aminothiazole derivatives as CDK inhibitors. The conventional and predictive correlation coefficients were found respectively to be 0.984 and 0.522. The models could be usefully employed to design CDK2 inhibitors and to find scaffolds through screening of chemical databases [162].

An ATP-competitive and CDK2 selective thiazole, SNS-032 (earlier BMS-387032) {N-[5-[[[5-(1,1-Dimethylethyl)-2-oxazolyl]methyl]thio]-2-thiazolyl]-4-piperidinecarboxamide} (**68**) has been selected to enter Phase 1 human clinical trials as an antitumor agent [163]. In a cell-free enzyme assay (**68**) showed a CDK2/cyclin E inhibition with IC_{50} = 0.048 μM and was 10- to 20-fold selective over CDK1/cyclin B and CDK4/cyclin D respectively. It was also highly selective over a panel of 12 unrelated kinases. Antiproliferative activity was established in an A2780 cellular cytotoxicity assay in which (**68**) showed an IC_{50} = 0.095 μM [164]. SAR studies were consistent with the solid-state structure of the inhibitor bound to CDK2 protein, which indicated that the acyl side chain of the molecule extended into the hydrophilic extra protein space and was amenable to modification [165].

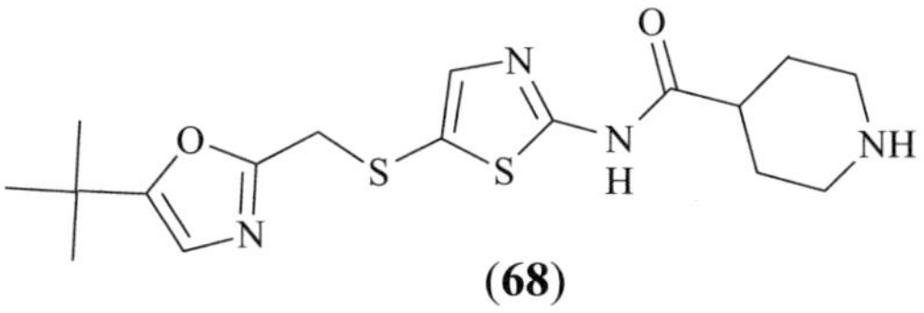

(68)

N-(5-Bromo-1,3-thiazol-2-yl)butanamide (**69**) was found active (IC_{50} = 0.808 μM) in a HTS for CDK2 inhibitors. By exploiting crystal structures of several complexes between CDK2 and inhibitors and applying Structure-Based Drug Design (SBDD), a very potent and selective CDK2 inhibitor 4-[(5-isopropyl-1,3-

thiazol-2-yl)amino]benzenesulfonamide (**70**) (IC_{50} = 0.02 μM) was found. The synthesis, structure-based analog design, kinases inhibition data and X-ray crystallographic structures of CDK2/inhibitor complexes are reported [166].

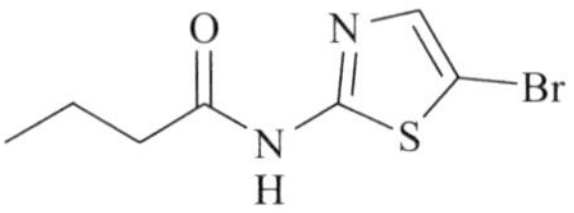

(69)

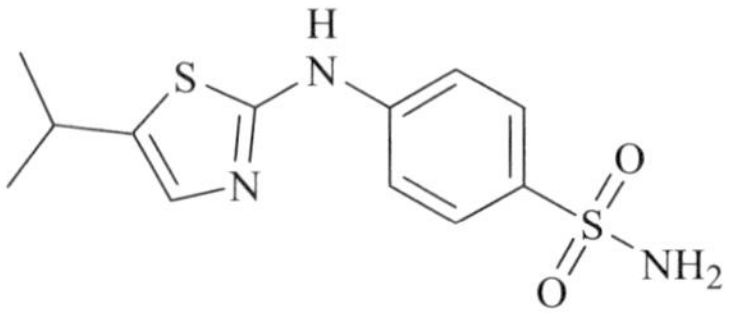

(70)

Following the recent discovery and development of 2-anilino-4-(thiazol-5-yl)pyrimidine cyclin dependent kinase (CDK) inhibitors, a program was initiated to evaluate related ring-constrained analogues, specifically, 2-methyl- and 2-amino-N-aryl-4,5-dihydrothiazolo[4,5-h]quinazolin-8-amines for inhibition of CDKs. Many of the analogues from this chemical series inhibit CDKs with very low nanomolar K_i values. The most potent compound (**71**) reported in this study inhibits CDK2 with an IC_{50} of 0.7 nM ([ATP] = 100 μM). Furthermore, an X-ray crystal structure of 2-methyl-N-(3-(nitro)phenyl)-4,5-dihydrothiazolo[4,5-h]quinazolin-8-amine (**71**), a representative from the chemical series in complex with cyclin A-CDK2, is reported, confirming the design rationale and expected binding mode within the CDK2 ATP binding pocket [167].

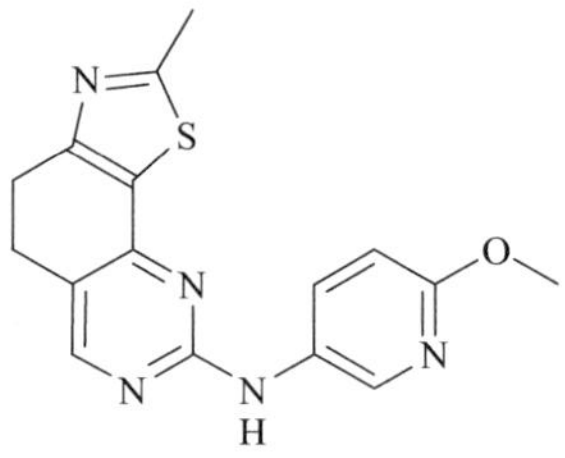

(71)

AG-012986 (**72**, 4-[4-amino-5-(2,6-difluoro-benzoyl)-thiazol-2-ylamino]-N-(2-dimethylamino-1R-methyl-ethyl)-benzamide) is a pan-CDK inhibitor that has *in vitro* and *in vivo* antitumor properties but was stopped in development due in part to rapid bone-marrow-independent white blood cell toxicity in preclinical studies and the potential for acute and delayed immunosuppression in humans. Recently it is reported that (**72**) could cause apoptosis of T-cells by targeting upstream kinases in the p38 pathway and impairing cellular survival [168].

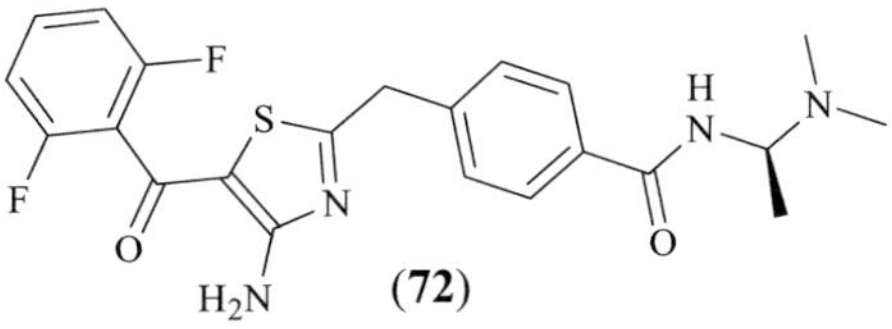

(72)

CDK1 is a nonredundant cyclin-dependent kinase (CDK) with an essential role in mitosis, but its multiple functions still are poorly understood at a molecular level. A selective small-molecule inhibitor of CDK1, compound (**73**) that reversibly arrests human cells at the G(2)/M border of the cell cycle and allows for effective cell synchronization in early mitosis is reported. Inhibition of CDK1 during cell division revealed that its activity is necessary and sufficient for maintaining the mitotic state of the cells, preventing replication origin licensing and premature cytokinesis. Although CDK1 inhibition for up to 24 h is well tolerated, longer exposure to the inhibitor induces apoptosis in tumor cells, suggesting that selective CDK1 inhibitors may have utility in cancer therapy [169].

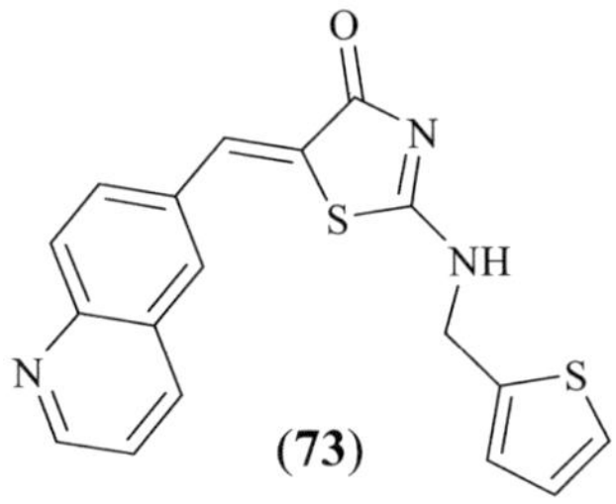

(73)

N-aryl aminothiazoles were prepared and found to be inhibitors *in vitro* of CDK1, CDK2, and CDK4. In cells they acted as potent cytotoxic agents. Selectivity for CDK1, CDK2, and CDK4 was dependent on the nature of the N-aryl group and was distinct from the CDK2 selective N-acyl analogues. An exemplary compound of the family, BMS-357075 (**74**) was a potent inhibitor of CDK1, CDK2, and CDK4 (IC_{50} = 0.018, 0.003, 0.026 μM, respectively) and produced a 56% increase in survival time *versus* untreated control against P388 murine leukemia in mice [170].

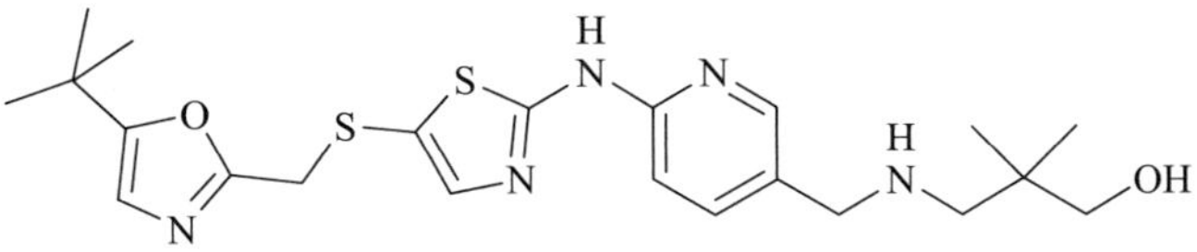

(74)

STG28 [(S)-5-(4-{[6-(Allyloxy)-2,5,7,8-tetramethylchroman-2-yl]methoxy}-3methoxybenzylidene)thiazolidine-2,4-dione] (**75**) is reported as exhibiting low micromolar potency in ablating cyclin D1 and inhibiting MCF-7 cell proliferation [171]. Compound (**75**) mediated the proteasomal degradation of cyclin D1 with a high degree of specificity. The pivotal role of cyclin D1 in promoting tumorigenesis and drug resistance, makes (**75**) a potent therapeutic in cancer therapy.

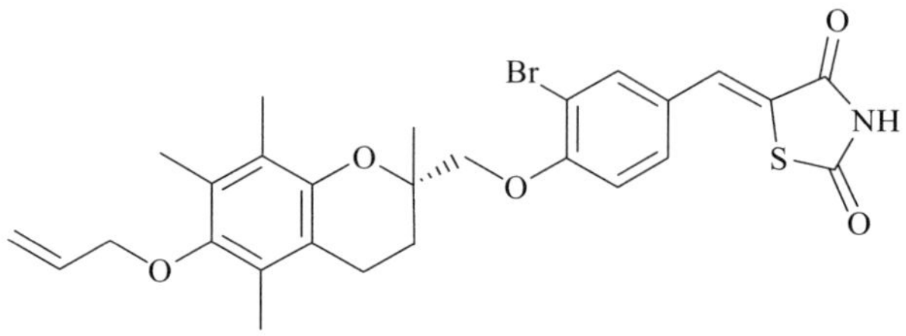

(75)

5-Pyrimidinyl-2-aminothiazole (**76**) was identified as an inhibitor of CDKs by a screening of the Merck sample repository [172]. Compound (**76**) exhibited significant selectivity for CDK4, 6 over CDK1, 2, 5, 7 and 9. It also inhibited pRb phosphorylation and BrdU incorporation in tumor cells.

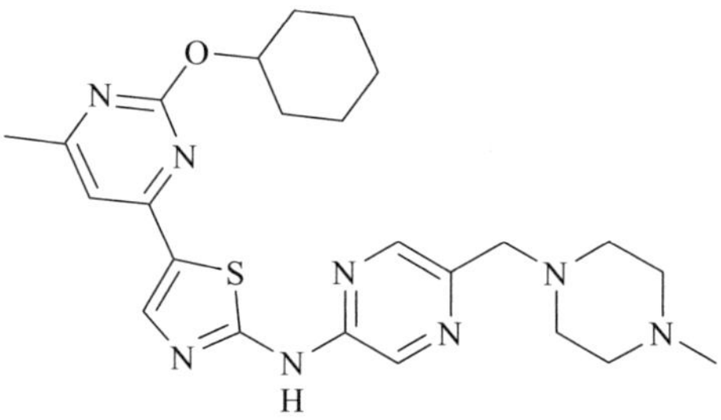

(76)

Paullones and Derivatives

Paullones are a class of molecules structurally based on the 7,12-dihydroindolo[3,2-d][1]benzazepin-6(5H)-one parent scaffold. Many of these structures are inhibitors of certain protein kinases, namely CDKs and GSK-3. A review gives an overview over the published reports regarding chemistry, biological activity and pharmacological applications of paullone derivatives [173]. CDK1 inhibitory activity of paullones depends on electronic properties of its 9-

substituents [174]. Initial studies demonstrated that paullones inhibit CDKs *in vitro*, thereby blocking cell-cycle progression. However, the exact mechanism for the antiproliferative effects of paullones was never explored. Recently, it was reported that the most potent paullone, Alsterpaullone (**77**) (IC_{50} CDK1 = 0.035 μM, CDK2 = 0.04 μM, GSK3β = 0.004 μM) induced apoptosis and promoted loss in clonogenicity in the Jurkat cell line [175]. The addition of side chains with epoxide motifs has improved the antiproliferative activity of 9-bromo derivative known as Kenpaullone (**78**) IC_{50} (CDK1/cyclin B = 0.40 μM, CDK5/p25 = 1.6 μM) and 9-trifluoromethylpaullone [176].

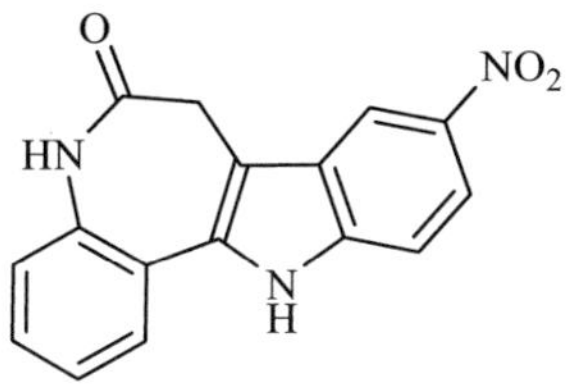

(77)

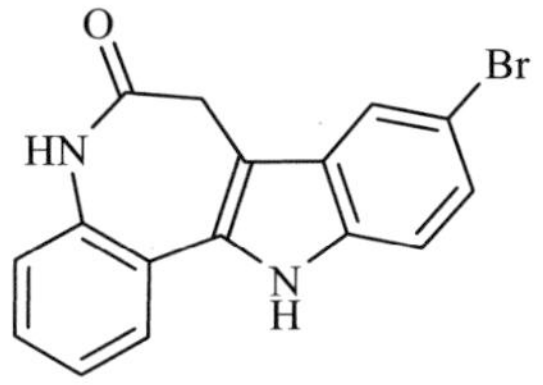

(78)

8-Bromo-6,11-dihydro-thieno-[3',2':2.3]azepino[4,5-*b*]indol-5(4H)-one (**79**), a thieno analogue of (**78**) shows antiproliferative activity in a drug sensitive cell line that led to cell accumulation in G2/M phase [177]. Aza derivatives of (**78**), 1-aza and 4-azakenpaullone (**80, 81**) are found to potent inhibitors of GSK3β as compared to CDK1 [178].

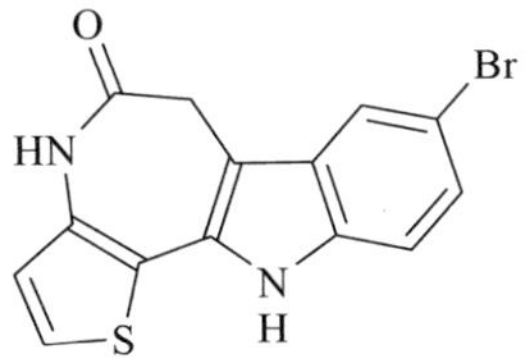

(79)

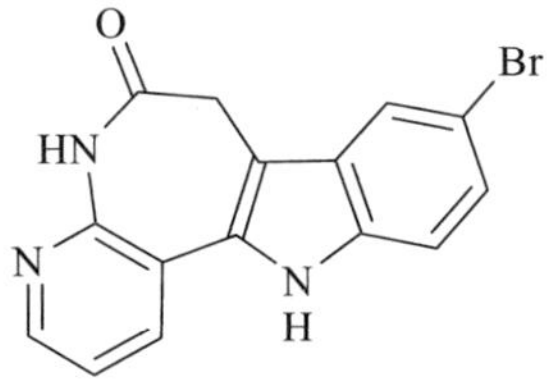

(80)

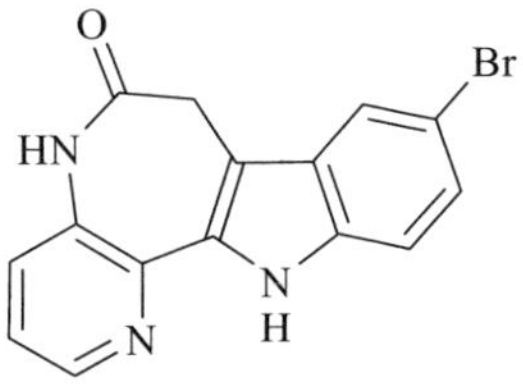

(81)

Hymenialdisine and Analogues

Hymenialdisine (HMD) [4-(2-amino-5-oxo-3H-imidazol-4-ylidene)-2-bromo-1,5,6,7-tetrahydropyrrolo[2,3-c]azepin-8-one] (**82a**) is a natural product, which was isolated from marine sponges including *Hymeniacidon aldis*, *Axinella verrucosa*, and *Aaurantiaca* in the early 1980s based on its antiproliferative effects on cultured lymphocytic canthella leukemia cells [179, 180]. It was shown to exhibit strong inhibitory activity against several closely related CDKs, such as CDK1/cyclin B (IC_{50} = 0.022 μM), CDK2/cyclin A (IC_{50} = 0.07 μM), CDK2/cyclin E (IC_{50} = 0.04 μM), and CDK5/p25 (IC_{50} = 0.028 μM), as well as against more distantly related kinases such as GSK3β (IC_{50} = 0.01 μM) and CK1 (Creatine kinase 1) (IC_{50} = 0.035 μM) [181]. Kinetic analysis has shown that HMD acts in an ATP-competitive fashion, and the co-crystal structure with CDK2 revealed that HMD occupies the ATP site and makes many of the hydrogen bonding interactions as seen in other CDK inhibitor complexes [182]. Despite potent activities against these kinases, HMD is relatively selective *in vitro* and exhibits only moderate to weak activity against many other kinases [181]. A number of HMD analogues have been synthesized with nano molar potency against CDKs [183] alongwith other kinases [184].

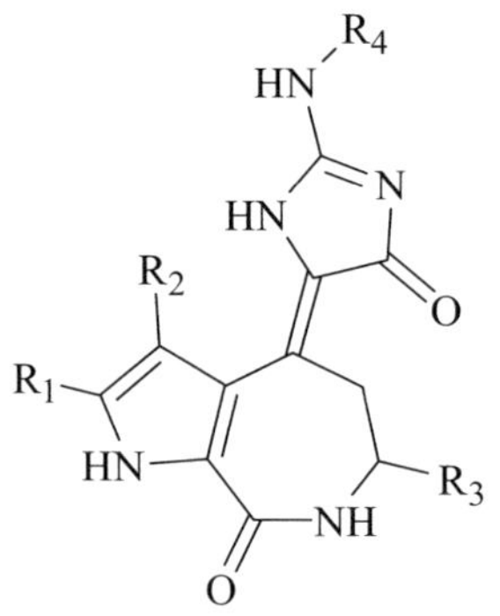

(82)

a. R_1 = Br; R_2 = R_3 = R_4 = H
b. R_1 = R_2 = Br; R_3 = R_4 = H
c. R_1 = R_3 = R_4 = H; R_2 = Br
d. R_1 = R_2 = Cl; R_3 = R_4 = H

Table 4: Inhibitory activities of Hymenialdisine and analogues (**82**). The values are IC_{50} in μM.

	R_1	**R_2**	**R_3**	**R_4**	**CDK1/B**	**CDK5/p25**	**GSK3β**
A	Br	H	H	H	0.022	0.028	0.01
B	Br	Br	H	H	0.53	0.056	0.051
C	H	Br	H	H	1.5	0.079	0.09
D	Cl	Cl	H	H	0.22	0.062	0.047

Miscellaneous Compounds

Butyrolactone, (**83**) a competitive inhibitor of ATP for binding and activation of CDKs was isolated from *Aspergillus* species F-25799. Compound (**83**) selectively inhibited CDK1 (IC_{50} = 0.68 μM) and CDK2 (IC_{50} = 0.82 μM) [185]. A series of its analogues were synthesized and their antitumor activities are reported [186]. The CDK inhibitior (**83**) is also reported as a potent inhibitor of p21 (WAF1/CIP1 expression) [187]. Compound (**83**) showed antineoplastic effect on non-small cell and small cell lung cancer lines with IC_{50} value ~ 50 μg/mL.

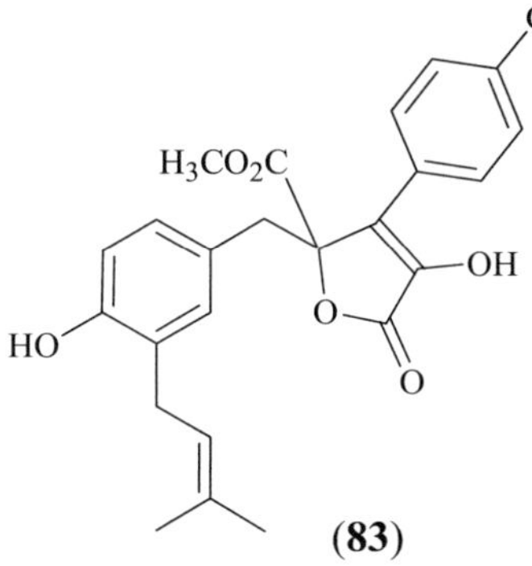

(**83**)

PAPU1 [84], [(E)-1-(3,4-dihydroxyphenethyl)-3-styrylurea] induced caspase-dependent apoptosis in melanoma cells. A study to examine the anti-proliferative effects of PAPU compounds on MCF-7 human breast cancer cells and explanation for the molecular mechanisms involved is reported. Treatment with PAPU compounds inhibited predominantly proliferation in these cells, where (**84**) was the most efficient form. Flow cytometric analysis showed that (**84**) blocked cell cycle progression in the G(0)/G(1) phase, and reduced the proportion of cells in G(2)/M phase. This was related to the inhibition of cell cycle regulatory factors, including cyclin D/E and CDK2/4, through induction of p21(Cip1) [188].

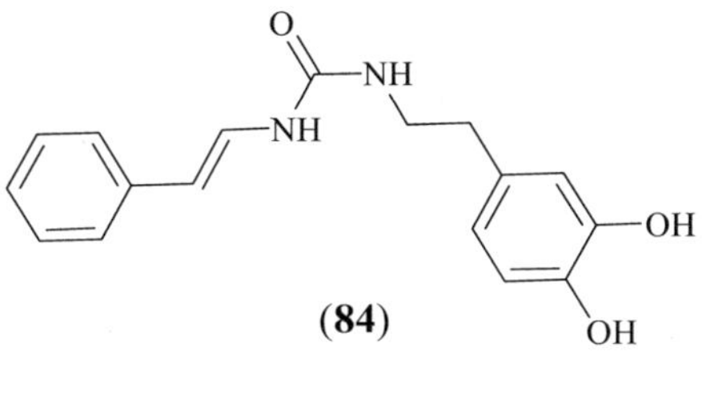

(**84**)

Fascaplysin (**85**), a marine natural product with selective CDK4 selective inhibition activity is also a natural angiogenesis inhibitor [189]. Synthesis and activity of various (**85**) based CDK4 selective inhibitors is reported [190, 191].

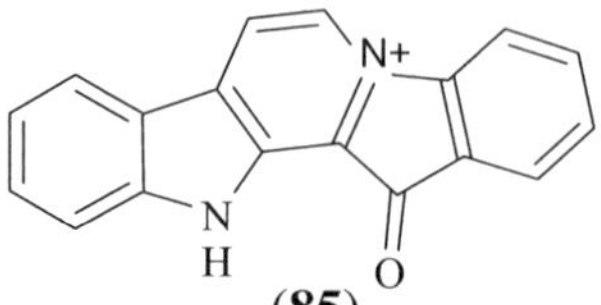

(85)

3-ATA (**86**, 3-amino thioacridone), a selective CDK4 inhibitor, attenuates kainic acid-induced apoptosis in cerebellar granule neurons. When neurons were pre-treated with (**86**) (10 μM for 24 h), they were less susceptible to damage induced by kainic acid (500 μM), since the number of dead cells decreased significantly [192].

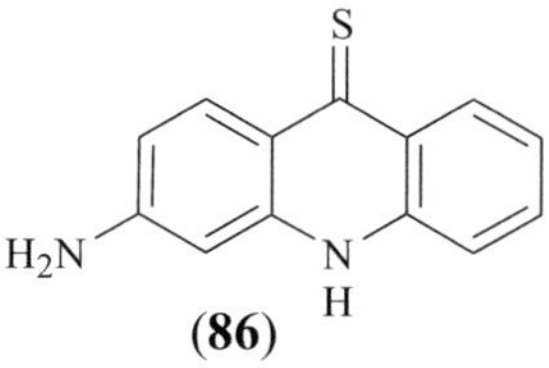

(86)

Diaryl urea derivatives were identified as highly selective and potent CDK4 inhibitors [193]. By constructing diaryl urea informer libraries based on the structural requirements of CDK inhibitors in the ATP binding pocket of the CDK4 model, a potent CDK4 inhibitor N-(9-oxo-9H-fluoren-4-yl)-N-pyridin-2-yl urea (**87**) with IC_{50} value of 0.10 μM was synthesised. Further modification based on the proposed binding mode provided an even more potent compound, N-(9bR)-5-oxo-2, 3,5,9b-tetrahydro-1H-pyrrolo-[2,1-a]isoindol-9-yl]-N-pyridin-2-ylurea (**88**) with IC_{50} CDK1 = 0.122 μM, CDK2 = 0.08 μM, CDK4 = 0.042 μM respectively [194]. Structure-based drug design and optimization from the starting point of diaryl urea, led to the discovery of potent CDK1, 2, 4, 6 inhibitor, (**89**) (IC_{50} CDK1 = 1.8 μM, CDK2 = 0.44 μM, CDK4 = 0.0023 μM) which is suitable for iv administration for *in vivo* study [195].

Selected selenium compounds have found use as anticancer agents [196]. The representative compound in this class, Methylselenocysteine (**90**) has been shown to inhibit CDK2 activity in synchronized mouse mammary epithelial tumor cells while having no impact on CDK4 activity. Compound (**90**) arrested cells in the S phase during the TM6 cell cycle [197]. In a separate study the gene array analysis suggested that c-Myc, cyclin C, proliferating cell nuclear antigen, CDK1, CDK2, CDK4, cyclin B and cyclin D2 mRNA levels were lower in selenium-deficient cells than in the cells supplemented with 0.25 μM selenomethionine. Furthermore, the phosphorylation state of total cellular protein was higher (57%) in selenium-supplemented cells than in selenium-deficient cells [198]. The group of genes significantly altered by selenium includes cyclin D1, CDK5, CDK4, CDK2, cdc25A and GADD [199].

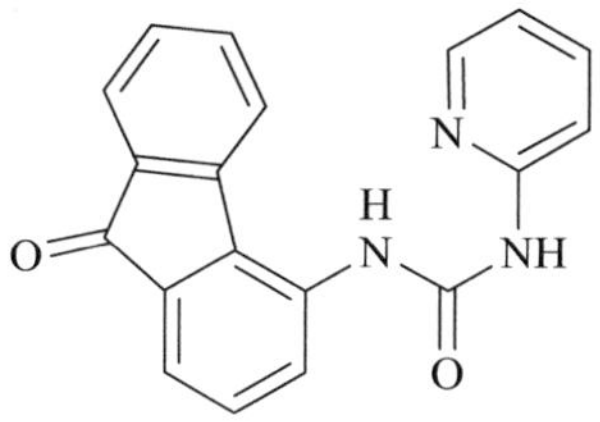

(**87**)

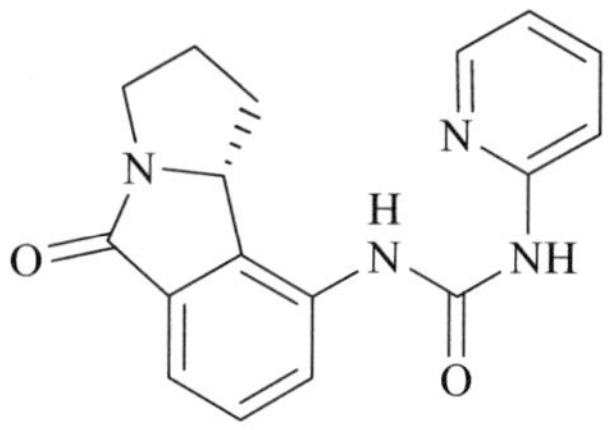

(**88**)

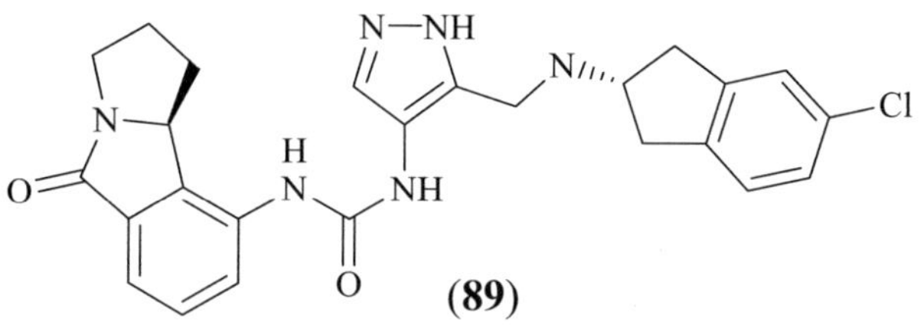

(**89**)

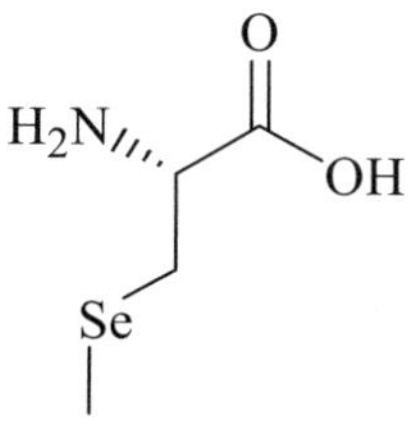

(**90**)

Trypatmine derivatives are reported as a new class of CDK4 inhibitors. CA199 (**91**) a trypamine analogue of fascaplysin, is a specific inhibitor of CDK4/cyclin D1 (IC_{50} CDK4/D1 = 20 μM, CDK2 > 500 μM) in enzyme assays that blocks G(0)/G(1) stages. It prevents pRb hyper-phosphorylation but does not bind or intercalate DNA like fascaplysin [200].

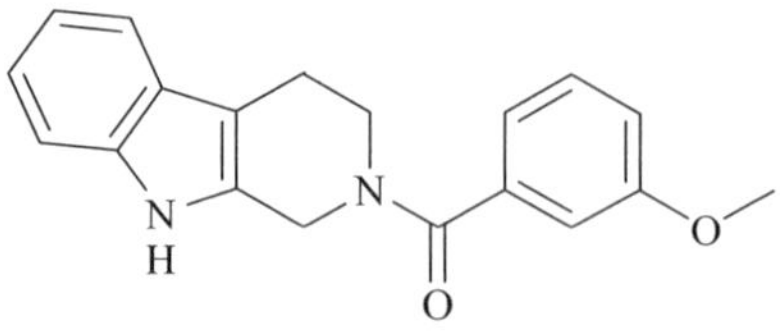

(91)

Pyrazolo[3,4-*c*]pyridazine (**92**) was identified in a HTS carried out by BASF Bioresearch Corp. (Worcester, MA) as a potent inhibitor of CDK1/cyclin B and has shown selectivity for the CDK family (IC_{50} CDK1/cyclin B = 6.1 μM, KDR > 50 μM, LCK > 50 μM). Analogues of the lead compound are synthesized and their antitumor activities are reported [201].

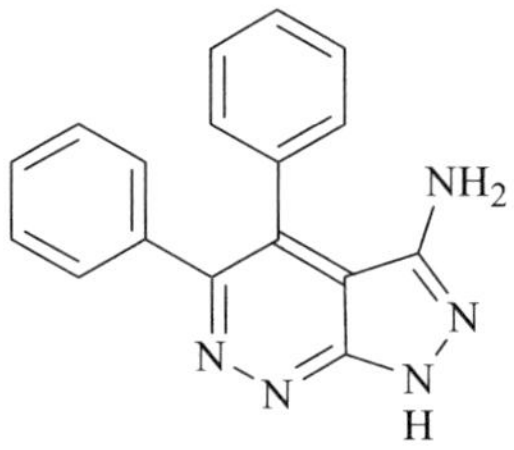

(92)

PHA-848125 (**93**, N,1,4,4-tetramethyl-8-{[4-(4-methylpiperazin-1-yl)phenyl] amino}-4,5-dihydro-1H-pyrazolo[4,3-h] quinazoline-3-carboxamide), a potent dual inhibitor of CDKs and Tropomyosin Receptor Kinase (TRKs) (IC_{50} CDK2, TRKA = 45, 53 nM, respectively), possesses significant antitumor activity. Compound (**93**) inhibits cell proliferation of a wide panel of tumoral cell lines with submicromolar IC_{50}, show cell cycle arrest in G(1), reduced DNA synthesis, accompanied by inhibition of pRb phosphorylation and modulation of other CDK-dependent markers. The compound additionally inhibits phosphorylation of TRKA and its substrates in cells, which functionally express this receptor. The dual CDK-TRK inhibitor (**93**) has the potential for being a novel and efficacious targeted drug for cancer treatment [202].

Aloisines, 6-phenyl[5H]pyrrolo[2,3-*b*]pyrazines (**94**) are reported as a novel potent CDK inhibitory scaffold. Kinetic studies as well as the resolution of a CDK2-aloisine co-crystallized structure demonstrate that aloisines act by competitive inhibition of ATP-binding to the catalytic subunit of the kinase [203].

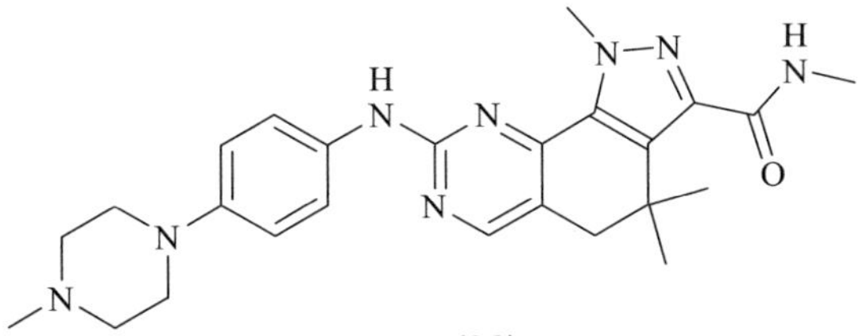

(93)

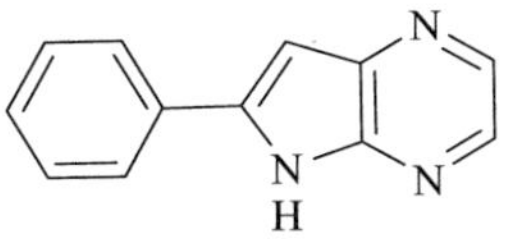

(94)

Meriolins (**97**) represent a chemical structural hybrid between Meridianins (**95**) and Variolins (**96**), two families of kinase inhibitors extracted from various marine invertebrates. Variolin B (**96b**) (IC_{50} CDK1/cyclin B = 0.06 μM, CDK2/cyclin A = 0.08 μM, CDK5/p25 = 0.09 μM and CDK9/cyclin T = 0.026 μM) is currently in preclinical evaluation as an antitumor agent. Compond (**97c**) showed enhanced specificity toward CDKs, with marked potency on CDK2/cyclin A (IC_{50} = 0.011 μM) and CDK9/cyclin T (IC_{50} = 0.006 μM) [204, 25]. The synthesis of new meridianin derivatives is reported [206, 207].

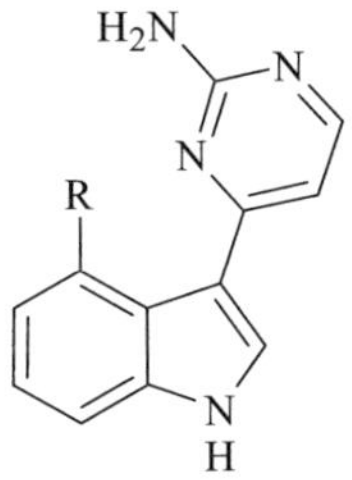

(95)

a. R = OH
b. R = H

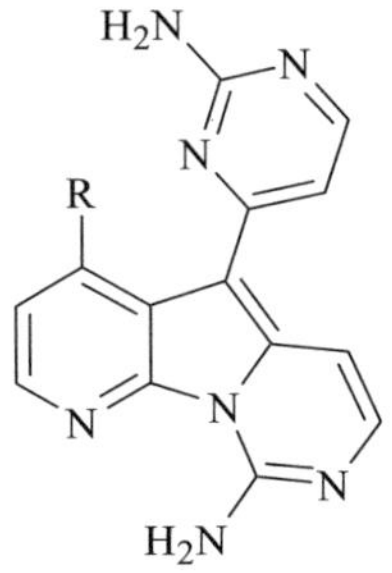

(96)

a. R = OH
b. R = H

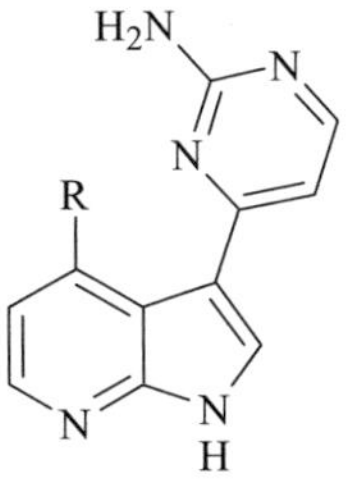

(97)

a. R = OH
b. R = H
c. R = OMe
d. R = OEt

Indisulam (E7070) [N-(3-chloro-7-indolyl)-1,4-benzenedisulphonamide] (**98**), a novel sulfonamide antitumor agent, was discovered from sulfonamide-focused libraries [208]. Compound (**98**) induced disturbance of the G1/S transition eventually led to G2 arrest in HCT116 human colon cancer cells and A549 human lung cancer cells. The study further clarified that (**98**) inhibited pRb phosphorylation, reduced the protein expression of cyclin A, cyclin B1, CDK2, and CDC2, and repressed CDK2 activity with the induction of p53 and p21 proteins only in the parental A549 cells [209]. The synthesis and antitumor activity of (**98**) and analogues are reported [210]. Phase trials of (**98**) are currently ongoing to assess its clinical efficacy against several solid tumors [211].

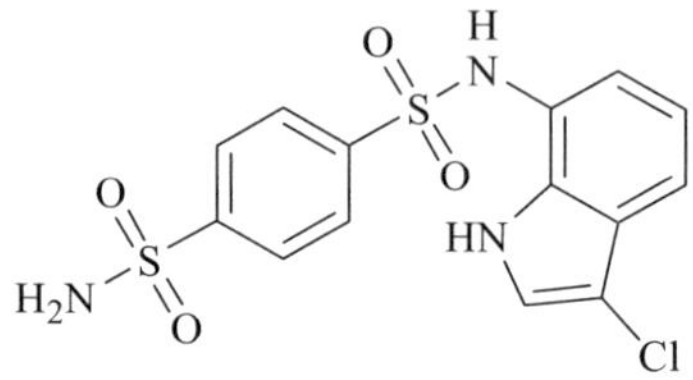

(**98**)

JNJ-7706621 (**99**) is a novel cell cycle inhibitor that showed potent inhibition of several CDKs (IC_{50} CDK1/cyclin B = 0.006 μM, CDK2/cyclin A = 0.002 μM and CDK4/cyclin D1 = 0.11 μM) [212, 213]. Compound (**99**) selectively blocked proliferation of tumor cells of various origins but was about 10-fold less effective at inhibiting normal human cell growth *in vitro* [214]. Compound (**99**) is currently under preclinical evaluation as an antitumor agent [215].

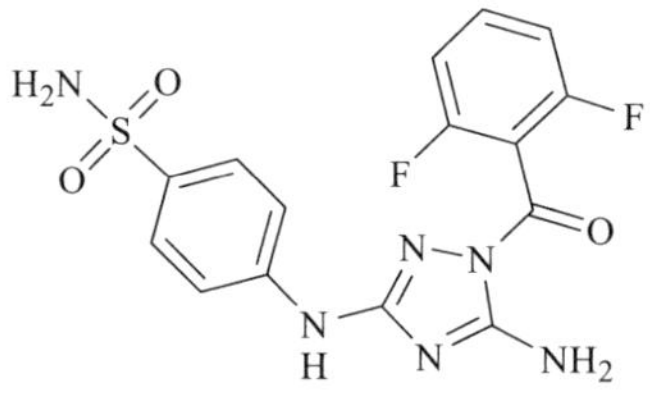

(**99**)

CDK inhibitor, CDKI-71 [**100**, 3-(5-cyano-4-(4-methyl-2-(methylamino)thiazol-5-yl)pyrimidin-2-ylamino)benzenesulfonamide] displayed potent cytotoxicity and caspase-dependent apoptosis induction that were closely associated with the inhibition of RNAPII phosphorylation at serine-2. This was caused by effective targeting of CDK9/cyclin T and resulted in the downstream inhibition of Mcl-1. No correlation between apoptosis and inhibition of cell-cycle CDKs 1 and 2 was observed [216].

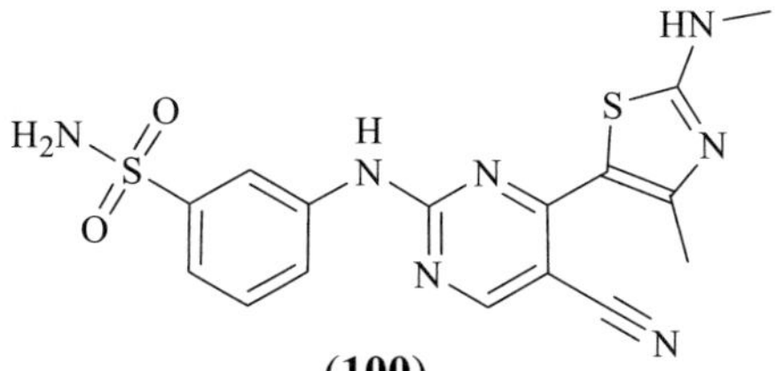

(100)

Table 5: Key CDK Inhibitors. The values are IC_{50} in μM.

Compound Name	**Compound No.**	**CDK1/B**	**CDK2/A**	**CDK2/E**	**CDK4/D**	**Clinical Trials**
Staurosporine	**2**	-	0.007	-	3-10	-
UCN-1	**3**	0.031	0.03	-	-	Phase I
Flavopiridol	**6**	0.4	0.1	-	0.4	Phase II
Olomucine II	**14**	0.02	-	-	-	-
R-Roscovitine, CYC202, Seliciclib	**15**	0.7	-	0.7	-	Phase II
Purvalanol B	**19b**	-	0.006	0.009	-	-
SB-210878	**27**	-	-	-	0.54	-
SCH 727965	**31**	0.001	0.001	-	-	-
AZ703	**34**	0.006	0.003	0.004	3.058	-
CGP-60474	**36**	0.02	-	0.05	-	-
PD 0332991	**40**	-	> 5	-	0.011	Phase I
BS-194	**46**	0.03	0.003	-	-	-
AZD5438	**53**					
R547*	**57**	0.001-0.003	-	0.001-0.003	0.001-0.003	Phase I
Indirubin-3'-monoxime	**60**	0.18	-	-	-	-
PNU292137	**63**	-	0.037	-	-	-
PHA-533533	**64**	-	0.037	-	-	-
AT7519	**66**	-	0.047	-	-	-
SNS-032, BMS-387032	**68**	-	-	0.048	-	Phase I
Alsterpaullone	**77**	0.035	-	-	-	-

Table 5: cont....

Kenpaullone	**78**	0.4	-	-	-	-
Hymenialdisine	**82a**	0.022	0.07	0.04	-	-
Variolin B	**96b**	0.06	0.08	-	-	Preclinical
Indisulam, E7070	**98**	-	-	-	-	Phase II
JNJ-770662	**99**	0.006	0.002	-	0.11	Preclinical

* The values are binding constants K_i in μM.

CONCLUSION

The importance of CDKs in cell cycle regulation and the frequent documented deregulation of CDKs and their modulators in neurodegenerative diseases have stimulated great research effort in cancer treatment. Although the clinical trials have provided excellent *in vitro* activity for few of these inhibitors but the essential requirement of specificity is still missing. As most of the inhibitors inhibit CDK1, 2, 4 and 6 with nearly the same potency, the search for a specific inhibitor still is on.

ACKNOWLEDGEMENT

The authors would like to thanks ChemAxon for academic version of Instant JChem.

CONFLICT OF INTEREST

The author(s) confirm that this chapter content has no conflict of interest.

DISCLOSURE

The chapter submitted for the eBook Series entitled **"Advances in Cancer Drug Targets, Volume 1"** is an update of our article in **Current Cancer Drug Targets, Volume 8, Issue 1, 2008,** with additional text and references.

REFERENCES

[1] Foye, W. O., Ed. *Cancer Chemotherapeutic Agent*; American Chemical Society: Washington DC, **1995**.

[2] Morgan, D. O. Principles of CDK Regulation. *Nature* **1995**, *374(6518)*, 131-134.

[3] Manning, G.; Whyte, D. B.; Martinez, R.; Hunter, T.; Sudarsanan, S. The Protein Kinase Complement of the Human Genome. *Science* **2002**, *298(5600)*, 1912-1934.

[4] Harper, J. W.; Adams, P. D. Cyclin-Dependent Kinases. *Chem. Rev.* **2001**, *101(8)*, 2511-2526.

[5] Hunter, T.; Pines, J. Cyclins and Cancer. II: Cyclin D and CDK Inhibitors Come of Age. *Cell* **1994**, *79(4)*, 573-582.

[6] Legraverend, M.; Grierson, D. S. The Purines: Potent and Versatile Small Molecule Inhibitors and Modulators of Key Biological Targets. *Bioorg. Med. Chem.* **2006**, *14(12)*, 3987-4006.

[7] Uhlmann, F.; Bouchoux, C.; López-Avilés, S. A. Quantitative Model for Cyclin-dependent Kinase Control of the Cell Cycle: Revisited. *Philos. Trans. R. Soc. Lond. B. Biol. Sci.* **2011**, *366(1584)*, 3572-3583.

[8] Wang, Q.; Su, L.; Liu, N.; Zhang, L.; Xu, W.; Fang, H. Cyclin Dependent Kinase 1 Inhibitors: A Review of Recent Progress. *Curr. Med. Chem.* **2011**, *18(13)*, 2025-43.

[9] Sharma, P. S.; Sharma, R.; Tyagi, R. Inhibitors of Cyclin Dependent Kinases: Useful Targets for Cancer Treatment. *Curr. Cancer. Drug Targets* **2008**, *8(1)*, 53-75.

[10] Zhang, J.; Yang, P. L.; Gray, N. S. Targeting Cancer with Small Molecule Kinase Inhibitors. *Nat. Rev. Cancer.* **2009**, *9(1)*, 28-39.

[11] Fabbro, D.; Cowan-Jacob, S. W.; Möbitz, H.; Martiny-Baron, G. Targeting Cancer with Small-molecular-weight Kinase Inhibitors. *Methods Mol. Biol.* **2012**, *795*, 1-34.

[12] Anastassiadis, T.; Deacon, S. W.; Devarajan, K.; Ma, H.; Peterson J. R. Comprehensive Assay of Kinase Catalytic Activity Reveals Features of Kinase Inhibitor Selectivity. *Nat. Biotechnol.* **2011**, *29(11)*, 1039-1045.

[13] Davis, M. I.; Hunt, J. P.; Herrgard, S.; Ciceri, P.; Wodicka, L. M.; Pallares, G.; Hocker, M.; Treiber, D. K.; Zarrinkar, P. P. Comprehensive Analysis of Kinase Inhibitor Selectivity. *Nat. Biotechnol.* **2011**, *29(11)*, 1046-1051.

[14] Stone, A.; Sutherland, R. L.; Musgrove, E. A. Inhibitors of Cell Cycle Kinases: Recent Advances and Future Prospects as Cancer Therapeutics. *Crit. Rev. Oncog.* **2012**, *17(2)*, 175-198.

[15] Posy, S. L.; Hermsmeier, M. A.; Vaccaro, W.; Ott, K. H.; Todderud, G.; Lippy, J. S.; Trainor, G. L.; Loughney, D. A.; Johnson, S. R. Trends in Kinase Selectivity: Insights for Target Class-focused Library Screening. *J. Med. Chem.* **2011**, *54(1)*, 54-66.

[16] Wesierska-Gadek, J.; Chamrád, I.; Kryštof, V. Novel Potent Pharmacological Cyclin-dependent Kinase Inhibitors. *Future Med. Chem.* **2009**, *1(9)*, 1561-81.

[17] Nakayama, K.; Nakayama K. Cip/Kip Cyclin-Dependent Kinase Inhibitors: Brakes of the Cell Cycle Engine During Development. *BioEssays* **1998**, *20(12)*, 1020-1029.

[18] Chim, C. S.; Fung, T. K.; Wong, K. F.; Lau, J. S.; Law, M.; Liang, R. Methylation of INK4 and CIP/KIP Families of Cyclin-Dependent Kinase Inhibitor in Chronic Lymphocytic Leukaemia in Chinese Patients. *J. Clin. Pathol.* **2006**, *59(9)*, 921-926.

[19] Maddika, S.; Ande, S. R.; Panigrahi, S.; Paranjothy, T.; Weglarczyk, K.; Zuse, A.; Eshraghi, M.; Manda, K. D.; Wiechec, E.; Los, M. Cell Survival, Cell Death and Cell Cycle Pathways are Interconnected: Implications for Cancer Therapy. *Drug Resist. Updat.* **2007**, *10(1-2)*, 13-29.

[20] Peter, M.; Herskowitz, I. Joining the Complex: Cyclin-Dependent Kinase Inhibitory Proteins and the Cell Cycle. *Cell* **1994**, *79 (2)*, 181-184.

[21] Denicourt, C.; Dowdy, S. F. Cip/Kip Proteins: More than Just CDKs Inhibitors. *Genes Dev.* **2004**, *18(8)*, 851-855.

[22] Xiong, Y.; Hannon, G. J.; Zhang, H.; Casso, D.; Kobayashi, R.; Beach, D. p21 is a Universal Inhibitor of Cyclin Kinases. *Nature* **1993**, *366(6456)*, 701-704.

[23] Janicke, R. U.; Sohn, D.; Essmann, F.; Schulze-Osthoff, K. The Multiple Battles Fought by Anti-Apoptotic p21. *Cell Cycle* **2007**, *6(4)*, 407-413.

[24] Russo, A. A.; Jeffrey, P. D.; Patten, A. K.; Massague, J.; Pavletich, N. P. Crystal Structure of $p27^{Kip1}$ Cyclin-Dependent Kinase Inhibitor Bound to the Cyclin A-CDK2 Complex. *Nature* **1996**, *382(6589)*, 325-331.

[25] Hall, M.; Bates, S.; Peters, G. Evidence for Different Modes of Action of Cyclin Dependent Kinase Inhibitors: p15 and p16 Bind to Kinases, p21 and p27 Bind to Cyclins. *Oncogene* **1995**, *11(8)*, 1581-1588.

[26] Hengst, L.; Gopfert, U.; Lashuel, H. A.; Reed, S. I. Complete Inhibition of CDK/cyclin by One Molecule of $p21^{Cip1}$. *Genes Dev.* **1998**, *12(24)*, 3882-3888.

[27] Gao, C. Y.; Zalenka, P. S. Cyclins, Cyclin-Dependent Kinases and Differentiation. *BioEssays* **1997**, *19(4)*, 307-315.

[28] Carnero, A.; Hannon, G. J. In *Cyclin Dependent Kinase (CDK) Inhibitors*; Vogt, P. K.; Reed, S. I.; Eds.; Springer: New York, **1997**, pp. 43-55.

[29] Guan, K. L.; Jenkins, C. W.; Li, Y.; Nichols, M. A.; Wu, X.; O'Keefe, C. L.; Matera, A. G.; Xiong, Y. Growth Suppression by p18, a $p16^{INK4/MTS1}$- and $p14^{INK4B/MTS2}$-Related CDK6 Inhibitor, Correlates with Wild-Type pRb Function. *Genes Dev.* **1994**, *8(24)*, 2939-2952.

[30] Hannon, G. J.; Beach, D. $p15^{INK4B}$ is a Potential Effector of TGFβ-Induced Cell Cycle Arrest. *Nature* **1994**, *371(6494)*, 257-261.

[31] Reynisdottir, I.; Polyak, K.; Iavarone, A.; Massague, J. Kip/Cip and INK4 CDK Inhibitors Cooperate to Induce Cell Cycle Arrest in Response to TFGβ. *Genes Dev.* **1995**, *9(15)*, 1831-1845.

[32] Li, J.; Poi, M. J.; Qin, D.; Selby, T. L.; Byeon, I. J.; Tsai, M. D. Tumor Suppressor INK4: Quantitative Structure-Function Analyses of $p18^{INK4C}$ as an Inhibitor of Cyclin-Dependent Kinase 4. *Biochemistry* **2000**, *39(4)*, 649-657.

[33] Brotherton, D. H.; Dganaraj, V.; Wick, S.; Brizula, L.; Domaille, P. J.; Volyanik, E.; Xu, X.; Parisin, E.; Smith, B. O.; Archer, S. J.; Serrano, M.; Brenner, S. L.; Blundell, T. L.; Laue, E. D. Crystal Structure of the Complex of the Cyclin-Dependent Kinase CDK6 Bound to the Cell-Cycle Inhibitor $p19^{INK4d}$. *Nature* **1998**, *395(6699)*, 244-250.

[34] Kim, S. H. Structure-Based Inhibitor Design for CDK2, a Cell Cycle Controlling Protein Kinase. *Pure Appl. Chem.* **1998**, *70(3)*, 555-565.

[35] Furusaki, A.; Hashiba, N.; Matsumoto, T.; Hirano, A.; Iwai, Y.; Omura, S. The Crystal and Molecular Structure of Staurosporine, a New Alkaloid from a *Streptomyces* Strain. *Bull. Chem. Soc. Jpn.* **1982**, *55*, 3681-3685.

[36] Meijer, L. Chemical Inhibitors of Cyclin-Dependent Kinases. *Trends Cell. Biol.* **1996**, *6(10)*, 393-397.

[37] Meijer, L. Chemical Inhibitors of Cyclin-Dependent Kinases. In *Progress in Cell Cycle Research*; Meijer, L., Guidet, S., Tung, H. Y. L., Eds.; Plenum Press: New York, **1995**, pp 351-361.

[38] Gani, O. A.; Engh, R. A. Protein Kinase Inhibition of Clinically Important Staurosporine Analogues. *Nat. Prod. Rep.* **2010**, *27(4)*, 489-498.

[39] Grosios, K. UCN-01 Kyowa Hakko Kogyo Co. *Curr. Opin. Investig. Drugs* **2001**, *2(2)*, 287-297.

[40] Li, T.; Christensen, S. D.; Frankel, P. H.; Margolin, K. A.; Agarwala, S. S.; Luu, T.; Mack, P. C.; Lara, P. N. Jr.; Gandara, D. R. A Phase II Study of Cell Cycle Inhibitor UCN-01 in Patients with Metastatic Melanoma: a California Cancer Consortium Trial. *Invest. New Drugs.* **2012**, 30(2), 741-748.

[41] Kummar, S.; Gutierrez, M. E.; Gardner, E. R.; Figg, W. D.; Melillo, G.; Dancey, J.; Sausville, E. A.; Conley, B. A.; Murgo, A. J.; Doroshow, J. H. A Phase I Trial of UCN-01 and Prednisone in Patients with Refractory Solid Tumors and Lymphomas. *Cancer Chemother. Pharmacol.* **2010**, *65(2)*, 383-389.

[42] Abe, S.; Kubota, T.; Otani, Y.; Furukawa, T.; Watanabe, M.; Kumai, K.; Kitajima, M. Sensitivity of UCN-01 Lies in the Balance of CDK2 Kinase and p21. *Gan To Kagaku Ryoho.* **2000**, *27(8)*, 1260-1266.

[43] Chin, L. S.; Murray, S. F.; Doherty, P. F.; Singh, S. K. K252a Induces Cell Cycle Arrest and Apoptosis by Inhibiting Cdc2 and Cdc25c. *Cancer Invest.* **1999**, *17(6)*, 391-395.

[44] Takai, N.; Ueda, T.; Nishida, M.; Nasu, K.; Fukuda, J.; Miyakawa, I. K252a Inhibits Proliferation of Ovarian Cancer Cells by Upregulating $p21^{WAF1}$. *Oncol. Rep.* **2005**, *14(1)*, 141-143.

[45] Link, J. T.; Raghavan, S.; Gallant, M.; Danishefsky, S. J.; Chou, T. C.; Ballas, L. M. Staurosporine and ent-Staurosporine: The First Total Syntheses, Prospects for a Regioselective Approach, and Activity Profiles. *J. Am. Chem. Soc.* **1996**, *118(12)*, 2825-2842.

[46] Pereira, E. R.; Belin, L.; Sancelme, M.; Prudhomme, M.; Ollier, M.; Rapp, M.; Severe, D.; Riou, J.-F.; Fabbro, D.; Meyer, T. Structure-Activity Relationships in a Series of Substituted Indolocarbazoles: Topoisomerase I and Protein Kinase C Inhibition and Antitumoral and Antimicrobial Properties. *J. Med. Chem.* **1996**, *39(22)*, 4471-4477.

[47] Wood, J. L.; Stoltz, B. M.; Goodman, S. N.; Onwueme, K. Design and Implementation of an Efficient Synthetic Approach to Pyranosylated Indolocarbazoles: Total Synthesis of (+)-RK286c, (+)-MLR-52, (+)-Staurosporine, and (-)-TAN-1030a. *J. Am. Chem. Soc.* **1997**, *119(41)*, 9652-9661.

[48] Kuo, P. C.; Liu, H. F.; Chao, J. I. Survivin and p53 Modulate Quercetin-Induced Cell Growth Inhibition and Apoptosis in Human Lung Carcinoma Cells. *J. Biol. Chem.* **2004**, *279(53)*, 55875-55885.

[49] Jeong, J. H.; An, J. Y.; Kwon, Y. T.; Rhee, J. G.; Lee, Y. J. Effects of Low Dose Quercetin: Cancer Cell-specific Inhibition of Cell Cycle Progression. *J. Cell. Biochem.* **2009**, *106(1)*, 73-82.

[50] Wirger A.; Perabo F. G.; Burgemeister, S.; Haase, L.; Schmidt, D. H.; Doehn, C.; Mueller, S. C.; Jocham, D. Flavopiridol, an Inhibitor of Cyclin-Dependent Kinases, Induces Growth Inhibition and Apoptosis in Bladder Cancer Cells *in vitro and in vivo*. *Anticancer Res.* **2005**, *25(6B)*, 4341-4347.

[51] Dickson, M. A.; Shah, M. A.; Rathkopf, D.; Tse, A.; Carvajal, R. D.; Wu, N.; Lefkowitz, R. A.; Gonen, M.; Cane, L. M.; Dials, H. J.; Schwartz, G. K. A Phase I Clinical Trial of FOLFIRI in Combination with the Pan Cyclin-dependent Kinase (CDK) Inhibitor Flavopiridol. *Cancer Chemother. Pharmacol.* **2010**, *66(6)*, 1113-1121.

[52] Sedlacek, H. H.; Czech, J.; Naik, R.; Kaur, G.; Worland, P.; Losiewich, M.; Parker, B.; Carlson, B.; Smith, A. Flavopiridol (L86-8275; NSC 649890), a New Kinase Inhibitor for Tumor Therapy. *Int. J. Oncol.* **1996**, *9*, 1143-1168.

[53] Losiewicz, M. D.; Carlson, B. A.; Kaur, G.; Sausville, E. A.; Worland, P. J. Potent Inhibition of Cdc2 Kinase Activity by the Flavonoid L86-8275. *Biochem. Biophys. Res. Commun.* **1994**, *201(2)*, 589-595.

[54] Czech, J.; Hoffman, D.; Naik, R.; Sedlacek, H. Antitumoral Activity of Flavone L86-8275. *Int. J. Oncol.* **1995**, *6*, 31-36.

[55] Holkova, B.; Perkins, E. B.; Ramakrishnan, V.; Tombes, M. B.; Shrader, E.; Talreja, N.; Wellons, M. D.; Hogan, K. T.; Roodman, G. D.; Coppola, D.; Kang, L.; Dawson, J.; Stuart, R. K.; Peer, C.; Figg, W. D. Sr.; Kolla, S.; Doyle, A.; Wright, J.; Sullivan, D. M.; Roberts, J. D.; Grant, S. Phase I Trial of Bortezomib (PS-341; NSC 681239) and Alvocidib (Flavopiridol; NSC 649890) in Patients with Recurrent or Refractory B-cell Neoplasms. *Clin. Cancer Res.* **2011**, *17(10)*, 3388-3397.

[56] Ahn, Y. M.; Vogeti, L.; Liu, C. J.; Santhapuram, H. K.; White, J. M.; Vasandani, V.; Mitscher, L. A.; Lushington, G. H.; Hanson, P. R.; Powell, D. R.; Himes, R. H.; Roby, K. F.; Ye, Q.; Georg, G. I. Design, Synthesis, and Antiproliferative and CDK2-Cyclin a Inhibitory Activity of Novel Flavopiridol Analogues. *Bioorg. Med. Chem.* **2007**, *15(2)*, 702-713.

[57] Polier, G.; Ding, J.; Konkimalla, B. V.; Eick, D.; Ribeiro, N.; Köhler, R.; Giaisi, M.; Efferth, T.; Desaubry, L.; Krammer, P. H.; Li-Weber, M. Wogonin and Related Natural Flavones are Inhibitors of CDK9 that Induce Apoptosis in Cancer Cells by Transcriptional Suppression of Mcl-1. *Cell Death Dis.* **2011**, *2*, e182.

[58] Joshi, K. S.; Rathos, M. J.; Joshi, R. D.; Sivakumar, M.; Mascarenhas, M.; Kamble, S.; Lal, B.; Sharma, S. *In vitro* Antitumor Properties of a Novel Cyclin-dependent Kinase Inhibitor, P276-00. *Mol. Cancer Ther.* **2007**, *6(3)*, 918-925.

[59] Raje, N.; Hideshima, T.; Mukherjee, S.; Raab, M.; Vallet, S.; Chhetri, S.; Cirstea, D.; Pozzi, S.; Mitsiades, C.; Rooney, M.; Kiziltepe, T.; Podar, K.; Okawa, Y.; Ikeda, H.; Carrasco, R.; Richardson, P. G.; Chauhan, D.; Munshi. N. C.; Sharma, S.; Parikh, H.; Chabner, B.; Scadden, D.; Anderson, K. C. Preclinical Activity of P276-00, a Novel Small-molecule Cyclin-dependent Kinase Inhibitor in the Therapy of Multiple Myeloma. *Leukemia.* **2009**, *23(5)*, 961-970.

[60] Lee, D. E.; Lee, K. W.; Jung, S. K.; Lee, E. J.; Hwang, J. A.; Lim, T. G.; Kim, B. Y.; Bode, A. M.; Lee, H. J.; Dong, Z. 6,7,4'-Trihydroxyisoflavone Inhibits HCT-116 Human Colon Cancer Cell Proliferation by Targeting CDK1 and CDK2. *Carcinogenesis.* **2011**, *32(4)*, 629-635.

[61] Lu, H.; Chang, D. J.; Baratte, B.; Meijer, L.; Schulze-Gahmen, S. Crystal Structure of a Human Cyclin-Dependent Kinase 6 Complex with a Flavonol Inhibitor, Fisetin. *J. Med. Chem.* **2005**, *48(3)*, 737-743.

[62] Lee, A. J.; Park, T.; Jeong, S.; Kim, K. H.; Hong, C. 3-Hydroxychromones as Cyclin-Dependent Kinase Inhibitors: Synthesis and Biological Evaluation. *Bioorg. Med. Chem. Lett.* **2007**, *17(5)*, 1284-1287.

[63] Vesely, J.; Havlicek, L.; Strnad, M.; Blow, J. J.; Donella-Deana, A.; Pinna, L.; Letham, D. S.; Kato, J. Y.; Detivaud, L.; LeClerc, S.; Meijer, L. Inhibition of Cyclin Dependent Kinases by Purine Analogues. *Eur. J. Biochem.* **1994**, *224(2)*, 771-786.

[64] Raynaud, F. I.; Whittaker, S. R.; Fischer, P. M.; McClue, S.; Walton, M. I.; Barrie, S. E.; Garrett, M. D.; Rogers, P.; Clarke, S. J.; Kelland, L. R.; Valenti, M.; Brunton, L.; Eccles, S.; Lane, D. P.; Workman, P. *In vitro* and *in vivo* Pharmacokinetic-Pharmacodynamic

Relationships for the Trisubstituted Aminopurine Cyclin-Dependent Kinase Inhibitors Olomucine, Bohemine and CYC202. *Clin. Cancer Res.* **2005**, *11(13)*, 4875-4887.

[65] Boutis, A.; Papazisis, K.; Pistevou-Gompaki. K.; Lambropoulos, A.; Sofroniadis, I.; Papageorgiou, A.; Destouni, E.; Kortsaris, A. Cyclin-Dependent Kinase (CDK) Inhibitor Olomoucine Enhances Gamma-Irradiation-Induced Apoptosis and Cell Cycle Arrest in Raji Cells. *Anticancer Res.* **2006**, *26(5A)*, 3493-3498.

[66] Krystof, V.; Lenobel, R.; Havlicek, L.; Kuzma, M.; Strnad, M. Synthesis and Biological Activity of Olomoucine II. *Bioorg. Med. Chem. Lett.* **2002**, *12(22)*, 3283-3286.

[67] Krystof, V.; McNae, I. W.; Walkinshaw, M. D.; Fischer, P. M.; Muller, P.; Vojtesek, B.; Orsag, M.; Havlicek, L.; Strnad, M. Antiproliferative Activity of Olomoucine II, a Novel 2,6,9-Trisubstituted Purine Cyclin-Dependent Kinase Inhibitor. *Cell. Mol. Life Sci.* **2005**, *62(15)*, 1763-1771.

[68] Bach, S.; Knockaert, M.; Reinhardt, J.; Lozach, O.; Schmitt, S.; Baratte, B.; Koken, M.; Coburn, S. P.; Tang, L.; Jiang, T.; Liang, D. C.; Galons, H.; Dierick, J. F.; Pinna, L. A.; Meggio, F.; Totzke, F.; Schachtele, C.; Lerman, A. S.; Carnero, A.; Wan, Y.; Gray, N.; Meijer, L. Roscovitine Targets, Protein Kinases and Pyridoxal Kinase. *J. Biol. Chem.* **2005**, *280(35)*, 31208-31219.

[69] Mapelli, M.; Massimiliano, L.; Crovace, C.; Seeliger, M. A.; Tsai, L.-H.; Meijer, L.; Musacchio, A. Mechanism of CDK5/p25 Binding by CDK Inhibitors. *J. Med. Chem.* **2005**, *48(3)*, 671-679.

[70] Hassan, M.; Sallam, H.; Hassan, Z. The Role of Pharmacokinetics and Pharmacodynamics in Early Drug Development with Reference to the Cyclin-dependent Kinase (Cdk) Inhibitor - Roscovitine. *Sultan Qaboos Univ. Med. J.* **2011**, *11(2)*, 165-178.

[71] Nair, B. C.; Vallabhaneni, S.; Tekmal, R. R.; Vadlamudi, R. K. Roscovitine Confers Tumor Suppressive Effect on Therapy-resistant Breast Tumor Cells. *Breast Cancer Res.* **2011**, *13(3)*, R80.

[72] Liebl, J.; Krystof, V.; Vereb, G.; Takács, L.; Strnad, M.; Pechan, P.; Havlicek, L.; Zatloukal, M.; Fürst, R.; Vollmar, A. M.; Zahler, S. Anti-angiogenic Effects of Purine Inhibitors of Cyclin Dependent Kinases. *Angiogenesis.* **2011**, *14(3)*, 281-291.

[73] Cho, S. J.; Kim, Y. J.; Surh, Y. J.; Kim, B. M.; Lee, S. K. Ibulocydine is a Novel Prodrug CDK Inhibitor that Effectively Induces Apoptosis in Hepatocellular Carcinoma Cells. *J. Biol. Chem.* **2011**, *286(22)*, 19662-19671.

[74] Adona, P. R.; Lima Verde Leal, C. Meiotic Inhibition with Different Cyclin- Dependent Kinase Inhibitors in Bovine Oocytes and its Effects on Maturation and Embryo Development. *Zygote* **2004**, *12(3)*, 197-204.

[75] Liskova, B.; Zerzankova, L.; Novakova, O.; Kostrhunova, H.; Travnicek, Z.; Brabec, V. Cellular Response to Antitumor cis-Dichlorido Platinum(II) Complexes of CDK inhibitor Bohemine and its Analogues. *Chem. Res. Toxicol.* **2012**, *25(2)*, 500-509.

[76] Raynaud, F. I.; Fischer, P. M.; Nutley, B. P.; Goddard, P. M.; Lane, D. P.; Workman, P. Cassette Dosing Pharmacokinetics of a Library of 2,6,9-Trisubstituted Purine Cyclin-Dependent Kinase 2 Inhibitors Prepared by Parallel Synthesis. *Mol. Cancer Ther.* **2004**, *3(3)*, 353-362.

[77] Hikita, T.; Oneyama, C.; Okada, M. Purvalanol A, a CDK Inhibitor, Effectively Suppresses Src-mediated Transformation by Inhibiting both CDKs and c-Src. *Genes Cells* **2010**, *15(10)*, 1051-1062.

[78] Ringer, L.; Sirajuddin, P.; Heckler, M.; Ghosh, A.; Suprynowicz, F.; Yenugonda, V. M.; Brown, M. L.; Toretsky, J. A.; Uren, A.; Lee, Y.; MacDonald, T. J.; Rodriguez, O.; Glazer, R. I.; Schlegel, R.; Albanese, C. VMY-1-103 is a Novel CDK Inhibitor that Disrupts Chromosome Organization and Delays Metaphase Progression in Medulloblastoma Cells. *Cancer Biol. Ther.* **2011**, *12(9)*, 818-826.

[79] Wilson, S. C.; Atrash, B.; Barlow, C.; Eccles, S.; Fischer, P. M.; Hayes, A.; Kelland, L.; Jackson, W.; Jarman, M.; Mirza, A.; Moreno, J.; Nutley, B. P.; Raynaud, F. I.; Sheldrake, P.; Walton, M.; Westwood, R.; Whittaker, S.; Workman, P.; McDonald, E. Design, Synthesis and Biological Evaluation of 6-Pyridylmethylaminopurines as CDK Inhibitors. *Bioorg. Med. Chem.* **2011**, *19(22)*, 6949-6965.

[80] Vandromme, L; Piguel, S.; Lozach, O.; Meijer, L.; Legraverend, M.; Griersona, D. S. Suzuki-Type Pd(0) Coupling Reactions in the Synthesis of 2-Arylpurines as CDK Inhibitors. *Bioorg. Med. Chem. Lett.* **2006**, *16(12),* 3144-3146.

[81] Hardcastle, I. R.; Ian, R.; Arris, C. E.; Bentley, J.; Boyle, F. T.; Chen, Y.; Curtin, N. J.; Endicott, J. A.; Gibson, A. E.; Golding, B. T.; Griffin, R. J.; Jewsbury, P.; Menyerol, J.; Mesguiche, V.; Newell, D. R.; Noble, M. E. M.; Pratt, D. J.; Wang, L.-Z.; Whitfield, H. J. N^2-Substituted O^6-Cyclohexylmethyl-guanine Derivatives: Potent Inhibitors of Cyclin-Dependent Kinases 1 and 2. *J. Med. Chem.* **2004**, *47(15)*, 3710-3722.

[82] Davies, T. G.; Bentley, J.; Arris, C. E.; Boyle, F. T.; Curtin, N. J.; Endicott, J. A.; Gibson, A. E.; Golding, B. T.; Griffin, R. J.; Hardcastle, I. R.; Jewsbury, P.; Johnson, L. N.; Mesguiche, V.; Newell, D. R.; Noble, M. E.; Tucker, J. A.; Wang, L.; Whitfield, H. J. Structure-Based Design of a Potent Purine-Based Cyclin-Dependent Kinase Inhibitor. *Nat. Struct. Biol.* **2002**, *9*, 745-749.

[83] Oumata, N.; Bettayeb, K.; Ferandin, Y.; Demange, L.; Lopez-Giral, A.; Goddard, M. L.; Myrianthopoulos, V.; Mikros, E.; Flajolet, M.; Greengard, P.; Meijer, L.; Galons, H. Roscovitine-derived, Dual-specificity Inhibitors of Cyclin-dependent Kinases and Casein Kinases 1. *J. Med. Chem.* **2008**, *51(17)*, 5229-5242.

[84] Trova, M. P.; Barnes, K. D.; Alicea, L.; Benanti, T.; Bielaska, M.; Bilotta, J.; Bliss, B.; Duong, T. N.; Haydar, S.; Herr, R. J.; Hui, Y.; Johnson, M.; Lehman, J. M.; Peace, D.; Rainka, M.; Snider, P.; Salamone, S.; Tregay, S.; Zheng, X.; Friedrich, T. D. Heterobiaryl Purine Derivatives as Potent Antiproliferative Agents: Inhibitors of Cyclin Dependent Kinases. Part II. *Bioorg. Med. Chem. Lett.* **2009**, *19(23)*, 6613-6617.

[85] Trova, M. P.; Barnes, K. D.; Barford, C.; Benanti, T.; Bielaska, M.; Burry, L.; Lehman, J. M.; Murphy, C.; O'Grady, H.; Peace, D.; Salamone, S.; Smith, J.; Snider, P.; Toporowski, J.; Tregay, S.; Wilson, A.; Wyle, M.; Zheng, X.; Friedrich, T. D. Biaryl Purine Derivatives as Potent Antiproliferative Agents: Inhibitors of Cyclin Dependent Kinases. Part I. *Bioorg. Med. Chem. Lett.* **2009**, *19(23)*, 6608-6612.

[86] Dolezal, K.; Popa, I.; Krystof, V.; Spíchal, L.; Fojtíková, M.; Holub, J.; Lenobel, R.; Schmülling, T.; Strnad, M. Preparation and Biological Activity of 6-Benzylaminopurine Derivatives in Plants and Human Cancer Cells. *Bioorg. Med. Chem.* **2006**, *14(3)*, 875-884.

[87] Havlicek, L.; Fuksova, K.; Krystof, V.; Orsag, M.; Vojtesek, B.; Strnad, M. 8-Azapurines as New Inhibitors of Cyclin-dependent Kinases. *Bioorg. Med. Chem.* **2005**, *13(18)*, 5399-5407.

[88] Moravec, J.; Krystof, V.; Hanus, J.; Havlícek, L.; Moravcová, D.; Fuksová, K.; Kuzma, M.; Lenobel, R.; Otyepka, M.; Strnad, M. 2,6,8,9-Tetrasubstituted Purines as New CDK1 Inhibitors. *Bioorg. Med. Chem. Lett.* **2003**, *13(18)*, 2993-2996.

[89] Orzáez, M.; Gortat, A.; Mondragón, L.; Bachs, O.; Pérez-Payá, E. ATP-noncompetitive Inhibitors of CDK-cyclin Complexes. *ChemMedChem.* **2009**, *4(1)*, 19-24.

[90] Trávnícek, Z.; Starha, P.; Popa, I.; Vrzal, R.; Dvorák, Z. Roscovitine-based CDK Inhibitors Acting as N-donor Ligands in the Platinum(II) Oxalato Complexes: Preparation, Characterization and *in vitro* Cytotoxicity. *Eur. J. Med. Chem.* **2010**, *45(10)*, 4609-4614.

[91] Travnicek, Z.; Krystof, V.; Sipl, M. Zinc(II) Complexes with Potent Cyclin-Dependent Kinase Inhibitors Derived from 6-Benzylaminopurine: Synthesis, Characterization, X-ray Structures and Biological Activity. *J. Inorg. Biochem.* **2006**, *100(2)*, 214-225.

[92] Bramson, H. N.; Corona, J.; Davis, S. T.; Dickerson, S. H.; Edelstein, M.; Frye, S. V.; Gampe, R. T. Jr.; Harris, P. A.; Hassell, A.; Holmes, W. D.; Hunter, R. N.; Lackey, K. E.; Lovejoy, B.; Luzzio, M. J.; Montana, V.; Rocque, W. J.; Rusnak, D.; Shewchuk, L.; Veal, J. M.; Walker, D. H.; Kuyper, L. F. Oxindole-Based Inhibitors of Cyclin-Dependent Kinase 2 (CDK2): Design, Synthesis, Enzymatic Activities, and X-ray Crystallographic Analysis. *J. Med. Chem.* **2001**, *44(25)*, 4339-4358.

[93] Singh, S. K.; Dessalew, N.; Bharatam, P. V. 3D-QSAR CoMFA Study on Oxindole Derivatives as Cyclin Dependent Kinase 1 (CDK1) and Cyclin Dependent Kinase 2 (CDK2) Inhibitors. *Med. Chem.* **2007**, *3(1)*, 75-84.

[94] Luk, K. C.; Simcox, M. E.; Schutt, A.; Rowan, K.; Thompson, T.; Chen, Y.; Kammlott, U.; DePinto, W.; Dunten, P.; Dermatakis, A. A new series of potent oxindole inhibitors of CDK2. *Bioorg. Med. Chem. Lett.* **2004**, *14(4)*, 913-917.

[95] Xiong, X.; Zhang, Y.; Gao, X.; Dong, Z.; Li, L.; Ji, C.; Fu, L.; Luo, X.; Liu, H.; Mei, C. B5, a novel pyrrole-substituted indolinone, exerts potent antitumor efficacy through G2/M cell cycle arrest. *Invest. New Drugs* **2010**, *28(1)*, 26-34.

[96] Guengerich, F. P.; Sorrells, J. L.; Schmitt, S.; Krauser, J. A.; Aryal, P.; Meijer, L. Generation of New Protein Kinase Inhibitors Utilizing Cytochrome P450 Mutant Enzyme for Indigoid Synthesis. *J. Med. Chem.* **2004**, *47(12)*, 3236-3241.

[97] Zhu, G.; Conner, S. E.; Zhou, X.; Shih, C.; Li, T.; Anderson, B. D.; Brooks, H. B.; Campbell, R. M.; Considine, E.; Dempsey, J. A.; Faul, M. M.; Ogg, F. C.; Patel, B.; Schultz, R. M.; Spencer, C. D.; Teicher, B.; Watkins, S. A. Synthesis, Structure-Activity Relationship, and Biological Studies of Indolocarbazoles as Potent Cyclin D1-CDK4 Inhibitor. *J. Med. Chem.* **2003**, *46(11)*, 2027-2030.

[98] Sanchez-Martinez, C.; Shih, C.; Zhu, G.; Li, T.; Brooks, H. B.; Patel, B. K.; Schultz, R. M.; DeHahn, T. B.; Spencer, C. D.; Watkins, S. A.; Ogg, C. A.; Considine, E.; Dempsey, J. A.; Zhang, F. Studies on Cyclin-Dependent Kinase Inhibitors: Indolo-[2,3-a]pyrrolo[3,4-c]carbazoles *versus* Bis-indolylmaleimides. *Bioorg. Med. Chem. Lett.* **2003**, *13(21)*, 3841-3846.

[99] Sun, Y.; Li, Y. X.; Wu, H. J.; Wu, S. H.; Wang, Y. A.; Luo, D. Z.; Liao, D. J. Effects of an Indolocarbazole-derived CDK4 Inhibitor on Breast Cancer Cells. *J Cancer.* **2011**, *2*, 36-51.

[100] Sun, Y.; Li, Y. X.; Wu, H. J.; Wu, S. H.; Wang, Y. A.; Luo, D. Z.; Liao, D. J. Effects of an Indolocarbazole-Derived CDK4 Inhibitor on Breast Cancer Cells. *J. Cancer.* **2011**, *2*, 36-51.

[101] Zhou, H.; Shen, T.; Luo, Y.; Liu, L.; Chen, W.; Xu, B.; Han, X.; Pang, J.; Rivera, C. A.; Huang, S. The Antitumor Activity of the Fungicide Ciclopirox. *Int. J. Cancer* **2010**, *127(10)*, 2467-2477.

[102] Parry, D.; Guzi, T.; Shanahan, F.; Davis, N.; Prabhavalkar, D.; Wiswell, D.; Seghezzi, W.; Paruch, K.; Dwyer, M. P.; Doll, R.; Nomeir, A.; Windsor, W.; Fischmann, T.; Wang, Y.;

Oft, M.; Chen, T.; Kirschmeier, P.; Lees, E. M. Dinaciclib (SCH 727965), a Novel and Potent Cyclin-dependent Kinase Iinhibitor. *Mol. Cancer Ther.* **2010**, *9(8)*, 2344-2353.

[103] Feldmann, G.; Mishra, A.; Bisht, S.; Karikari, C.; Garrido-Laguna, I.; Rasheed, Z.; Ottenhof, N. A.; Dadon, T.; Alvarez, H.; Fendrich, V.; Rajeshkumar, N. V.; Matsui, W.; Brossart, P.; Hidalgo, M.; Bannerji, R.; Maitra, A.; Nelkin, B. D. Cyclin-dependent Kinase Inhibitor Dinaciclib (SCH727965) Inhibits Pancreatic Cancer Growth and Progression in Murine Xenograft Models. *Cancer Biol. Ther.* **2011**, *12(7)*, 598-609.

[104] Kassis, P.; Brzeszcz, J.; Bénéteau, V.; Lozach, O.; Meijer, L.; Le Guével, R.; Guillouzo, C,; Lewinski, K.; Bourg, S.; Colliandre, L.; Routier, S.; Mérour, J. Y. Synthesis and Biological Evaluation of New 3-(6-Hydroxyindol-2-yl)-5-(phenyl) Pyridine or Pyrazine V-Shaped Molecules as Kinase Inhibitors and Cytotoxic Agents. *Eur. J. Med. Chem.* **2011**, *46(11)*, 5416-5434.

[105] Lin, R.; Connolly, P. J.; Lu, Y.; Chiu, G.; Li, S.; Yu, Y.; Huang, S.; Li, X.; Emanuel, S. L.; Middleton, S. A.; Gruninger, R. H.; Adams, M.; Fuentes-Pesquera, A. R.; Greenberger, L. M. Synthesis and Evaluation of Pyrazolo[3,4-b]pyridine CDK1 Inhibitors as Anti-tumor Agents. *Bioorg. Med. Chem. Lett.* **2007**, *17(15)*, 4297-4302.

[106] Huang, S.; Lin, R.; Yu, Y.; Lu, Y.; Connolly, P. J.; Chiu, G.; Li, S.; Emanuel, S. L.; Middleton, S. A. Synthesis of 3-(1H-Benzimidazol-2-yl)-5-isoquinolin-4-ylpyrazolo[1,2-b]pyridine, a Potent CDK1 Inhibitor. *Bioorg. Med. Chem. Lett.* **2007**, *17(5)*, 1243-1245.

[107] Byths, K. F.; Geh, C.; Forder, C. L.; Oakes, S. E.; Thomas, A. P. The Cellular Phenotype of AZ703, a Novel Selective Imidazo[1,2-a]pyridine Cyclin-Dependent Kinase Inhibitor. *Mol. Cancer Ther.* **2006**, *5(3)*, 655-664.

[108] Martínez-Urbina, M. A.; Zentella, A.; Vilchis-Reyes, M. A.; Guzmán, A.; Vargas, O.; Ramírez-Apan. M. T.; Ventura-Gallegos, J. L.; Díaz, E. 6-Substituted 2-(N-trifluoroacetylamino)imidazopyridines induce cell cycle arrest and apoptosis in SK-LU-1 human cancer cell line. *Eur. J. Med. Chem.* **2010**, *45(3)*, 1211-1219.

[109] Kuo, G. H.; Deangelis, A.; Emanuel, S.; Wang, A.; Zhang, Y.; Connolly, P. J.; Chen, X.; Gruninger, R. H.; Rugg, C.; Fuentes-Pesquera, A.; Middleton, S. A.; Jolliffe, L.; Murray, W. V. Synthesis and Identification of [1,3,5]Triazine-Pyridine Biheteroaryl as a Novel Series of Potent Cyclin-Dependent Kinase Inhibitors. *J. Med. Chem.* **2005**, *48(14)*, 4535-4546.

[110] Tu, S.; Zhang, J.; Zhu, X.; Xu, J.; Zang, Y.; Wang, Q.; Jia, R.; Jiang, B.; Zhang, J. New Potential Inhibitors of Cyclin-Dependent Kinase 4: Design and Synthesis of Pyrido[2,3-d]pyrimidine Derivatives Under Microwave Irradition. *Bioorg. Med. Chem. Lett.* **2006**, *16(13)*, 3578-3581.

[111] Barvian, M.; Boschelli, D. H.; Cossrow, J.; Dobrusin, E.; Fattaey, A.; Fritsch, A.; Fry, D.; Harvey P.; Keller, P.; Garrett, M.; La, F.; Leopold, W.; McNamara, D.; Quin, M.; Trumpp-Kallmeyer, S.; Toogood, P.; Wu, Z.; Zhang, E. Pyrido-[2,3-d]pyrimidin-7-one Inhibitors of Cyclin-Dependent Kinases. *J. Med. Chem.* **2000**, *43*, 4606-4616.

[112] VanderWel, S. N.; Harvey, P. J.; McNamara, D. J.; Repine, J. T.; Keller, P. R.; Quin J. III; Booth, R. J.; Elliott, W. L.; Dobrusin, E. M.; Fry, D. W.; Toogood, P. L. Pyrido[2,3-d]pyrimidin-7-ones as Specific Inhibitors of Cyclin-Dependent Kinase 4. *J. Med. Chem.* **2005**, *48(7)*, 2371-2387.

[113] Toogood, P. L.; Harvey, P. J.; Repine, J. T.; Sheehan, D. J.; VanderWel, S. N.; Zhou, H.; Keller, P. R.; McNamara, D. J.; Sherry, D.; Zhu, T.; Brodfuehrer, J.; Choi, C.; Barvian, M. R.; Fry, D. W. Discovery of a Potent and Selective Inhibitor of Cyclin-Dependent Kinase 4/6. *J. Med. Chem.* **2005**, *48(7)*, 2388-2406.

[114] Flaherty, K. T.; Lorusso, P. M.; Demichele, A.; Abramson, V. G.; Courtney, R.; Randolph, S. S.; Shaik, M. N.; Wilner, K. D.; O'Dwyer, P. J.; Schwartz, G. K. Phase I, Dose-escalation Trial of the Oral Cyclin-dependent Kinase 4/6 Inhibitor PD 0332991, Administered Using a 21-day Schedule in Patients with Advanced Cancer. *Clin. Cancer Res.* **2012**, *18(2)*, 568-576.

[115] Markwalder, J. A.; Arnone, M. R.; Benfield, P. A.; Boisclair, M.; Burton, C. R.; Chang, C. H.; Cox, S. S.; Czerniak, P. M.; Dean, C. L.; Doleniak, D.; Grafstrom, R.; Harrison, B. A.; Kaltenbach, R. F. III.; Nugiel, D.; Rosi, K. A.; Sherk, S. R.; Sisk, L. M.; Stouten, P.; Trainor, G. L.; Worland, P.; Seitz, S. P. Synthesis and Biological Evaluation of 1-Aryl-4,5-dihydro-1H-pyrazolo[3,4-d]pyrimidin-4-one Inhibitors of Cyclin-Dependent Kinases. *J. Med. Chem.* **2004**, *47(24)*, 5894-5911.

[116] El-Moghazy, S. M.; Ibrahim, D. A.; Abdelgawad, N. M.; Farag, N. A.; El-Khouly, A. S. Design, Synthesis and Biological Evaluation of Novel Pyrimido[4,5-d]pyrimidine CDK2 Inhibitors as Anti-Tumor Agents. *Sci. Pharm.* **2011**, *79(3)*, 429-447.

[117] Wang, S.; Meades, C.; Wood, G.; Osnowski, A.; Anderson, S.; Yuill, R.; Thomas, M.; Mezna, M.; Jackson, W.; Midgley, C.; Griffiths, G.; Fleming, I.; Green, S.; McNae, I.; Wu, S. Y.; McInnes, C.; Zheleva, D.; Walkinshaw, M. D.; Fischer, P. M. 2-Anilino-4-(thiazol-5-yl)pyrimidine CDK Inhibitors: Synthesis, SAR Analysis, X-ray Crystallography, and Biological Activity. *J. Med. Chem.* **2004**, *47(7),* 1662-1675.

[118] William, A. D.; Lee, A. C.; Goh, K. C.; Blanchard, S.; Poulsen, A.; Teo, E. L.; Nagaraj, H.; Lee, C. P.; Wang H, Williams, M.; Sun, E. T.; Hu, C.; Jayaraman, R.; Pasha, M. K.; Ethirajulu, K.; Wood, J. M.; Dymock, B. W. Discovery of kinase spectrum selective macrocycle (16E)-14-methyl-20-oxa-5,7,14,26-tetraazatetracyclo[19.3.1.1(2,6).1(8,12)]heptacosa-1(25),2(26),3,5,8(27),9,11,16,21,23-decaene (SB1317/TG02), a Potent Inhibitor of Cyclin Dependent Kinases (CDKs), Janus Kinase 2 (JAK2), and Fms-like Tyrosine Kinase-3 (FLT3) for the Treatment of Cancer. *J. Med. Chem.* **2012**, *55(1)*, 169-196.

[119] Goh, K. C.; Novotny-Diermayr, V.; Hart, S.; Ong, L. C.; Loh, Y. K.; Cheong, A.; Tan, Y. C.; Hu. C.; Jayaraman, R.; William, A. D.; Sun, E. T.; Dymock, B. W.; Ong, K. H.; Ethirajulu, K.; Burrows, F.; Wood, J. M. TG02, a Novel Oral Multi-kinase Inhibitor of CDKs, JAK2 and FLT3 with Potent Anti-leukemic Properties. *Leukemia.* **2012**, *26(2)*, 236-243.

[120] Wang, S.; Griffiths, G.; Midgley, C. A.; Barnett, A. L.; Cooper, M.; Grabarek, J.; Ingram, L.; Jackson, W.; Kontopidis, G.; McClue, S. J.; McInnes, C.; McLachlan, J.; Meades, C.; Mezna, M.; Stuart, I.; Thomas, M. P.; Zheleva, D. I.; Lane, D. P.; Jackson, R. C.; Glover, D. M.; Blake, D. G.; Fischer, P. M. Discovery and Characterization of 2-Anilino-4-(thiazol-5-yl)pyrimidine Transcriptional CDK Inhibitors as Anticancer Agents. *Chem. Biol.* **2010**, *17(10)*, 1111-1121.

[121] Heathcote, D. A.; Patel, H.; Kroll, S. H.; Hazel, P.; Periyasamy, M.; Alikian, M.; Kanneganti, S. K.; Jogalekar, A. S.; Scheiper, B.; Barbazanges, M.; Blum, A.; Brackow, J.; Siwicka, A.; Pace, R. D.; Fuchter, M. J.; Snyder, J. P.; Liotta, D. C.; Freemont, P. S.; Aboagye, E. O.; Coombes, R. C.; Barrett, A. G.; Ali, S. A Novel Pyrazolo[1,5-a]pyrimidine is a Potent Inhibitor of Cyclin-dependent Protein Kinases 1, 2, and 9, Which Demonstrates Antitumor Effects in Human Tumor Xenografts Following Oral Administration. *J. Med. Chem.* **2010**, *53(24)*, 8508-8522.

[122] Huang, S.; Li, R.; Connolly, P. J.; Emanuel, S.; Middleton, S. A. Synthesis of 2-Amino-4-(7-azaindol-3-yl)pyrimidines as Cyclin Dependent Kinase 1 (CDK1) Inhibitors. *Bioorg. Med. Chem. Lett.* **2006**, *16(18)*, 4818-4821.

[123] Richardson, C. M.; Williamson, D. S.; Parratt, M. J.; Borgognoni, J.; Cansfield, A. D.; Dokurno, P.; Francis, G. L.; Howes, R.; Moore, J. D.; Murray, J. B.; Robertson, A.; Surgenor, A. E.; Torrance, C. J. Triazolo[1,5-a]pyrimidines as Novel CDK2 Inhibitors: Protein Structure-Guided Design and SAR. *Bioorg. Med. Chem. Lett.* **2006**, *16(5)*, 1353-1357.

[124] Jorda, R.; Havlícek, L.; McNae, I. W.; Walkinshaw, M. D.; Voller, J.; Sturc, A.; Navrátilová, J.; Kuzma, M.; Mistrík, M.; Bártek, J.; Strnad, M.; Krystof, V. Pyrazolo[4,3-d]pyrimidine Bioisostere of Roscovitine: Evaluation of a Novel Selective Inhibitor of Cyclin-dependent Kinases with Antiproliferative Activity. *J. Med. Chem.* **2011**, *54(8)*, 2980-2993.

[125] Marchetti, F.; Cano, C.; Curtin, N. J.; Golding, B. T.; Griffin, R. J.; Haggerty, K.; Newell, D. R.; Parsons, R. J.; Payne, S. L.; Wang, L. Z.; Hardcastle, I. R. Synthesis and Biological Evaluation of 5-Substituted O^4-alkylpyrimidines as CDK2 Inhibitors. *Org. Biomol. Chem.* **2010**, *8(10)*, 2397-2407.

[126] Ali, S.; Heathcote, D. A.; Kroll, S. H.; Jogalekar, A. S.; Scheiper, B.; Patel, H.; Brackow, J.; Siwicka, A.; Fuchter, M. J.; Periyasamy, M.; Tolhurst, R. S.; Kanneganti, S. K.; Snyder, J. P.; Liotta, D. C.; Aboagye, E. O.; Barrett, A. G.; Coombes, R. C. The Development of a Selective Cyclin-dependent Kinase Inhibitor that Shows Antitumor Activity. *Cancer Res.* **2009**, *69(15)*, 6208-6215.

[127] Byth, K. F.; Thomas, A.; Hughes, G.; Forder, C.; McGregor, A.; Geh, C.; Oakes, S.; Green, C.; Walker, M.; Newcombe, N.; Green, S.; Growcott, J.; Barker, A.; Wilkinson, R. W. AZD5438, a Potent Oral Inhibitor of Cyclin-dependent Kinases 1, 2, and 9, Leads to Pharmacodynamic Changes and Potent Antitumor Effects in Human Tumor Xenografts. *Mol. Cancer Ther.* **2009**, *8(7)*, 1856-1866.

[128] Boss, D. S.; Schwartz, G. K.; Middleton, M. R.; Amakye, D. D.; Swaisland, H.; Midgley, R. S.; Ranson, M.; Danson, S.; Calvert, H.; Plummer, R.; Morris, C.; Carvajal, R. D.; Chirieac, L. R.; Schellens, J. H.; Shapiro, G. I. Safety, Tolerability, Pharmacokinetics and Pharmacodynamics of the Oral Cyclin-dependent Kinase Inhibitor AZD5438 When Administered at Intermittent and Continuous Dosing Schedules in Patients with Advanced Solid Tumours. *Ann. Oncol.* **2010**, *21(4)*, 884-894.

[129] Jones, C. D.; Andrews, D. M.; Barker, A. J.; Blades, K.; Daunt, P.; East, S.; Geh, C.; Graham, M. A.; Johnson, K. M.; Loddick, S. A.; McFarland, H. M.; McGregor, A.; Moss, L.; Rudge, D. A.; Simpson, P. B.; Swain, M. L.; Tam, K. Y.; Tucker, J. A.; Walker, M. The Discovery of AZD5597, a Potent Imidazole Pyrimidine Amide CDK Inhibitor Suitable for Intravenous Dosing. *Bioorg. Med. Chem. Lett.* **2008**, *18(24)*, 6369-6373.

[130] Cho, S. J.; Lee, S. S.; Kim, Y. J.; Park, B. D.; Choi, J. S.; Liu, L.; Ham, Y. M.; Moon Kim, B.; Lee, S. K. Xylocydine, a Novel CDK Inhibitor, is an Effective Inducer of Apoptosis in Hepatocellular Carcinoma Cells *in vitro* and *in vivo*. *Cancer Lett.* **2010**, *287(2)*, 196-206.

[131] Xiao, C.; Sun, C.; Han, W.; Pan, F.; Dan, Z.; Li, Y.; Song, Z. G.; Jin, Y. H. Synthesis of 6-(Het) Ary Xylocydine Analogues and Evaluating their Inhibitory Activities of CDK1 and CDK2 *in vitro*. *Bioorg. Med. Chem.* **2011**, *19(23)*, 7100-7110.

[132] Jones, C. D.; Andrews, D. M.; Barker, A. J.; Blades, K.; Byth, K. F.; Finlay, M. R.; Geh, C.; Green, C. P.; Johannsen, M.; Walker, M.; Weir, H. M. Imidazole Pyrimidine Amides as

Potent, Orally Bioavailable Cyclin-dependent Kinase Inhibitors. *Bioorg. Med. Chem. Lett.* **2008**, *18(24)*, 6486-6489.

[133] Chu, X. J.; DePinto, W.; Bartkovitz, D.; So, S. S.; Vu, B. T.; Packman, K.; Lukacs, C.; Ding, Q.; Jiang, N.; Wang, K.; Goelzer, P.; Yin, X.; Smith, M. A.; Higgins, B. X.; Chen, Y.; Xiang, Q.; Moliterni, J.; Kaplan, G.; Graves, B.; Lovey, A.; Fotouhi, N. Discovery of [4-Amino-2-(1-methanesulfonylpiperidin-4-ylamino)pyrimidin-5-yl](2,3-difluoro-6-methoxyphenyl)methanone (R547), a Potent and Selective Cyclin-Dependent Kinase Inhibitor with Significant *in vivo* Antitumor Activity. *J. Med. Chem.* **2006**, *49(22)*, 6549-6560.

[134] Berkofsky-Fessler, W.; Nguyen, T. Q.; Delmar, P.; Molnos, J.; Kanwal, C.; DePinto, W.; Rosinski, J.; McLoughlin, P.; Ritland, S.; DeMario, M.; Tobon, K.; Reidhaar-Olson, J. F.; Rueger, R.; Hilton, H. Preclinical Biomarkers for a Cyclin-dependent Kinase Inhibitor Translate to Candidate Pharmacodynamic Biomarkers in Phase I Patients. *Mol. Cancer Ther.* **2009**, *8(9)*, 2517-2525.

[135] Sondhi, S. M.; Goyal, R. N.; Lahoti, A. M.; Singh, N.; Shukla, R.; Raghubir, R. Synthesis and Biological Evaluation of 2-Thiopyrimidine Derivatives. *Bioorg. Med. Chem.* **2005**, *13(9)*, 3185-3195.

[136] Lücking, U.; Siemeister, G.; Schäfer, M.; Briem, H.; Krüger, M.; Lienau, P.; Jautelat, R. Macrocyclic Aminopyrimidines as Multitarget CDK and VEGF-R Inhibitors with Potent Antiproliferative Activities. *ChemMedChem.* **2007**, *2(1)*, 63-77.

[137] Jones, C. D.; Andrews, D. M.; Barker, A. J.; Blades, K.; Byth, K. F.; Finlay, M. R.; Geh, C.; Green, C. P.; Johannsen, M.; Walker, M.; Weir, H. M. Imidazole pyrimidine amides as potent, orally bioavailable cyclin-dependent kinase inhibitors. *Bioorg. Med. Chem. Lett.* **2008**, *18(24)*, 6486-6489.

[138] Mascarenhas, N. M.; Bhattacharyya, D.; Ghoshal, N. Why Pyridine Containing Pyrido[2,3-d]pyrimidin-7-ones Selectively Inhibit CDK4 than CDK2: Insights from Molecular Dynamics Simulation. *J. Mol. Graph. Model.* **2010**, *28(7)*, 695-706.

[139] Wang, F.; Ma, Z.; Li, Y.; Zhu, S.; Xiao, Z.; Zhang, H.; Wang, Y. Development of *in silico* Models for Pyrazoles and Pyrimidine Derivatives as Cyclin-dependent Kinase 2 Inhibitors. *J. Mol. Graph. Model.* **2011**, *30*, 67-81.

[140] Xiao, Z.; Hao, Y.; Liu, B.; Qian, L. Indirubin and Meisoindigo in the Treatment of Chronic Myelogenous Leukemia in China. *Leuk. Lymphoma* **2002**, *43(9)*, 1763-1768.

[141] Moon, M. J.; Lee, S. K.; Lee, J. W.; Song, W. K.; Kim, S. W.; Kim, J. I.; Cho, C.; Choi, S. J.; Kim, Y. C. Synthesis and Structure-activity Relationships of Novel Indirubin Derivatives as Potent Anti-proliferative Agents with CDK2 Inhibitory Activities. *Bioorg. Med. Chem.* **2006**, *14(1)*, 237-246.

[142] Mapelli, M.; Massimiliano, L.; Crovace, C.; Seeliger, M. A.; Tsai, L. H.; Meijer, L.; Musacchio, A. Mechanism of CDK5/p25 binding by CDK inhibitors. *J. Med. Chem.* **2005**, *48(3)*, 671-679.

[143] Marko, D.; Schatzle, S.; Friedel, A.; Genzlinger, A.; Zankl, H.; Meijer, L.; Eisenbrand, G. Inhibition of Cyclin-Dependent Kinase 1 (CDK1) by Indirubin Derivatives in Human Tumour Cells. *Br. J. Cancer* **2001**, *84(2)*, 283-289.

[144] Kosmopoulou, M. N.; Leonidas, D. D.; Chrysina, E. D.; Bischler, N.; Eisenbrand, G.; Sakarellos, C. E.; Pauptit, R.; Oikonomakos, N. G. Binding of the Potential Antitumour Agent Indirubin-5-sulphonate at the Inhibitor Site of Rabbit Muscle Glycogen

Phosphorylase b. Comparison with Ligand Binding to pCDK2/cyclin A Complex. *Eur. J. Biochem.* **2004**, *271(11)*, 2280-90.

[145] Polychronopoulos, P.; Magiatis, P.; Skaltsounis, A. L.; Myrianthopoulos, V.; Mikros, E.; Tarricone, A.; Musacchio, A.; Roe, S. M.; Pearl, L.; Leost, M.; Greengard, P.; Meijer, L. Structural Basis for the Synthesis of Indirubins as Potent and Selective inhibitors of Glycogen Synthase Kinase-3 and Cyclin- Dependent Kinases. J. Med. Chem. 2004, 47(4), 935-946.

146] Kim, S. H.; Choi, S. J.; Kim, Y. C.; Kuh, H. J. Anti-tumor Activity of Noble Indirubin Derivatives in Human Solid Tumor Models *in vitro*. *Arch. Pharm. Res.* **2009**, *32(6)*, 915-922.

[147] Zhang, B.; Tan, V. B.; Lim, K. M.; Tay, T. E.; Zhuang, S. Study of the Inhibition of Cyclin-Dependent Kinases with Roscovitine and Indirubin-3'- oxime from Molecular Dynamics Simulations. *J. Mol. Model.* **2007**, *13(1)*, 79-89.

[148] Choi, S. J.; Lee, J. E.; Jeong, S. Y.; Im, I.; Lee, S. D.; Lee, E. J.; Lee, S. K.; Kwon, S. M.; Ahn, S. G.; Yoon, J. H.; Han, S. Y.; Kim, J. I.; Kim, Y. C. 5,5'-Substituted indirubin-3'-oxime Derivatives as Potent Cyclin-dependent Kinase Inhibitors with Anticancer Activity. *J. Med. Chem.* **2010**, *53(9)*, 3696-3706.

[149] Ribas, J.; Bettayeb, K.; Ferandin, Y.; Knockaert, M.; Garrofe-Ochoa, X.; Totzke, F.; Schachtele, C.; Mester, J.; Polychronopoulos, P.; Magiatis, P.; Skaltsounis, A. L. Boix, J.; Meijer, L. 7-Bromoindirubin-3'-oxime Induces Caspase-Independent Cell Death. *Oncogene* **2006**, *25(47)*, 6304-6318.

[150] Beauchard, A.; Ferandin, Y.; Frere, S.; Lozach, O.; Blairvacq, M.; Meijer, L.; Thierya, V.; Bessona, T. Synthesis of Novel 5-Substituted Indirubins as Protein Kinases Inhibitors. *Bioorg. Med. Chem.* **2006**, *14(18)*, 6434-6443.

[151] Samanta, S.; Debnath, B.; Basu, A.; Gayen, S.; Srikanth, K.; Jha, T. Exploring QSAR on 3-Aminopyrazoles as Antitumor Agents for their Inhibitory Activity of CDK2/cyclin A. *Eur. J. Med. Chem.* **2006**, *41(10)*, 1190-1195.

[152] Pevarello, P.; Brasca, M. G.; Amichi, R.; Orsini, P.; Traquandi, G.; Corti, L.; Piutti, C.; Sansonna, P.; Villa, M.; Pierce, B. S.; Pulici, M.; Giordano, P.; Martina, K.; Fritzen, E. L.; Nugent, R. A.; Casale, E.; Cameron, A.; Ciomei, M.; Roletto, F.; Isacchi, A.; Fogliatto, G. P.; Pesenti, F.; Pastori, W.; Marsiglio, A.; Leach, K. L.; Clare, P. M.; Fiorentini, F.; Varasi, M.; Vulpetti, A. 3-Aminopyrazole Inhibitors of CDK2/cyclin A as Antitumor Agents. 1. Lead Finding. *J. Med. Chem.* **2004**, *47(13)*, 3367-3380.

[153] Pevarello, P.; Brasca, M. G.; Orsini, P.; Traquandi, G.; Longo, A.; Nesi, M.; Orzi, F.; Piutti, C.; Sansonna, P.; Varasi, M.; Cameron, A.; Vulpetti, A.; Roletto, F.; Alzani, R.; Ciomei, M.; Albanese, C.; Pastori, W.; Marsiglio, A.; Pesenti, E.; Fiorentini, F.; Bischoff, J. R.; Mercurio, C. 3-Aminopyrazole Inhibitors of CDK2/cyclin A as Antitumor Agents. 2. Lead Optimization. *J. Med. Chem.* **2005**, *48(8)*, 2944-2956.

[154] Nesi, M.; Borghi, D.; Brasca, M. G.; Fiorentini, F.; Pevarello, P. A Practical Synthesis of the Major 3-Hydroxy-2-pyrrolidinone Metabolite of a Potent CDK2/cyclin A Inhibitor. *Bioorg. Med. Chem. Lett.* **2006**, *16(12)*, 3205- 3208.

[155] Brasca, M. G.; Albanese, C.; Alzani, R.; Amici, R.; Avanzi, N.; Ballinari, D.; Bischoff, J.; Borghi, D.; Casale, E.; Croci, V.; Fiorentini, F.; Isacchi, A.; Mercurio, C.; Nesi, M.; Orsini, P.; Pastori, W.; Pesenti, E.; Pevarello, P.; Roussel, P.; Varasi, M.; Volpi, D.; Vulpetti, A.; Ciomei, M.; Brasca, M. G.; Albanese, C.; Alzani, R.; Amici, R.; Avanzi, N.; Ballinari, D.; Bischoff, J.; Borghi, D.; Casale, E.; Croci, V.; Fiorentini, F.; Isacchi, A.; Mercurio, C.; Nesi, M.; Orsini, P.; Pastori, W.; Pesenti, E.; Pevarello, P.; Roussel, P.; Varasi, M.; Volpi,

D.; Vulpetti, A.; Ciomei, M. Optimization of 6,6-Dimethyl pyrrolo[3,4-c]pyrazoles: Identification of PHA-793887, a Potent CDK Inhibitor Suitable for Intravenous Dosing. *Bioorg. Med. Chem.* **2010**, *18(5)*, 1844-1853.

[156] Massard, C.; Soria, J. C.; Anthoney, D. A.; Proctor, A.; Scaburri, A.; Pacciarini, M. A.; Laffranchi, B.; Pellizzoni, C.; Kroemer, G.; Armand, J. P.; Balheda, R.; Twelves, C. J. A First in Man, Phase I Dose-escalation Study of PHA-793887, an Inhibitor of Multiple Cyclin-dependent Kinases (CDK2, 1 and 4) Reveals Unexpected Hepatotoxicity in Patients with Solid Tumors. *Cell Cycle* **2011**, *10(6)*, 963-970.

[157] Wyatt, P. G.; Woodhead, A. J.; Berdini, V.; Boulstridge, J. A.; Carr, M. G.; Cross, D. M.; Davis, D. J.; Devine, L. A.; Early, T. R.; Feltell, R. E.; Lewis, E. J.; McMenamin, R. L.; Navarro, E. F.; O'Brien, M. A.; O'Reilly, M.; Reule, M.; Saxty, G.; Seavers, L. C.; Smith, D. M.; Squires, M. S.; Trewartha, G.; Walker, M. T.; Woolford, A. J. Identification of N-(4-Piperidinyl)-4-(2,6-dichlorobenzoylamino)-1H-pyrazole-3-carboxamide (AT7519), a Novel Cyclin Dependent Kinase Inhibitor Using Fragment-based X-ray Crystallography and Structure Based Drug Design. *J. Med. Chem.* **2008**, *51(16)*, 4986-4999.

[158] Mahadevan, D.; Plummer, R.; Squires, M. S.; Rensvold, D.; Kurtin, S.; Pretzinger, C.; Dragovich, T.; Adams, J.; Lock, V.; Smith, D. M.; Von Hoff, D.; Calvert, H. A Phase I Pharmacokinetic and Pharmacodynamic Study of AT7519, a Cyclin-dependent Kinase Inhibitor in Patients with Refractory Solid Tumors. *Ann. Oncol.* **2011**, *22(9)*, 2137-2143.

[159] Yue, E. W.; DiMeo, S. V.; Higley, C. A.; Markwalder, J. A.; Burton, C. R.; Benfield, P. A.; Grafstrom, R. H.; Cox, S.; Muckelbauer, J. K.; Smallwood, A. M.; Chen, H.; Chang, C. H.; Trainor, G. L.; Seitz, S. P. Synthesis and Evaluation of Indenopyrazoles as Cyclin-dependent Kinase Inhibitors. Part 4: Heterocycles at C3. *Bioorg. Med. Chem. Lett.* **2004**, *14(2)*, 343-346.

[160] Singh, S. K.; Dessalew, N.; Bharatam, P. V. 3D-QSAR CoMFA Study on Indenopyrazole Derivatives as Cyclin Dependent Kinase 4 (CDK4) and Cyclin Dependent Kinase 2 (CDK2) Inhibitors. *Eur. J. Med. Chem.* **2006**, *41(11)*, 1310-1319.

[161] Hirai, H.; Shimomura, T.; Kobayashi, M.; Eguchi, T.; Taniguchi, E.; Fukasawa, K.; Machida, T.; Oki, H.; Arai, T.; Ichikawa, K.; Hasako, S.; Haze, K.; Kodera, T.; Kawanishi, N.; Takahashi-Suziki, I.; Nakatsuru, Y.; Kotani, H.; Iwasawa, Y. Biological Characterization of 2-Aminothiazole-derived CDK4/6 Selective Inhibitor *in vitro* and *in vivo*. *Cell Cycle* **2010**, *9(8)*, 1590-1600.

[162] Dessalew, N.; Bharatama, P. V.; Singh, S. K. 3D-QSAR CoFMA Study on Aminothiazole Derivatives as Cyclin-Dependent Kinase 2. QSAR & Combinatorial *Science* **2006**, *26(1)*, 85-91.

[163] Wu, Y.; Chen, C.; Sun, X.; Shi, X.; Jin, B.; Ding, K.; Yeung, S. C.; Pan, J. Cyclin-Dependent Kinase 7/9 Inhibitor SNS-032 Abrogates FIP1-like-1 Platelet-Derived Growth Factor Receptor a and Bcr-Abl Oncogene Addiction in Malignant Hematologic Cells. *Clin. Cancer Res.* **2012**, *18(7)*, 1966-1978.

[164] Misra, R. N.; Xiao H. Y.; Kim, K. S.; Lu, S.; Han W. C.; Barbosa, S. A.; Hunt, J. T.; Rawlins, D. B.; Shan, W.; Ahmed, S. Z.; Qian, L.; Chen, B. C.; Zhao, R.; Bednarz, M. S.; Kellar, K. A.; Mulheron, J. G.; Batorsky, R.; Roongta, U.; Kamath, A.; Marathe, P.; Ranadive, S. A.; Sack, J. S.; Tokarski, J. S; Pavletich, N. P.; Lee, F. Y.; Webster, K. R.; Kimball, S. D. N- (Cycloalkylamino)acyl-2-aminothiazole Inhibitors of Cyclin-Dependent Kinase 2. N-[5-[[[5-(1,1-dimethylethyl)-2-oxazolyl]methyl]thio]-2- thiazolyl]-4-piperidinecarboxamide (BMS-387032), a Highly Efficacious and Selective Antitumor Agent. *J. Med. Chem.* **2004**, *47(7)*, 1719-1728.

[165] Fan, J.; Fahr, B.; Stockett, D.; Chan, E.; Cheeti, S.; Serafimova, I.; Lu, Y.; Pham, P.; Walker, D. H.; Hoch, U.; Choong, I. C. Modifications of the Isonipecotic Acid Fragment of SNS-032: Analogs with Improved Permeability and Lower Efflux Ratio. *Bioorg. Med. Chem. Lett.* **2008**, *18(23)*, 6236-6239.

[166] Vulpetti, A.; Casale, E.; Roletto, F.; Amici, R.; Villa, M.; Pevarello, P. Structure-Based Drug Design to the Discovery of New 2-Aminothiazole CDK2 Inhibitors. *J. Mol. Graphics Model.* **2006**, *24(5)*, 341-348.

[167] McIntyre, N. A.; McInnes, C.; Griffiths, G.; Barnett, A. L.; Kontopidis, G.; Slawin, A. M.; Jackson, W.; Thomas, M.; Zheleva, D. I.; Wang, S.; Blake, D. G.; Westwood, N. J.; Fischer, P. M. Design, Synthesis, and Evaluation of 2-Methyl- and 2-Amino-N-aryl-4,5-dihydrothiazolo[4,5-h]quinazolin-8-amines as Ring-constrained 2-Anilino-4-(thiazol-5-yl)pyrimidine Cyclin-dependent Kinase Inhibitors. *J. Med. Chem.* **2010**, *53(5)*, 2136-2145.

[168] Lee, D. U.; Jessen, B. Off-target Immune Cell Toxicity Caused by AG-012986, a Pan-CDK Inhibitor, is Associated with Inhibition of p38 MAPK Phosphorylation. *J. Biochem. Mol. Toxicol.* **2012**, *26(3)*, 101-108.

[169] Vassilev, L. T.; Tovar, C.; Chen, S.; Knezevic, D.; Zhao, X.; Sun, H.; Heimbrook, D. C.; Chen, L. Selective Small-molecule Inhibitor Reveals Critical Mitotic Functions of Human CDK1. *Proc. Natl. Acad. Sci. U S A* **2006**, *103(28)*, 10660-10665.

[170] Misra, R. N.; Xiao, H. Y.; Williams, D. K.; Kim, K. S.; Lu, S.; Keller, K. A.; Mulheron, J. G.; Batorsky, R.; Tokarski, J. S.; Sack, J. S.; Kimball, S. D.; Lee, F. Y.; Webster, K. R. Synthesis and Biological Activity of N-Aryl-2-aminothiazoles: Potent Pan Inhibitors of Cyclin-dependent Kinases. *Bioorg. Med. Chem. Lett.* **2004**, *14(11)*, 2973-2977.

[171] Huang, J. W.; Shiau, C. W.; Yang, J.; Wang, D. S.; Chiu, H. C.; Chen, C. Y.; Chen, C. S. Development of Small-Molecule Cyclin D1-Ablative Agents. *J. Med. Chem.* **2006**, *49(15)*, 4684-4689.

[172] Shimamura, T.; Shibata, J.; Kurihara, H.; Mita, T.; Otsuki, S.; Sagara, T.; Hirai, H.; Iwasawa, Y. Identification of Potent 5-Pyrimidinyl-2- aminothiazole CDK4, 6 Inhibitors with Significant Selectivity over CDK1, 2, 5, 7, and 9. *Bioorg. Med. Chem. Lett.* **2006**, *16(14)*, 3751-3754.

[173] Tolle, N.; Kunick, C. Paullones as Inhibitors of Protein Kinases. *Curr. Top. Med. Chem.* **2011**, *11(11)*, 1320-1332.

[174] Sharma, P. S.; Tyagi, R.; Sharma, R. Semi-empirical Calculations on Paullones, a Promising Class of Cyclin-dependent Kinase Inhibitors. *Indian J. Biochem. Biophys.* **2008**, *45(6)*, 416-420.

[175] Kunick, C.; Lauenroth, K.; Wieking, K.; Xie, X.; Schultz, C.; Gussio, R.; Zaharevitz, D.; Leost, M.; Meijer, L.; Weber, A.; Jorgensen, F. S.; Lemcke, T. Evaluation and Comparison of 3D-QSAR CoMSIA Models for CDK1, CDK5, and GSK-3 Inhibition by Paullones. *J. Med. Chem.* **2004**, *47(1)*, 22- 36

[176] Xie, X.; Lemcke, T.; Gussio, R.; Zaharevitz, D. W.; Leost, M.; Meijer, L.; Kunick, C. Epoxide-Containing Side Chains Enhance Antiproliferative Activity of Paullones. *Eur. J. Med. Chem.* **2005**, *40(7)*, 655-661.

[177] Brault, L.; Migianu, E.; Neguesque, A.; Battaglia, E.; Bagrel, D.; Kirsch, G. New Thiophene Analogues of Kenpaullone: Synthesis and Biological Evaluation in Breast Cancer Cells. *Eur. J. Med. Chem.* **2005**, *40(8)*, 757-763.

[178] Power, D. P.; Lozach, O.; Meijer, L.; Grayson, D. H.; Connon, S. J. Concise Synthesis and CDK/GSK Inhibitory Activity of the Missing 9-Azapaullones. *Bioorg. Med. Chem. Lett.* **2010**, *20(16)*, 4940-4944.

[179] Cimino, G.; De Rosa, S.; De Stefano, S.; Mazzarella, L.; Puliti, R.; Sodano, G. Isolation and X-ray Crystal Structure of a Novel Bromo Compound from Two Marine Sponges. *Tetrahedron Lett.* **1982**, *23(7)*, 767-768.

[180] Schmitz, F. J.; Gunasekera, S. P.; Lakshmi, V.; Tillekeratne, L. M. V. Marine Natural Products: Pyrrololactams from Several Sponges. *J. Nat. Prod.* **1985**, *48(1)*, 47-53.

[181] Meijer, L.; Thunnissen, A. -M. W. H.; White, A. W.; Garnier, M.; Nikolic, M.; Tsai, L. -H.; Walter, J.; Cleverley, K. E.; Salinas, P. C.; Wu, Y. -Z.; Biernat, J.; Mandelkow, E. -M.; Kim, S. -H.; Pettit, G. R. Inhibition of Cyclin-Dependent Kinases, GSK-3β and CK1 by Hymenialdisine, a Marine Sponge. *Chem. Biol.* **2000**, *7(1)*, 51-63.

[182] Tasdemir, D.; Mallon, R.; Greenstein, M.; Feldberg, L. R.; Kim, S. C.; Collins, K.; Wojciechowicz, D.; Mangalindan, G. C.; Concepción, G. P.; Harper, M. K.; Ireland, C. M. Aldisine alkaloids from the Philippine Sponge Stylissa massa are Potent Inhibitors of Mitogen-Activated Protein Kinase Kinase-1 (MEK-1). *J. Med. Chem.* **2002**, *45(2)*, 529-532.

[183] Wan, Y.; Hur, W.; Cho, C. Y.; Liu, Y.; Adrian, F. J.; Lozach, O.; Bach, S.; Mayer, T.; Fabbro, D.; Meijer, L.; Gray, N. S. Synthesis and Target Identification of Hymenialdisine Analogs. *Chem. Biol.* **2004**, *11(2)*, 247-259.

[184] Nguyen, T. N.; Tepe, J. J. Preparation of Hymenialdisine, Analogues and Their Evaluation as Kinase Inhibitors. *Curr. Med. Chem.* **2009**, *16(24)*, 3122-43.

[185] Kitagawa, M.; Okabe, T.; Ogino, H.; Matsumoto, H.; Suzuki-Takahashi, I.; Kokubo, T.; Higashi,H.; Saitoh, S.; Taya, Y.; Yasuda, H. Butyrolactone I, a Selective Inhibitor of CDK2 and Cdc2 Kinase. *Oncogene* **1993**, *8(9)*, 2425-2432.

[186] Brana, M. F.; Garcia, M. L.; Lopez, B.; de Pascual-Teresa, B.; Ramos, A.; Pozuelo, J. M.; Dominguez, M. T. Synthesis and Biological Evaluation of Analogues of Butyrolactone I and Molecular Model of its Interaction with CDK2. *Org. Biomol. Chem.* **2004**, *2(13),* 1864-1871.

[187] Sax, J. K.; Dash, B. C.; Hong, R.; Dicker, D. T.; El-Deiry, W. S. The Cyclin-Dependent Kinase Inhibitor Butyrolactone is a Potent Inhibitor of $p21^{WAF1/CIP1}$ expression. *Cell Cycle* **2002,** *1(1),* 90-96.

[188] Yu, J. Y.; Kim, J. H.; Kim, T. G.; Kim, B. T.; Jang, Y. S.; Lee, J. C. (E)-1-(3,4-Dihydroxyphenethyl)-3-styrylurea Inhibits Proliferation of MCF-7 Cells Through G1 Cell Cycle Arrest and Mitochondria-mediated Apoptosis. *Mol. Cells* **2010**, *30(4)*, 303-310.

[189] Lin, J.; Yan, X. J.; Chen, H. M. Fascaplysin, a Selective CDK4 Inhibitor, Exhibit Anti-angiogenic Activity *in vitro* and *in vivo*. *Cancer Chemother. Pharmacol.* **2007**, *59(4)*, 439-445.

[190] Aubry, C.; Wilson, A. J.; Emmerson, D.; Murphy, E.; Chan, Y. Y.; Dickens, M. P.; García, M. D.; Jenkins, P. R.; Mahale, S.; Chaudhuri, B. Fascaplysin-inspired Diindolyls as Selective Inhibitors of CDK4/cyclin D1. *Bioorg. Med. Chem.* **2009**, *17(16)*, 6073-6084.

[191] García, M. D.; Wilson, A. J.; Emmerson, D. P.; Jenkins, P. R.; Mahale, S.; Chaudhuri, B. Synthesis, Crystal Structure and Biological Activity of Beta-carboline Based Selective CDK4-cyclin D1 Inhibitors. *Org. Biomol. Chem.* **2006**, *4(24)*, 4478-4484.

[192] Verdaguer, E.; Jordà, E. G.; Canudas, A. M.; Jiménez, A.; Sureda, F. X.; Rimbau, V.; Pubill, D.; Escubedo, E.; Camarasa, J.; Pallàs, M.; Camins, A. 3-Amino Thioacridone, a Selective Cyclin-dependent Kinase 4 Inhibitor, Attenuates Kainic Acid-induced Apoptosis in Neurons. *Neuroscience* **2003**, *120(3)*, 599-603.

[193] Honma, T.; Yoshizumi, T.; Hashimoto, N.; Hayashi, K.; Kawanishi, N.; Fukasawa, K.; Takaki, T.; Ikeura, C.; Ikuta, M.; Suzuki-Takahashi, I.; Hayama, T.; Nishimura, S.; Morishima, H. A Novel Approach for the Development of Selective CDK4 Inhibitors: Library Design Based on Locations of CDK4 Specific Amino Acid Residues. *J. Med. Chem.* **2001**, *44(26)*, 4628-4640.

[194] Honma, T.; Hayashi, K.; Aoyama, T.; Hashimoto, N.; Machida, T.; Fukasawa, K.; Iwama, T.; Ikeura, C.; Ikuta, M.; Suzuki-Takahashi, I.; Iwasawa, Y.; Hayama, T.; Nishimura, S.; Morishima, H. Structure-Based Generation of a New Class of Potent CDK4 Inhibitors: New *de Novo* Design Strategy and Library Design. *J. Med. Chem.* **2001**, *44(26),* 4615-4627.

[195] Kawanishi, N.; Sugimoto, T.; Shibata, J.; Nakamura, K.; Masutani, K.; Ikuta, M.; Hirai, H. Structure-Based Drug Design of a Highly Potent CDK1,2,4,6 Inhibitor with Novel Macrocyclic Quinoxalin-2-one Structure. *Bioorg. Med. Chem. Lett.* **2006**, *16(19)*, 5122–5126.

[196] El-Bayoumy, K.; Sinha, R. Molecular Chemoprevention by Selenium: a Genomic Approach. *Mutat. Res.* **2005**, *591(1-2)*, 224-236.

[197] Sinha, R.; Medina, D. Inhibition of CDK2 Kinase Activity by Methylselenocysteine in Synchronized Mouse Mammary Epithelial Tumor Cells. *Carcinogenesis* **1997**, *18(8)*, 1541-1547.

[198] Zeng, H. Selenite and Selenomethionine Promote HL-60 Cell Cycle Progression. *J. Nutr.* **2002**, *132(4)*, 674-679.

[199] Narayanan, B. A. Chemopreventive Agents Alters Global Gene Expression Pattern: Predicting their Mode of Action and Targets. *Current Cancer Drug Targets* **2006**, *6(8)*, 711-727.

[200] Mahale, S.; Aubry, C.; Jenkins, P. R.; Marechal, J. D.; Sutcliffe, M. J.; Chaudhuri, B. Inhibition of Cancer Cell Growth by Cyclin Dependent Kinase 4 Inhibitors Synthesized Based on the Structure of Fascaplysin. *Bioorg. Chem.* **2006**, *34(5)*, 287-297.

[201] Brana, M. F.; Cacho, M.; Garcia, M. L.; Mayoral, E. P.; Lopez, B.; de Pascual-Teresa, B.; Ramos, A.; Acero, N.; Llinares, F.; Munoz-Mingarro, D.; Lozach, O.; Meijer, L. Pyrazolo[3,4-c]pyridazines as Novel and Selective Inhibitors of Cyclin-Dependent Kinases. *J. Med. Chem.* **2005**, *48(22)*, 6843-6854.

[202] Albanese, C.; Alzani, R.; Amboldi, N.; Avanzi, N.; Ballinari, D.; Brasca, M. G.; Festuccia, C.; Fiorentini, F.; Locatelli, G.; Pastori, W.; Patton, V.; Roletto, F.; Colotta, F.; Galvani, A.; Isacchi, A.; Moll, J.; Pesenti, E.; Mercurio, C.; Ciomei, M. Dual Targeting of CDK and Tropomyosin Receptor Kinase Families by the Oral Inhibitor PHA-848125, an Agent with Broad-spectrum Antitumor Efficacy. *Mol. Cancer Ther.* **2010**, *9(8)*, 2243-2254.

[203] Mettey, Y.; Gompel, M.; Thomas, V.; Garnier, M.; Leost, M.; Ceballos- Picot, I.; Noble, M.; Endicott, J.; Vierfond, J. M.; Meijer, L. Aloisines, a New Family of CDK/GSK-3 Inhibitors. SAR study, Crystal Structure in Complex with CDK2, Enzyme Selectivity, and Cellular Effects. *J. Med. Chem.* **2003**, *46(2)*, 222-236.

[204] Echalier, A.; Bettayeb, K.; Ferandin, Y.; Lozach, O.; Clément, M.; Valette, A.; Liger, F.; Marquet, B.; Morris, J. C.; Endicott, J. A.; Joseph, B.; Meijer, L. Meriolins (3-(Pyrimidin-4-yl)-7-azaindoles): Synthesis, Kinase Inhibitory Activity, Cellular Effects, and Structure of a CDK2/Cyclin A/Meriolin Complex. *J. Med. Chem.* **2008**, *51(4)*, 737-751.

[205] Bettayeb, K.; Tirado, O. M.; Marionneau-Lambot, S.; Ferandin, Y.; Lozach, O.; Morris, J. C.; Mateo-Lozano, S.; Drueckes, P.; Schächtele, C.; Kubbutat, M. H.; Liger, F.; Marquet, B.; Joseph, B.; Echalier, A.; Endicott, J. A.; Notario, V.; Meijer, L. Meriolins, a New Class

of Cell Death Inducing Kinase Inhibitors with Enhanced Selectivity for Cyclin-Dependent Kinases. *Cancer Res.* **2007**, *67(17)*, 8325-8334.

[206] Akue-Gedu, R.; Debiton, E.; Ferandin, Y.; Meijer, L.; Prudhomme, M.; Anizon, F.; Moreau, P. Synthesis and Biological Activities of Aminopyrimidyl-indoles Structurally Related to Meridianins. *Bioorg. Med. Chem.* **2009**, *17(13)*, 4420-4424.

[207] Giraud, F.; Alves, G.; Debiton, E.; Nauton, L.; Théry, V.; Durieu, E.; Ferandin, Y.; Lozach, O.; Meijer, L.; Anizon, F.; Pereira, E.; Moreau, P. Synthesis, Protein Kinase Inhibitory Potencies, and *in vitro* Antiproliferative Activities of Meridianin Derivatives. *J. Med. Chem.* **2011**, *54(13)*, 4474-4489.

[208] Supuran, C. T. Indisulam: an Anticancer Sulfonamide in Clinical Development. *Expert Opin. Investig. Drugs* **2003**, *12(2)*, 283-287.

[209] Fukuoka, K.; Usuda, J.; Iwamoto, Y.; Fukumoto, H.; Nakamura, T.; Yoneda, T.; Narita, N.; Saijo, N.; Nishio, K. Mechanisms of Action of the Novel Sulfonamide Anticancer Agent E7070 on Cell Cycle Progression in Human Non-Small Cell Lung Cancer Cells. *Invest. New Drugs* **2001**, *19(3)*, 219-227.

[210] Owa, T.; Yoshino, H.; Okauchi, T.; Okabe, T.; Ozawa, Y.; Hata Sugi, N.; Yoshimatsu, K.; Nagasu, T.; Koyanagi, N.; Kitoh, K. Synthesis and Biological Evaluation of N-(7-indolyl)-3-pyridinesulfonamide Derivatives as Potent Antitumor Agents. *Bioorg. Med. Chem. Lett.* **2002**, *12(16)*, 2097-2100.

[211] Zandvliet, A. S.; Karlsson, M. O.; Schellens, J. H.; Copalu, W.; Beijnen, J. H.; Huitema, A. D. Two-stage Model-based Clinical Trial Design to Optimize Phase I Development of Novel Anticancer Agents. *Invest. New Drugs* **2010**, *28(1)*, 61-75.

[212] Lin, R.; Connolly, P. J.; Huang, S.; Wetter, S. K.; Lu, Y.; Murray, W. V.; Emanuel, S. L.; Gruninger, R. H.; Fuentes-Pesquera, A. R.; Rugg, C. A.; Middleton, S. A.; Jolliffe, L. K. 1-Acyl-1H-[1,2,4] triazole-3,5-diamine Analogues as Novel and Potent Anticancer Cyclin-Dependent Kinase Inhibitors: Synthesis and Evaluation of Biological Activities. *J. Med. Chem.* **2005**, *48(13)*, 4208-4211.

[213] Huang, S.; Connolly, P. J.; Lin, R.; Emanuel, S.; Middleton, S. A. Synthesis and Evaluation of N-acyl Sulfonamides as Potential Prodrugs of Cyclin-dependent Kinase Inhibitor JNJ-7706621. *Bioorg. Med. Chem. Lett.* **2006**, *16(14)*, 3639-3641.

[214] Emanuel, S.; Rugg, C. A.; Gruninger, R. H.; Lin, R.; Fuentes-Pesquera, A.; Connolly, P. J.; Wetter, S. K.; Hollister, B.; Kruger, W. W.; Napier, C.; Jolliffe, L.; Middleton, S. A. The *in vitro* and *in vivo* Effects of JNJ-7706621: a Dual Inhibitor of Cyclin-Dependent Kinases and Aurora Kinases. *Cancer Res.* **2005**, *65(19)*, 9038-9046.

[215] Danhier, F.; Ucakar, B.; Magotteaux, N.; Brewster, M. E.; Préat, V. Active and Passive Tumor Targeting of a Novel Poorly Soluble Cyclin Dependent Kinase Inhibitor, JNJ-7706621. *Int. J. Pharm.* **2010**, *392(1-2)*, 20-28.

[216] Liu, X.; Shi, S.; Lam, F.; Pepper, C.; Fischer, P. M.; Wang, S. CDKI-71, a Novel CDK9 Inhibitor, is Preferentially Cytotoxic to Cancer Cells Compared to Flavopiridol. *Int. J. Cancer* **2012**, *130(5)*, 1216-1226.

Send Orders of Reprints at bspsaif@emirates.net.ae

Advances in Cancer Drug Targets, Vol. 1, 2013, 120-145

CHAPTER 4

Cellular FLICE-Like Inhibitory Protein (c-FLIP): A Key Anti-Apoptotic Factor and a Target for Cancer Therapy

Ahmad R. Safa*

Department of Pharmacology and Toxicology, Indiana University Simon Cancer Center, Indiana University School of Medicine, 980 W. Walnut St., Indianapolis, IN 46202

Abstract: Cellular FLICE-like inhibitory protein (c-FLIP) has been identified as a protease-dead, procaspase-8-like regulator of apoptosis. c-FLIP impedes tumor necrosis factor-α (TNF-α), Fas-L, TNF-related apoptosis-inducing ligand (TRAIL), and chemotherapy-induced apoptosis by binding to FADD and/or caspase-8 or -10 in a ligand-dependent fashion, which in turn prevents death-inducing signaling complex (DISC) formation. c-FLIP is a family of alternatively spliced variants, and primarily exists as long (c-FLIP$_L$) and short (c-FLIP$_S$) splice variants in human cells. Accumulating evidence indicates an anti-apoptotic role for c-FLIP in various types of human cancers. For example, small interfering RNAs (siRNAs) that specifically knocked down expression of c-FLIP$_L$ in diverse human cancer cell lines, *e.g.*, lung and cervical cancer cells, augmented TRAIL-induced DISC recruitment, and thereby enhanced effector caspase stimulation and apoptosis. Therefore, the outlook for the therapeutic index of c-FLIP-targeted drugs appears excellent, not only from the efficacy observed in experimental models of cancer therapy, but also because the current understanding of dual c-FLIP action in normal tissues supports the notion that c-FLIP-targeted cancer therapy will be well tolerated. Interestingly, several chemotherapeutic agents induce c-FLIP downregulation in neoplastic cells. Moreover, numerous small molecule inhibitors have been found which cause degradation of c-FLIP variants and decrease mRNA and protein levels of c-FLIP$_L$ and c-FLIP$_S$. In this chapter, I assess the outlook for improving cancer therapy through c-FLIP-targeted therapeutics.

Keywords: Taxol, apoptosis, caspase-8, caspase-10, c-FLIP, leukemia, death receptors.

INTRODUCTION

Resistance to chemotherapeutics is a major clinical problem and an important cause of treatment failure in cancer. Various molecular mechanisms have been found to cause resistance to chemotherapeutic agents in neoplastic cells *in vitro* [1-5]. Identifying novel mechanisms of resistance to chemotherapeutic agents will assist in the design of more effective strategies to overcome resistance in cancer

***Address correspondence to Ahmad R. Safa:** Department of Pharmacology and Toxicology and Indiana University Simon Cancer Center, 980 W. Walnut St. R3-C524, Indianapolis, IN 46202. Tel: 317-278-4952; Fax: 317-274-8046; E-mail: asafa@iupui.edu

Atta-ur-Rahman (Ed)

cells. Defects in apoptotic signaling in malignant cells contribute to the drug resistance in various cancer types [3, 6]. Furthermore, death receptor-mediated apoptosis is deficient in some drug resistant cancer cells. Therefore, strategies to lower the thresholds for triggering apoptosis in various cancers may lead to new and more effective therapeutic regimens. The death-inducing cytokine tumor necrosis factor-related apoptosis-inducing ligand (TRAIL) holds enormous promise as a cancer therapeutic due to its highly selective apoptosis-inducing action on neoplastic *versus* normal cells [7-10]. However, to exploit this opportunity, the problems of TRAIL resistance in cancer must first be overcome [3, 11-15]. Cellular FLICE-like inhibitory protein (c-FLIP), a catalytically inactive caspase-8/-10 homologue, is involved in TRAIL and chemotherapeutic drug resistance in a wide range of human malignancies [12-20]. Substantial levels of c-FLIP are expressed in deadly human cancers such as ovarian, colon, glioblastoma, breast, colorectal, and prostate cancers, and it is implicated in the TRAIL resistance owing to its overexpression in a substantial proportion of these malignancies [3, 11, 12, 21-24]. Furthermore, interference with c-FLIP expression sensitizes tumor cells to TRAIL and other tumor necrosis factor-related death ligands, such as FAS ligand, in experimental models [11, 17, 20, 25, 26]. c-FLIP is an important modulator of the initiator procaspases-8 and -10 and thereby regulates life and death in normal cells and tissues, and renders resistance to death receptor-mediated apoptosis in various cancer cells. In addition to its function as an apoptosis modulator, c-FLIP exerts other cellular functions including increased cell proliferation and tumorigenesis [3, 11, 12, 27]. Moreover, dysregulation of c-FLIP expression has been associated with diseases such as cancer and autoimmune diseases [3, 11, 28, 29]. Therefore, c-FLIP is a critical target for therapeutic intervention. In this review, we assess the outlook for improving the outcome of cancer therapy by targeting c-FLIP and exploring the possibility of its degradation and/or decreasing its expression in order to provide a potentially safe approach to the treatment of cancer. The possibility of developing novel modalities of cancer therapy that improve the efficacy and lessen the toxicity of cancer chemotherapy by targeting specific c-FLIP isoforms is discussed.

APPOPTOSIS SIGNALING PATHWAYS

Two well-studied pathways regulate apoptosis, the mitochondrion-initiated pathway (Fig. **1**) and the cell surface death receptors pathway (Fig. **2**) [3, 11, 12, 30-32]. In the mitochondrial pathway, cytochrome *c*, certain caspases, apoptosis-inducing factor, Smac/DIABLO, an inhibitor of apoptosis protein (IAP)-binding protein, and other apoptosis-inducing factors are released from the mitochondrial intramembrane space to the cytosol [33]. Once released, cytochrome *c* and dATP bind to apoptotic proteinase-activating factor-1 (Apaf-1), and this complex along with adenine nucleotides promotes procaspase-9 autoactivation [34], which in turn activates caspases-2, -3, -6, -7, -8, and -10. In the death receptor-mediated apoptosis pathway (*e.g.* Fas/Fas ligand interaction and cell death), the initiator caspases-8 and -10 activate the downstream caspases including caspase-3. Active caspases-8 and -10 are known to cleave a pro-apoptotic Bcl-2 family member, Bid, and the truncated Bid induces mitochondrial cytochrome *c* release [32-35], thereby linking the two pathways. After activation, both caspases-8 and -9 activate caspase-3, which in turn cleaves other caspases and numerous cellular proteins [36-38].

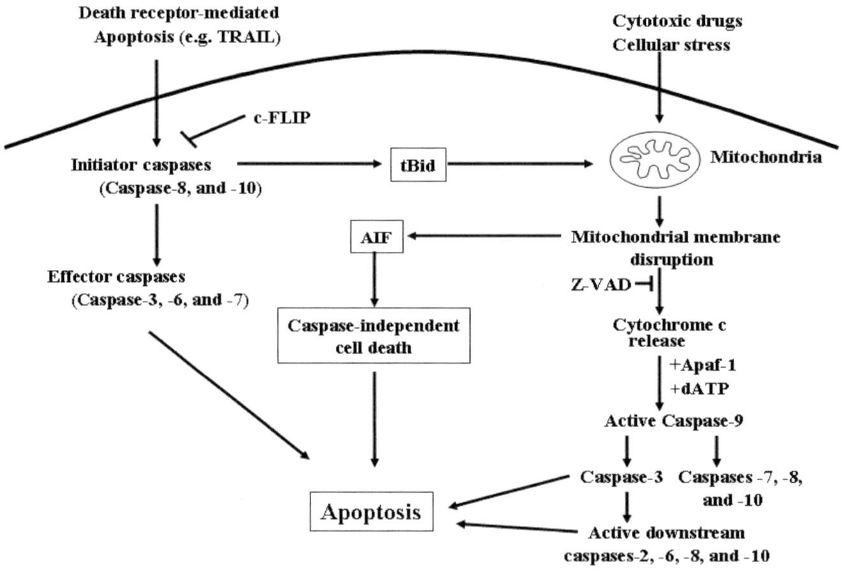

Figure 1: Mitochondrial Death Pathway. The mitochondrial pathway of apoptosis is usually caused by disruption of mitochondrial membrane potential ($\Delta\Psi m$), release of cytochrome *c*, activation of caspase-9, and subsequent activation of downstream caspases-2, -3, -6, -7, -8 and -10, which eventually leads to apoptosis. On the other hand, caspase-dependent apoptosis induced by death receptor ligation (*e.g.*, Fas ligand/Fas or TNF-α/TNF-α receptor) can function independently of the mitochondria by caspase-8 activation, which directly activates caspase-3, -6 and -7, or by causing proteolytic cleavage of the pro-apoptotic protein Bid to a truncated form (tBid), which in turn is inserted in the mitochondrial membrane and induces release of cytochrome *c*. Release of the apoptosis inducing factor (AIF) from mitochondria causes caspase-independent apoptosis.

c-FLIP AND THE DEATH RECEPTOR APOPTOSIS PATHWAY

The superfamily of TNF receptor (TNFR) consists of cell surface receptors that are activated by cognate ligands and signal proliferation, differentiation, and apoptosis (Fig. **2**). Death receptors in the TNFR superfamily include the TNF-α receptor, Fas (APO-1/CD95), and TRAIL receptors DR4 (also known as TRAIL receptor 1) and DR5 (also known as TRAIL receptor 2). Other TNFR superfamily members protect against apoptosis by serving as cell surface decoy receptors that compete for death ligand binding but cannot induce apoptosis [39, 40]. The death receptors contain an intracellular death domain (DD) which is essential for inducing apoptosis upon receptor ligation; the decoy receptors cannot signal apoptosis for lack of a functional DD [40]. The DD is a canonical 80 amino acid cytoplasmic docking surface in death receptors, that upon ligand binding to the receptor, homotypically binds a similar domain in the death adaptor protein FADD or TRADD [41] (Fig. **2**). Death adaptor proteins also have a death effector domain (DED) that forms a distinct docking surface for homotypic binding of initiator (apical) caspases. Once the initiator caspases are recruited to death

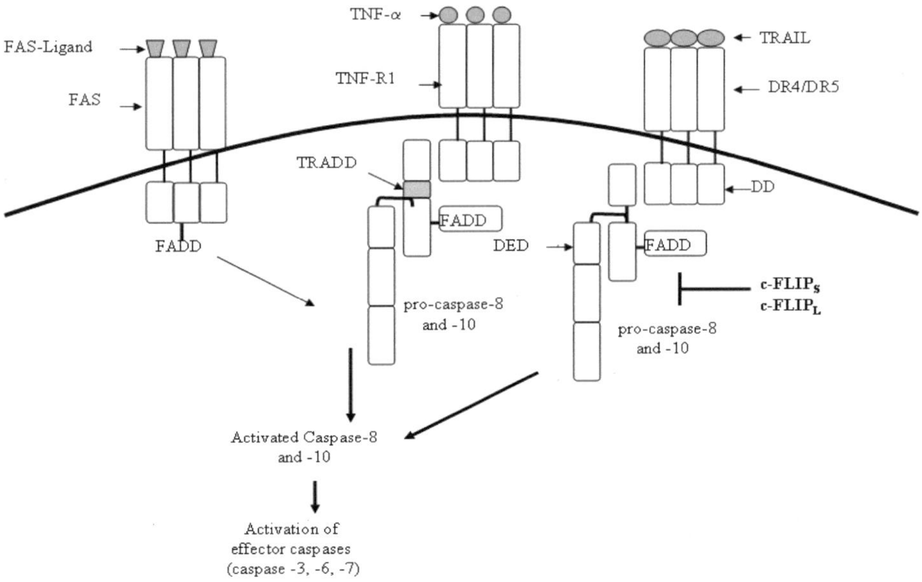

Figure 2: The Cell Death Receptor Pathway. FAS-ligand, TNF-α, and TRAIL bind to their respective receptors leading to the recruitment of FADD *via* a death domain (DD) interaction.

After FADD binding, the death effector domain (DED) of FADD interacts with the DEDs of procaspases-8 and -10 forming the death-inducing signaling compex (DISC). Following DISC formation, caspases-8 and -10 are activated, disassociate from the DISC, and activate downstream effector caspases. c-FLIP binds to procaspases-8, -10, and FADD, and inhibits DISC formation.

receptor-tethered FADD, the DISC (death-inducing signaling complex) is formed, whereupon the caspases are trans-proteolyzed, dimerized, and rendered active; executioner caspase activation and apoptosis ensues. An important regulator of death receptor-induced death is c-FLIP, which binds to procaspases-8, -10 and FADD, and when overexpressed, can protect tumor cells from apoptosis. This supports the notion that cancer therapeutics that target apical proteins in the death receptor pathway, *e.g.*, caspase-8 and -10 isoforms and c-FLIP variants (see below), may have a favorable therapeutic index. In the following sections we will discuss apoptosis induced by TRAIL and other chemotherapeutic agents such as Taxol (paclitaxel) and doxorubicin, through downregulation of c-FLIP variants, and address the possibilities for using c-FLIP as a therapeutic target.

STRUCTURE OF c-FLIP

Initially, viral FLICE-inhibitory proteins (v-FLIPs) were identified by a bioinformatic search for novel virus-encoded apoptotic regulatory molecules containing a DED [42-44]. Following the characterization of v-FLIPs, the mammalian cellular homologue was identified and called c-FLIP [45]. Animal models have revealed that c-FLIP plays an important role in T cell proliferation and heart development. Moreover, abnormal c-FLIP expression has been found in various diseases such as cancers, multiple sclerosis, Alzheimer's disease, diabetes mellitus, and rheumatoid arthritis. At the protein level, three distinct c-FLIP splice variants have been reported: the 26 kDa short form (c-FLIP$_S$), the 24 kDa form of c-FLIP (c-FLIP$_R$), and the 55 kDa c-FLIP$_L$ [3, 11, 12, 46, 47] (Fig. **3**). The structures of c-FLIP$_S$ and the v-FLIPs are similar, except that the two DEDs of c-FLIP$_S$ are followed by 20 amino acids that appear to be crucial for its ubiquitylation and targeting for proteasomal degradation [48]. c-FLIP$_R$ also contains two DEDs but lacks the additional carboxy (C)-terminal amino acids that are present in c-FLIP$_S$. The C-terminus of c-FLIP$_L$ is longer than that of c-FLIP$_S$ and closely resembles the structure of caspases-8 and -10 [47], but this region of c-FLIP$_L$ does not contain a functional caspase domain. This lack of caspase activity is the result of the substitution of several amino acids, particularly the crucial cysteine residue in the catalytic domain which is necessary for the catalytic activity of caspases [49]. Furthermore, c-FLIP$_L$ harbors a caspase-8 cleavage site at position Asp-376 (LEVD); c-FLIP$_L$ cleavage at this site produces the proteolytic fragment variant p43c-FLIP [50, 51].

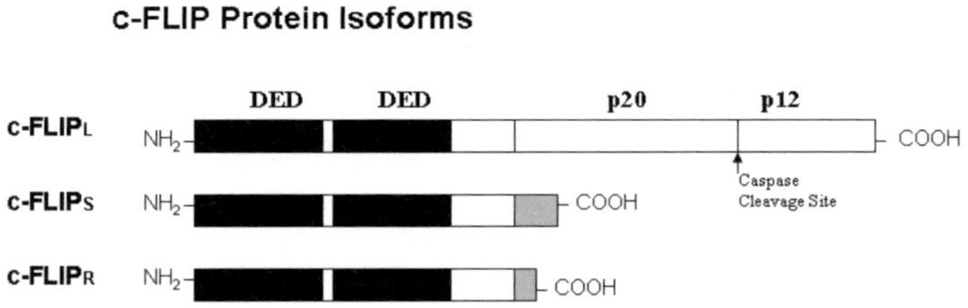

Figure 3: Structures of c-FLIP Variants. Three c-FLIP variants, c-FLIP$_L$, c-FLIP$_S$, and c-FLIP$_R$, contain two death effector domains (DEDs) at their N-termini. In addition to two DEDs, c-FLIP$_L$ contains a large (p20) and a small (p12) caspase-like domain without catalytic activity. c-FLIP$_S$ and c-FLIP$_R$ consist of two DEDs and a small C-terminus (adapted from [46]).

c-FLIP FUNCTION

c-FLIP is a protease-dead, procaspase-8-like regulator of apoptosis [27, 45, 52-54]. It has been shown that c-FLIP interferes with TNF-α, Fas-L, and TRAIL-induced signaling pathways by binding to FADD and/or caspase-8/10 in a ligand-dependent fashion, which in turn prevents DISC formation and subsequent activation of the caspase cascade [27, 53]. We have identified an apoptotic inhibitory complex (AIC) comprised of DR5, FADD, caspase-8, and c-FLIP$_L$ which exists in MCF-7 cells, and have shown that the absence of c-FLIP$_L$ from this complex induces ligand-independent DR5- and FADD-mediated caspase-8 activation in the death inducing signaling complex (DISC) [54]. However, studies using c-FLIP-deficient mice support a dual function for c-FLIP by confirming a role for c-FLIP in Fas L- and TNF-α-induced apoptosis, and revealing that c-FLIP has a similar function to caspase-8 in heart development [55]. Nonetheless, a now extensive literature encompassing diverse types of human cancer cells indicates that the action of c-FLIP is generally anti-apoptotic in cancer cells.

The structural differences between human c-FLIP variants clearly indicate distinct regulatory roles for c-FLIP$_L$ and c-FLIP$_S$ in apoptosis. In fact, c-FLIP$_S$ inhibits

TRAIL-induced DISC formation and apoptosis [56], while c-FLIP$_L$ is responsible for the above described dual functions whereby it inhibits Fas-induced caspase-8 activation when expressed at high levels, but enhances caspase-8 activation when its expression level is low [53-59]. These opposing c-FLIP$_L$ functions may reflect observations that c-FLIP$_L$ activates caspases-8 and -10 *in vitro* by forming heterodimeric enzyme molecules with catalytic activity similar to caspase-8 homodimers, despite the fact that c-FLIP$_L$ is protease dead [60]. Moreover, accumulating evidence has revealed that c-FLIP variants may be effectors that contribute to survival signaling by the Akt, ERK, and NF-κB signaling pathways [11, 12, 41, 57, 61, 62] (Fig. **4**).

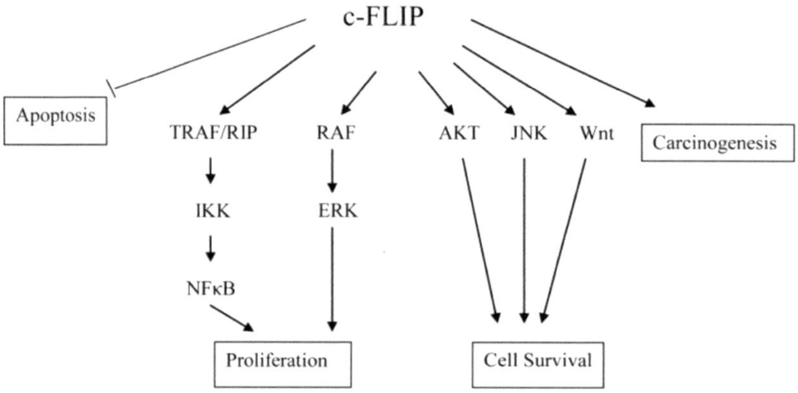

Figure 4: Model Depicting the Multifunctional Roles of c-FLIP on Various Signaling Pathways. As discussed in the text, in addition to its functional role in inhibiting apoptosis by binding to procaspases-8 and -10 and inhibiting their activation, c-FLIP also has the following functions: (1) initiating cell proliferation by recruiting and activating (a) downstream signaling proteins including TRAF, RIP, IKK, and NFκB, or (b) RAF and extracellular signal-regulated kinase (ERK), (2) controlling cell survival by activating Akt, JNK, and Wnt signaling pathways, and (3) participating in carcinogenesis.

It has been demonstrated that overexpression of c-FLIP$_L$ activates NF-κB and ERK signaling by binding to adaptor proteins in each pathway, such as TNFR-associated factors 1 (TRAF1) and 2 (TRAF2), receptor-interacting protein 1 (RIP), and Raf-1 [63, 64] (Fig. **4**). The caspase-8 processed N-terminal fragment of c-FLIP$_L$ (p43cFLIP) is more efficient than c-FLIP$_L$ at recruiting TRAF2 and RIP1, leading to more robust NF-κB activation [51, 52, 62-65]. In nonapoptotic cells, c-FLIP and the procaspase-8 heterodimer result in a novel NH_2-terminal fragment of c-FLIP (p22-FLIP) which is the key mediator of NF-κB activation by directly binding to the IKK complex [66]. These results provided a new mechanism of c-FLIP-mediated NF-κB activation. Recently, Chang *et al.* [67] demonstrated that TNF-α-mediated JNK activation increases turnover of the NF-κB-induced c-FLIP. This is not the result of direct c-FLIP phosphorylation, but rather depends on JNK-mediated phosphorylation and activation of the E3 ubiquitin ligase Itch which specifically ubiquitinates c-FLIP and induces its proteasomal degradation. Thus, JNK antagonizes NF-κB during TNF-α signaling by promoting the proteasomal elimination of c-$FLIP_L$.

In addition to inhibiting caspase-8 and -10 activation [68], c-$FLIP_L$ interacts with Daxx (a death domain-associated protein that has been implicated in proapoptosis and transcriptional regulation) and prevents Fas-induced JNK activation [69]. Thus, c-$FLIP_L$ acting on both the FADD- and Daxx-mediated signaling pathways may be involved in completely inhibiting Fas-induced cell death. Furthermore, Nakajima *et al.* [70] demonstrated that c-$FLIP_L$ directly interacts with a JNK activator, MAP kinase kinase 7 (MKK7), in a TNF-α-dependent manner and inhibits the interactions of MKK7 with MAP/ERK kinase kinase 1, apoptosis-signal-regulating kinase 1, and TGF-β-activated kinase 1. This interaction of c-$FLIP_L$ with MKK7 might selectively suppress JNK activation (Fig. **4**).

The calcium/calmodulin-dependent protein kinase II (CaMK II) has been shown to mediate the upregulation of c-FLIP, thereby protecting melanoma cells from TRAIL-induced apoptosis. Treating Fas resistant cells with the CaMK II inhibitor KN-93 inhibited CaMK II activity, reduced c-FLIP expression, inhibited c-FLIP phosphorylation, and rescued Fas agonistic antibody (CH-11) sensitivity [19, 71]. Targeting this pathway may provide novel therapeutic strategies in treating cancers with upregulated CaMK II. Interestingly, phosphorylation of c-FLIP variants by CaMK II appears to promote c-$FLIP_L$ recruitment to the DISC and inhibit TRAIL-induced apoptosis [19, 71], but phosphorylation of c-$FLIP_L$ by protein kinase C or the bile acid glycochenodeoxycholate results in decreased c-$FLIP_L$ recruitment to the DISC and increased sensitivity of hepatocellular carcinoma cells to TRAIL-triggered apoptosis [72]. Thus, it appears that the particular site of phosphorylation in c-$FLIP_L$ by different kinases influences the functional outcome of this protein in apoptosis.

c-FLIP$_S$ also suppress apoptosis by inhibiting caspase-8 activation, although at different levels of procaspase-8 processing [73, 74]. c-FLIP$_L$ induces a conformation of procaspase-8 that triggers partial but not complete proteolytic processing, while in contrast c-FLIP$_S$ even prevents partial procaspase-8 activation at the DISC [74].

Increased expression of c-FLIP can alter cell cycle progression and enhance cell proliferation and carcinogenesis. Overexpression of c-FLIP$_L$ inhibited the ubiquitinylation and proteasomal degradation of β-catenin, resulting in an increase of the target gene cyclin D1, colony formation, and invasive activity in prostate cancer cells. The FLIP/β-catenin/cyclin D1 signals contributing to colony formation and invasion were reversed by selective silencing of c-FLIP expression [41]. Similarly, c-FLIP$_L$, in cooperation with FADD, enhances canonical Wnt signaling by inhibiting proteasomal degradation of β-catenin, thus suggesting a new mechanism involved with tumorigenesis, in addition to inhibiting Fas signaling [75] (Fig. **4**). c-FLIP overexpression is also significantly related to the presence of HR-HPV infection during the progression of cervical squamous cell cancer and c-FLIP is an early marker of cervical carcinogenesis [76]. Moreover, c-FLIP overexpression accelerated progression to androgen independence by inhibiting apoptosis in LNCaP prostate tumors implanted in nude mice [77]. Similarly, c-FLIP is also an independent prognostic indicator in colorectal carcinomas [56], and its expression in Burkitt's lymphomas is also associated with a poor clinical outcome and could be a reliable prognostic factor in this type of cancer [78]. Furthermore, c-FLIP expression may contribute to the carcinogenesis and aggressiveness of endometrial carcinomas and may serve as a useful prognostic factor for this tumor [79, 80]. Overexpression of c-FLIP$_L$ also increases the hypoxia-inducible factor-1α (HIF1α) [81]. Overexpression of HIF1α can result in genes responsible for global changes in cell proliferation, metastasis, and invasion.

TRANSCRIPTION AND TRANSLATION REGULATION OF c-FLIP

Several transcription factors are known to downregulate c-FLIP$_L$ and c-FLIP$_S$ expression [12, 57] (Fig. **5**). c-FLIP$_S$ downregulation by E2F1 transcription factor occurs at the transcriptional level though its mechanism remains to be found. The specific overexpression of c-FLIP$_S$ is also seen in human lung adenocarcinomas with low levels of E2F1 [82].

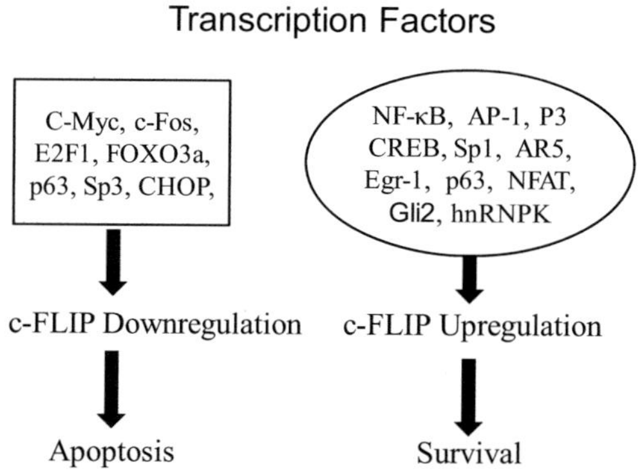

Figure 5: Transcription Factors Involved in the Regulation of c-FLIP Variant Expression. Many transcription factors bind to the promoter of c-FLIP, upregulate or downregulate c-FLIP expression leading to apoptosis or cell survival [12, 53, 128].

Androgen receptor (AR) is a ligand-activated transcription factor that mediates androgen action and is essential for the growth, function, and cell differentiation of the prostate gland. Gao *et al.* [77] demonstrated that the prostate apoptosis response factor-4 (Par-4) functions as an androgen receptor coactivator. This factor directly interacts with the DNA-binding domain of the androgen receptor, increases interaction of this receptor with DNA, and elevates androgen receptor-dependent transcription. Interestingly, Par-4 is recruited onto the c-FLIP promoter in the presence of androgens. The binding to Par-4 to the promoter enhanced c-FLIP expression and this elevated expression was reversed by the expression of a dominant-negative Par-4. Enhanced c-FLIP expression was associated with prostate cancer progression to the androgen-resistant stage [77].

Another regulator of c-FLIP expression is p53 tumor suppressor protein. p53 may exert transcriptional upregulating effects on the c-FLIP gene and also has potent effects on promoting the degradation of c-FLIP protein [83-85]. Moreover, the gene encoding c-FLIP is a direct target of c-myc-mediated transcriptional repression [86, 87]. Chromatin immunoprecipitation and luciferase reporter analyses have shown that c-myc binds and represses the c-*FLIP* promoter. Overexpression of c-myc or activation of myc-estrogen receptor (ER) decreased c-FLIP levels in both cell culture and mouse models of c-myc-induced tumorigenesis, while knocking down c-myc using siRNA increased c-FLIP expression [87].

Li *et al.* [88] reported that c-FLIP$_L$ is transcriptionally regulated by the activator protein-1 (AP-1) family member protein c-Fos and that MG-132, an inhibitor of the proteasome, sensitizes TRAIL-resistant prostate cancer cells by inducing c-Fos and repressing c-FLIP$_L$. Moreover, c-Fos, which is activated by MG-132, negatively regulates c-FLIP$_L$ by direct binding to the putative promoter region of the c-FLIP$_L$ gene. In addition to activating c-Fos, MG-132 activates c-Jun, another AP-1 family member. c-Fos heterodimerizes with c-Jun to form AP-1 and repress transcription of c-FLIP$_L$.

c-FLIP is also regulated at the translational level. Panner *et al.* [89, 90] showed that TRAIL resistance in glioblastoma multiforme cells (GBM) is the result of overexpression of c-FLIP$_S$, and that c-FLIP$_S$ expression is in turn translationally increased by activation of the Akt-mammalian target of rapamycin (mTOR)-p70 S6 kinase 1 (S6K1) pathway. Conversely, inhibition of mTOR or its target S6K1 suppressed polyribosomal accumulation of c-FLIP$_S$ mRNA, c-FLIP$_S$ protein expression, and promoted TRAIL resistance in GBM cells. An mTOR-independent pathway can also act through a Ral effector protein, RalBP1, to suppress cdc42-mediated activation of S6 kinase and the translation of c-FLIP$_S$ [90, 91]. However, not much is known about Ral except that it is an effector of Ras oncogenesis. The Ral proteins (RalA and RalB) are small GTPases and their activity is controlled by the RalGEF family of proteins: RalGDS, Rgl, and Rlf [92]. Activated Ral molecules interact with Ral effectors, including RalBP1 (a cdc42 GTPase-activating protein) [93]. Panner *et al.* [90] showed an mTOR-independent link between RalA and translation. These authors also demonstrated that RalBP1 serves in a membrane-bound, GTPase-activating protein (GAP)-dependent manner to link RalA activation to cdc42 suppression, thereby leading to a decrease in c-FLIP$_S$ expression and enhancing TRAIL-induced apoptosis.

c-FLIP DEGRADATION

c-FLIP is predominately degraded by the ubiquitin-proteasome degradation system [94]. Both c-FLIP isoforms can be degraded by the proteasome, but c-FLIP$_S$ appears to be particularly sensitive to ubiquitylation and proteasomal degradation, partly due to two crucial lysine residues in the C-terminal 20 amino acids that are unique to c-FLIP$_S$ [48]. The sensitivity of c-FLIP$_S$ to ubiquitin-mediated degradation adds a novel concept to DISC regulation and its control of apoptosis [48]. Downregulation of c-$FLIP_L$ and c-$FLIP_S$ due to degradation is observed in cells treated with various apoptosis-inducing agents. The cyclin-dependent kinase inhibitor flavopiridol degrades c-FLIP and increases apoptosis, which in turn can be reversed by an inhibitor of the ubiquitin-proteasome system [95]. Combined treatment with the anticancer agent 3,3'-diindolylmethane and TRAIL led to significant degradation of c-FLIP, predominantly *via* the ubiquitin-proteasome degradation system [94]. Moreover, Peroxisome Proliferator-Activated Receptor γ (PPARγ) agonists sensitize cancer cells to TRAIL by ubiquitination and proteasome-dependent c-FLIP degradation [96, 97].

Panner *et al.* [98] also described a ubiquitin-specific protease-8 (USP8) which is a downstream target of Akt, links Akt to the E3 ubiquitin ligase atrophin-interacting protein 4 (AIP4), and regulates c-$FLIP_S$ stability [98]. Overexpression of USP8 increased c-$FLIP_S$ ubiquitination, decreased c-$FLIP_S$ half-life, decreased c-$FLIP_S$ steady-state levels, and decreased TRAIL resistance.

Proteasome inhibitors are emerging class of drugs that decrease proliferation and induce apoptosis in a variety of malignancies. Interestingly, several proteasome inhibitors lead to the downregulation of c-$FLIP_L$ and c-$FLIP_S$ [99, 100].

c-FLIP VARIANTS AS TARGETS FOR CANCER THERAPY

Higher levels of c-FLIP in tumor tissue from patients with various cancers including colorectal cancer, bladder urothelial cancer, cervical cancer, Burkitt's lymphoma, non-Hodgkin's lymphoma, head and neck squamous cell carcinoma (HNSCC), and hepatocellular cancers have been reported [11, 101-104]. Moreover, these elevated expressions have been correlated with a poor clinical outcome and could be a reliable prognostic factor in these types of cancer.

Strategies to lower the threshold for triggering cancer cell apoptosis may lead to new and more effective therapeutic regimens for ovarian cancer. TRAIL holds enormous promise as a cancer therapeutic due to its highly selective apoptosis-inducing action on neoplastic *versus* normal cells [2]. However, to exploit this opportunity, the problem of TRAIL resistance in cancer must first be overcome.

While c-FLIP$_L$ may function as a fine-tuned regulator that manifests dual pro- and anti-apoptotic actions during development and in normal adult tissues, accumulating evidence indicates an anti-apoptotic role for c-FLIP in diverse types of human cancer [11, 16, 13, 18, 20, 101-105]. Notably, several reports demonstrated that small interfering RNAs (siRNAs) that specifically knocked down the expression of c-FLIP$_L$ or c-FLIP$_S$ in cancer cell lines of various types augmented TRAIL- and chemotherapy-induced apoptosis [12, 25, 17, 105]. Significantly, Piggott *et al.* [106] reported that c-FLIP is upregulated in breast cancer stem cells (BRSCs) and silencing c-FLIP by siRNA selectively eliminates breast cancer stem cells activity in response to TRAIL. Therefore, the outlook for the therapeutic index of c-FLIP-targeted drugs appears excellent, not only because of the therapeutic efficacy observed in models of c-FLIP targeting in cancer therapy with TRAIL, but also because the current understanding of c-FLIP action in normal tissues supports the notion that c-FLIP-targeted cancer therapy will be well tolerated.

There does not appear to be a "handle" to inhibit c-FLIP function with small molecule ligands, since the cytoprotective DISC binding is mediated by highly conserved DEDs which function by homotypic binding. However, small molecules that induce c-FLIP downregulation and sensitize neoplastic cells to apoptosis induction by TRAIL have been identified in global, unbiased chemical screens. Our results revealed that forced expression of c-FLIP$_L$ or c-FLIP$_S$ caused resistance to apoptosis in the CCRF-HSB-2 leukemia cell line [68]. Moreover, c-FLIP$_L$, but not c-FLIP$_S$ inhibited apoptosis induced by the fluoropyrimidine 5-fluorouracil (5-FU), the topoisomerase-1 inhibitor irinotecan (CPT-11), and the DNA damaging agent oxaliplatin (OXA) in HCT116 colorectal cancer cells, suggesting that c-FLIP$_L$ is the more important splice form in mediating chemoresistance [20]. Furthermore, c-FLIP inhibits TRAIL-independent, DR5- and caspase 8-dependent apoptosis in response to chemotherapy in colorectal cancer cells. We (Wu CH, Day TW, and Safa AR, unpublished results) have found that ectopic overexpression of c-FLIP$_L$ or c-FLIP$_S$ in MCF-7 induces resistant to Taxol. The c-FLIP$_L$ variant protects against apoptosis induced by a diverse group of chemotherapeutic drugs with different mechanisms of action [11, 12 102, 103, 107]. This interaction in turn prevents death-inducing signaling complex (DISC) formation and subsequent activation of the caspase cascade. c-FLIP also inhibits spontaneous death ligand-independent cell death [25, 102], further supporting the notion that targeting c-FLIP may have therapeutic potential for cancer treatment. Cisplatin, camptothecin, and etoposide were all shown to downregulate c-FLIP$_S$ expression in human malignant glioma cells [103, 108]. Moreover, doxorubicin decreased levels of c-FLIP, particularly c-FLIP$_S$ in prostate cancer cell lines, and sensitized these cells to TRAIL [109]. Overexpression of the c-FLIP$_L$ variant has been found in ovarian cancer cells resistance to cisplatin [110]. Interestingly, the damaged DNA-binding protein 2 (DDB2), a component involved in the genomic repair of UV damage, was recently shown to be involved in the cross-resistance of a cisplatin-selected HeLa cell line (HR3) to Fas-inducing antibody and tumor necrosis factor (TNF)-α-mediated apoptosis [110]. The HR3 cell line exhibits enhanced expression of DDB2 and cross-resistance to UV-induced activation of caspases and apoptosis. The overexpression of DDB2 was shown to increase both endogenous and exogenous c-FLIP mRNA levels, and inhibition of c-FLIP by antisense oligonucleotides suppressed DDB2 protection, revealing that DDB2 regulates TNF signaling-mediated apoptosis *via* c-FLIP. Therefore, therapeutics capable of modulating the death-inducing ligands and/or chemotherapeutic agents by downregulating c-FLIP variants should hold enormous promises in future clinical trials.

We reported that Taxol downregulates c-FLIP (both c-FLIP$_S$ and c-FLIP$_L$) in cancer cells [68], and that doses of the drug that induced concentration-dependent apoptosis were sufficient to abrogate the expression of both c-FLIP variants. The significance of these findings to paclitaxel-induced neoplastic cell apoptosis was demonstrated by our results showing that transfection with an antisense c-FLIP plasmid abrogated c-FLIP$_S$ and c-FLIP$_L$ expression and sensitized cancer cells to Taxol [68]. These results demonstrate that c-FLIP isoforms are major contributing factors to cancer cell resistance to paclitaxel-induced apoptosis.

AGENTS KNOWN TO DOWNREGULATE c-FLIP

c-FLIP can serve as a critical target for therapeutic intervention aimed at inhibiting its transcription and posttranscriptional changes and various small molecule inhibitors have been shown to reduce expression of the c-FLIP varians (reviewed in [12]). Many therapeutics capable of downregulating c-FLIP levels also enhance the expression of the TRAIL receptor DR5, and in some cases enhance levels of both the DR4 and DR5 TRAIL receptors. One such agent is lexatumumab, a humanized agonistic monoclonal antibody specific for the DR5 receptor, which is currently in Phase I/II clinical trials in patients with advanced malignancies. Recently, lexatumumab was shown to decrease the expression of c-$FLIP_L$ and increase the level of DR5 in primary and metastatic renal cell carcinoma [111]. Similarly, the induction of apoptosis by the proteasome inhibitors MG-132 and PS-341 (bortezomib, Velcade^R) in primary chronic lymphocytic leukemia (CLL) cells and the Burkitt lymphoma cell line BJAB was associated with upregulation of TRAIL and its death receptors, DR4 and DR5, and decreased c-FLIP protein expression [99]. As mentioned earlier, c-FLIP is degraded *via* a ubiquitin-proteosome system. Therefore, PS-341 should increase c-FLIP and prevent apoptosis. Interestingly, Zhao *et al.* have shown that PS-341 decreases c-FLIP at the gene level [112]. In contrast, Liu *et al.* reported that PS-341 up-regulates DR5 as well as c-FLIP and survivin in human non-small cell lung carcinomas (NSCLC) cells [113]. Thus, the effect of PS-341 on the regulation of c-FLIP expression may be cancer cell-type specific. A propos t ed central mechanism of action of PS-341 is he inhibition of NF-κB activation through inhibition of IκB degradation [114]. NF-κB activation results in upregulation of c-FLIP [115]. Thus, downregulation of the c-FLIP gene by PS-341 may be due to inhibition of NF-κB activation by this agent. PPARγ ligands exert PPARγ-independent effects on inducing DR5 expression and downregulating c-FLIP levels, leading to enhanced TRAIL-induced apoptosis [97]. Synthetic triterpenoids sensitize TRAIL-resistant T47D and MDA-MB-468 breast cancer cells to TRAIL-mediated apoptosis by downregulating c-$FLIP_L$, and up-regulate cell surface TRAIL receptors DR4 and DR5 in breast cancer cell [116]. Progesterone induces apoptosis in TRAIL-resistant ovarian cancer cells by circumventing c-$FLIP_L$ overexpression [12, 117].

Particularly impressive agents known to downregulate c-FLIP expression are the histone deacetylases inhibitors (HDACi). These compounds are considered to be among the most promising agents for the developing novel cancer therapeutics

[118, 119]. In diverse types of cancer cells, HDACi induce growth arrest, differentiation, and apoptosis. The results of clinical trials with several of these agents indicate that they are well tolerated at doses that have anti-tumor activity [119, 120]. Importantly, normal cells are almost always more resistant to HDACi than tumor cells [119, 120]. The mechanism of their antitumor activity and TRAIL sensitization are likely related at least in part to down-regulation of c-FLIP variants [12, 121-126] at the c-FLIP mRNA and protein levels. The HDACi Vorinostat, suberoylanilide hydroxamic acid (SAHA), sensitized cancer cells to TRAIL by downregulation of c-FLIP [121, 122]. Mawji *et al.* [123] showed that the 4-(4-chloro-2-methylphenoxy)-N-hydroxybutanamide (CMH) inhibited c-FLIP protein synthesis and suppressed anoikis, a process by which malignant metastatic epithelial cells resist apoptosis that normally occurs due to loss of anchorage from the extracellular matrix. This small molecule inhibitor of c-FLIP, also termed droxinostat, selectively inhibited HDAC3, HDAC6, and HDAC8 [124]. We demonstrated that CMH downregulates c-FLIP$_L$ and c-FLIP$_S$ mRNA and protein levels, caused poly(ADP-ribose) polymerase (PARP) degradation, reduced cell survival, and induced apoptosis in MCF-7 breast cancer cells [125]. Recently, Kerr *et al.* [126] reported that c-FLIP interacts with Ku70. Interestingly, Ku70 regulated c-FLIP protein stability by inhibiting its polyubiquitination. Moreover, these authors showed that the HDACi Vorinostat (SAHA) increased the acetylation of Ku70 and disrupted the FLIP/Ku70 complex, thereby initiating c-FLIP polyubiquitination and degradation by the proteasome.

Elucidating the mechanisms regulating c-FLIP expression in tumor cell population and cancer stem cells (CSCs) may lead to c-FLIP-downregulating targeted therapeutics that are efficacious and well tolerated in combination with TRAIL, conventional chemotherapeutic agents, or other therapies that activate the caspase-8/10-dependent apoptosis pathway. This approach may be especially effective in human malignancies that overexpress c-FLIP, *i.e.*, glioblastoma multiforme, prostate, colorectal, endometrial, ovarian, mesothelial, and lung cancer [11, 17, 20, 41, 79, 89, 101, 127].

Selective c-FLIP$_L$ and c-FLIP$_S$ knockdown strategies to sensitize cancer cells to TRAIL [105] may lead to combination therapies consisting of TRAIL plus innovative c-FLIP variant-selective gene therapy strategies. c-FLIP$_L$ and c-FLIP$_S$

knockdown could provide significant clinical advances in the use of TRAIL in treating lung cancer. Similarly, many agents abrogate the expression of c-FLIP variants [12], suggesting that these experimental therapeutics have potential value to reverse cancer cell resistance to death ligands and chemotherapeutic agents.

c-FLIP$_L$ and/or c-FLIP$_S$ serve as rational target(s) in various cancers for novel small molecule targeted therapeutics and/or gene therapy strategies., *e.g.*, small molecule therapeutics that selectively downregulate c-FLIP$_S$ or c-FLIP$_L$ and gene therapy strategies that knock down a specific c-FLIP variant. Developing these innovative therapeutic strategies in conjunction with TRAIL and chemotheraputic agents will potentially overcome the barrier of dose-limiting toxicity in cancer chemotherapy. Furthermore, rather than empirically combining cytotoxic drugs to attempt to enhance their therapeutic response, modulating specific targets in cancer cells based on rational preclinical design is a logical approach to eradicate cancer. TRAIL or chemotherapy resistance in diverse cancer cell types can be reversed by parallel treatment with other substances, such as agents known to downregulate c-FLIP variants.

The foregoing discussion in this article revealed that c-FLIP may represent an important clinical marker of drug resistance, and that targeting c-FLIP in combination with TRAIL or standard chemotherapies has therapeutic potential for treating cancer. The rapid progress in identifying c-FLIP inhibitors has provided optimism that future cancer therapy will be improved by innovations that replace current standard chemotherapy with targeted therapy or combined chemotherapy with drug resistance-reversing targeted therapy, *e.g.*, combination regimens of chemotherapy and small molecule drugs that downregulate c-FLIP variants.

ACKNOWLEDGEMENTS

We would like to thank Dr. Mary D. Kraeszig for her editorial assistance. The research in the author's laboratory was supported by research grants from the National Cancer Institute (CA 080734, CA 90878, and CA 101743), Department of Defense (DOD) (OC 06095), and the Indiana University Cancer Center Translational Research Acceleration Collaboration (ITRAC) initiative.

CONFLICT OF INTEREST

The author(s) confirm that this chapter content has no conflict of interest.

DISCLOSURE

The chapter submitted for the eBook Series entitled **"Advances in Cancer Drug Targets, Volume 1"** is an update of our article in **Current Cancer Drug Targets, Volume 8, Issue 1, 2008,** with additional text and references.

REFERENCES

[1] Clarke, R.; Leonessa, F.; Trock, B. Multidrug resistance/P-glycoprotein and breast cancer: review and meta-analysis. *Semin. Oncol.* **2005,** *32*, S9-15.

[2] Fojo, A. T.; Menefee, M. Microtubule targeting agents: basic mechanisms of multidrug resistance (MDR). *Semin. Oncol.* **2005,** *32*, S3-8.

[3] Safa, A.R; Day, T.W; Wu C.H. Cellular FLICE-like inhibitory protein (C-FLIP): a novel target for cancer therapy. *Curr Cancer Drug Targets.* **2008**, *8*, 37-46.

[4] Glavinas, H.; Krajcsi, P.; Cserepes, J.; Sarkadi, B. The role of ABC transporters in drug resistance, metabolism and toxicity. *Curt. Drug. Deliv.* **2004,** *1*, 27-42.

[5] Safa, A. R. Identification and characterization of the binding sites of P-glycoprotein for multidrug resistance-related drugs and modulators. *Curr. Med. Chem. Anticancer Agents.* **2004,** *4*, 1-17.

[6] Mashima, T.; Tsuruo, T. Defects of the apoptotic pathway as therapeutic target against cancer. *Drug Resist. Updat.* **2005,** *8*, 339-343.

[7] Yerbes, R.; Palacios, C; López-Rivas A. The therapeutic potential of TRAIL receptor signalling in cancer cells. *Clin. Transl. Oncol.* **2011**, *12*, 839-847.

[8] Duiker, E. W.; Mom, C. H.; de Jong, S.; Willemse, P. H.; Gietema, J. A.; van der Zee, A. G.; de Vries, E. G. The clinical trail of TRAIL. *Eur. J. Cancer.* **2006,** *42*, 2233-2240.

[9] Martinez-Lostao, L.; Marzo, I.; Anel, A.; Naval, J.; Targeting the Apo2L/TRAIL system for the therapy of autoimmune diseases and cancer. *Biochem. Pharmacol.* **2012,** *83,* 1475-83.

[10] Hellwig, C.T.; Rehm, M.; TRAIL signaling and synergy mechanisms used in TRAIL-based combination therapies. *Mol. Cancer Ther.* **2012,** *11*, 3-13.

[11] Lavrik, I.N.; Krammer, P.H. Regulation of CD95/Fas signaling at the DISC. *Cell Death Differ.* **2012,** *19*, 36-41.

[12] Safa, A.R.; Pollok, K.E. Targeting the anti-apoptotic protein c-FLIP for cancer therapy. *Cancers (Basel).* **2011**,1639-1671.

[13] Mathas, S.; Lietz, A.; Anagnostopoulos, I.; Hummel, F.; Wiesner, B.; Janz, M.; Jundt, F.; Hirsch, B.; Johrens-Leder, K.; Vornlocher, H. P.; Bommert, K.; Stein, H.; Dorken, B. c-FLIP mediates resistance of Hodgkin/Reed-Sternberg cells to death receptor-induced apoptosis. *J. Exp. Med.* **2004,** *199*, 1041-1052 Epub 2004 Apr 1012.

[14] Piggott L, Omidvar N, Martí Pérez S, Eberl M, Clarkson RW. Suppression of apoptosis inhibitor c-FLIP selectively eliminates breast cancer stem cell activity in response to the anti-cancer agent, TRAIL. *Breast Cancer Res.* **2011** Sep 14, 13(5), R88.

[15] Li Z, Xu X, Bai L, Chen W, Lin Y. Epidermal growth factor receptor-mediated tissue transglutaminase overexpression couples acquired tumor necrosis factor-related apoptosis-inducing ligand resistance and migration through c-FLIP and MMP-9 proteins in lung cancer cells. J Biol Chem. 2011 Jun 17;286(24):21164-72. Epub 2011 Apr 27.

[16] Plati. J.; Bucur, O.; Khosravi-Far, R.; Apoptotic cell signaling in cancer progression and therapy. *Integr. Biol. (Camb).* **2011,** *3*, 279-296.

[17] Galligan, L.; Longley, D. B.; McEwan, M.; Wilson, T. R.; McLaughlin, K.; Johnston, P. G. Chemotherapy and TRAIL-mediated colon cancer cell death: the roles of p53, TRAIL receptors, and c-FLIP. *Mol. Cancer Ther.* **2005,** *4*, 2026-2036.

[18] Logan, A.E.; Wilson, T.R.; Fenning, C.; Cummins, R.; Kay, E.; Johnston, P.G.; Longley, D.B. *In vitro* and *in vivo* characterisation of a novel c-FLIP-targeted antisense phosphorothioate oligonucleotide. *Apoptosis.* **2010**, *15,* 1435-1443.

[19] Xiao, C.; Yang, B. F.; Song, J. H.; Schulman, H.; Li, L.; Hao, C. Inhibition of CaMKII-mediated c-FLIP expression sensitizes malignant melanoma cells to TRAIL-induced apoptosis. *Exp. Cell. Res.* **2005,** *304*, 244-255 Epub 2004 Nov 2026.

[20] Longley, D. B.; Wilson, T. R.; McEwan, M.; Allen, W. L.; McDermott, U.; Galligan, L.; Johnston, P. G. c-FLIP inhibits chemotherapy-induced colorectal cancer cell death. *Oncogene.* **2005,** *25*, 838-848.

[21] Plissonnier, M.L.; Fauconnet, S.; Bittard, H.; Lascombe, I. Insights on distinct pathways of thiazolidinediones (PPARgamma ligand)-promoted apoptosis in TRAIL-sensitive or -resistant malignant urothelial cells. *Int. J. Cancer.* **2010,** *127*, 1769-1784.

[22] Mezzanzanica, D.; Balladore, E.; Turatti, F.; Luison, E.; Alberti, P.; Bagnoli, M.; Figini, M.; Mazzoni, A.; Raspagliesi, F.; Oggionni, M.; Pilotti, S.; Canevari, S. CD95-mediated apoptosis is impaired at receptor level by cellular FLICE-inhibitory protein (long form) in wild-type p53 human ovarian carcinoma. *Clin. Cancer Res.* **2004,** *10*, 5202-5214.

[23] Steele, L. P.; Georgopoulos, N. T.; Southgate, J.; Selby, P. J.; Trejdosiewicz, L. K. Differential susceptibility to TRAIL of normal *versus* malignant human urothelial cells. *Cell Death Differ.* **2006,** *13*, 1564-1576.

[24] Shin, E. C.; Seong, Y. R.; Kim, C. H.; Kim, H.; Ahn, Y. S.; Kim, K.; Kim, S. J.; Hong, S. S.; Park, J. H. Human hepatocellular carcinoma cells resist to TRAIL-induced apoptosis, and the resistance is abolished by cisplatin. *Exp. Mol. Med.* **2002,** *34*, 114-122.

[25] Sharp, D. A.; Lawrence, D. A.; Ashkenazi, A. Selective knockdown of the long variant of cellular FLICE inhibitory protein augments death receptor-mediated caspase-8 activation and apoptosis. *J. Biol. Chem.* **2005,** *280*, 19401-19409.

[26] Tao, R.H.; Berkova, Z.; Wise, J.F.; Rezaeian, A.H.; Daniluk, U.; Ao, X.; Hawke, D.H,; Karp, J.E.; Lin, H.K.; Molldrem, J.J.; Samaniego, F. PMLRARα binds to Fas and suppresses Fas-mediated apoptosis through recruiting c-FLIP *in vivo*. Blood. **2011,** *118*, 3107-3118.

[27] Kataoka, T. The caspase-8 modulator c-FLIP. *Crit. Rev. Immunol.* **2005,** *25*, 31-58.

[28] Baier, A.; Meineckel, I.; Gay, S.; Pap, T. Apoptosis in rheumatoid arthritis. *Curr. Opin. Rheumatol.* **2003,** *15*, 274-279.

[29] Thome, M.; Tschopp, J. Regulation of lymphocyte proliferation and death by FLIP. *Nat. Rev. Immunol.* **2001,** *1*, 50-58.

[30] Scatena, R. Mitochondria and cancer: a growing role in apoptosis, cancer cell metabolism and dedifferentiation. *Adv. Exp. Med. Biol.* **2012**, *942*, 287-308.

[31] Wenner, C.E. Targeting mitochondria as a therapeutic target in cancer. *J. Cell. Physiol.* **2012,** *227*, 450-456.

[32] Gogvadze, V.; Orrenius, S. Estaquier J, Vallette F, Vayssiere JL, Mignotte B. Mitochondrial pathways of apoptosis. *Adv Exp Med Biol.* **2012**, *942,* 157-183.

[33] Ferri, K. F.; Jacotot, E.; Blanco, J.; Este, J. A.; Zamzami, N.; Susin, S. A.; Xie, Z.; Brothers, G.; Reed, J. C.; Penninger, J. M.; Kroemer, G. Apoptosis control in syncytia induced by the HIV type 1-envelope glycoprotein complex: role of mitochondria and caspases. *J. Exp. Med.* **2000,** *192*, 1081-1092.

[34] Liu, X.; Kim, C. N.; Yang, J.; Jemmerson, R.; Wang, X. Induction of apoptotic program in cell-free extracts: requirement for dATP and cytochrome c. *Cell.* **1996,** *86*, 147-157.

[35] Li, H.; Zhu, H.; Xu, C. J.; Yuan, J. Cleavage of BID by caspase 8 mediates the mitochondrial damage in the Fas pathway of apoptosis. *Cell.* **1998,** *94*, 491-501.

[36] Kurokawa, M.; Kornbluth, S.; Caspases and kinases in a death grip. Cell. **2009,** *138*, 838-854.

[37] Gordy, C. He, Y.W. The crosstalk between autophagy and apoptosis: where does this lead? *Protein Cell.* **2012,** *3*, 17-27.

[38] Tadokoro, D.; Takahama, S.; Shimizu, K.; Hayashi, S.; Endo, Y.; Sawasaki, T.; Characterization of a caspase-3-substrate kinome using an N- and C-terminally tagged protein kinase library produced by a cell-free system. *Cell Death Dis.* **2010,** *28,* 1:e89.

[39] Krueger, A.; Baumann, S.; Krammer, P. H.; Kirchhoff, S. FLICE-inhibitory proteins: regulators of death receptor-mediated apoptosis. *Mol. Cell. Biol.* **2001,** *21*, 8247-8254.

[40] Ashkenazi, A. Targeting death and decoy receptors of the tumour-necrosis factor superfamily. *Nat. Rev. Cancer.* **2002,** *2*, 420-430.

[41] Shimada, K.; Nakamura, M.; Matsuyoshi, S.; Ishida, E.; Konishi, N. Specific positive and negative effects of FLIP on cell survival in human prostate cancer. *Carcinogenesis.* **2006,** *27*, 1349-1357 Epub 2006 Mar 1314.

[42] Thome, M.; Schneider, P.; Hofmann, K.; Fickenscher, H.; Meinl, E.; Neipel, F.; Mattmann, C.; Burns, K.; Bodmer, J. L.; Schroter, M.; Scaffidi, C.; Krammer, P. H.; Peter, M. E.; Tschopp, J. Viral FLICE-inhibitory proteins (FLIPs) prevent apoptosis induced by death receptors. *Nature.* **1997,** *386*, 517-521.

[43] Hu, S.; Vincenz, C.; Buller, M.; Dixit, V. M. A novel family of viral death effector domain-containing molecules that inhibit both CD-95- and tumor necrosis factor receptor-1-induced apoptosis. *J. Biol. Chem.* **1997,** *272*, 9621-9624.

[44] Bertin, J.; Armstrong, R. C.; Ottilie, S.; Martin, D. A.; Wang, Y.; Banks, S.; Wang, G. H.; Senkevich, T. G.; Alnemri, E. S.; Moss, B.; Lenardo, M. J.; Tomaselli, K. J.; Cohen, J. I. Death effector domain-containing herpesvirus and poxvirus proteins inhibit both Fas- and TNFR1-induced apoptosis. *Proc. Natl. Acad. Sci. U S A.* **1997,** *94*, 1172-1176.

[45] Irmler, M.; Thome, M.; Hahne, M.; Schneider, P.; Hofmann, K.; Steiner, V.; Bodmer, J. L.; Schroter, M.; Burns, K.; Mattmann, C.; Rimoldi, D.; French, L. E.; Tschopp, J. Inhibition of death receptor signals by cellular FLIP. *Nature.* **1997,** *388*, 190-195.

[46] Golks, A.; Brenner, D.; Fritsch, C.; Krammer, P. H.; Lavrik, I. N. c-FLIPR, a new regulator of death receptor-induced apoptosis. *J. Biol. Chem.* **2005,** *280*, 14507-14513.

[47] Tschopp, J.; Irmler, M.; Thome, M. Inhibition of fas death signals by FLIPs. *Curr. Opin. Immunol.* **1998,** *10*, 552-558.

[48] Poukkula, M.; Kaunisto, A.; Hietakangas, V.; Denessiouk, K.; Katajamaki, T.; Johnson, M. S.; Sistonen, L.; Eriksson, J. E. Rapid turnover of c-FLIPS is determined by its unique C-terminal tail. *J. Biol. Chem.* **2005,** *10*, 10.

[49] Cohen, G. M. Caspases: the executioners of apoptosis. *Biochem. J.* **1997,** *326*, 1-16.

[50] Krueger, A.; Schmitz, I.; Baumann, S.; Krammer, P. H.; Kirchhoff, S. Cellular FLICE-inhibitory protein splice variants inhibit different steps of caspase-8 activation at the CD95 death-inducing signaling complex. *J. Biol. Chem.* **2001,** *276*, 20633-20640. Epub 22001 Mar 20605.

[51] Kataoka, T.; Tschopp, J. N-terminal fragment of c-FLIP(L) processed by caspase 8 specifically interacts with TRAF2 and induces activation of the NF-kappaB signaling pathway. *Mol. Cell. Biol.* **2004,** *24*, 2627-2636.

[52] Srinivasula, S. M.; Ahmad, M.; Ottilie, S.; Bullrich, F.; Banks, S.; Wang, Y.; Fernandes-Alnemri, T.; Croce, C. M.; Litwack, G.; Tomaselli, K. J.; Armstrong, R. C.; Alnemri, E. S. FLAME-1, a novel FADD-like anti-apoptotic molecule that regulates Fas/TNFR1-induced apoptosis. *J. Biol. Chem.* **1997,** *272*, 18542-18545.

[53] Oztürk, S.; Schleich, K.; Lavrik, I.N.; Cellular FLICE-like inhibitory proteins (c-FLIPs): fine-tuners of life and death decisions. *Exp. Cell. Res.* **2012,** *318*, 1324-3131.

[54] Day, T.W.; Huang, S.; Safa, A.R.; c-FLIP knockdown induces ligand-independent DR5-, FADD-, caspase-8-, and caspase-9-dependent apoptosis in breast cancer cells. *Biochem. Pharmacol.* **2008,** *76*; 1694-704.

[55] Yeh, W. C.; Itie, A.; Elia, A. J.; Ng, M.; Shu, H. B.; Wakeham, A.; Mirtsos, C.; Suzuki, N.; Bonnard, M.; Goeddel, D. V.; Mak, T. W. Requirement for Casper (c-FLIP) in regulation of death receptor-induced apoptosis and embryonic development. *Immunity.* **2000,** *12*, 633-642.

[56] Burns, T. F.; El-Deiry, W. S. Identification of inhibitors of TRAIL-induced death (ITIDs) in the TRAIL-sensitive colon carcinoma cell line SW480 using a genetic approach. *J. Biol. Chem.* **2001,** *276*, 37879-37886.

[57] Bagnoli, M.; Canevari, S.; Mezzanzanica, D.; Cellular FLICE-inhibitory protein (c-FLIP) signalling: a key regulator of receptor-mediated apoptosis in physiologic context and in cancer. *Int. J. Biochem. Cell. Biol.* **2010**, *42*, 210-213.

[58] Micheau, O.; Thome, M.; Schneider, P.; Holler, N.; Tschopp, J.; Nicholson, D. W.; Briand, C.; Grutter, M. G. The long form of FLIP is an activator of caspase-8 at the Fas death-inducing signaling complex. *J. Biol. Chem.* **2002,** *277*, 45162-45171

[59] Chang, D. W.; Xing, Z.; Pan, Y.; Algeciras-Schimnich, A.; Barnhart, B. C.; Yaish-Ohad, S.; Peter, M. E.; Yang, X. c-FLIP(L) is a dual function regulator for caspase-8 activation and CD95-mediated apoptosis. *Embo J.* **2002,** *21*, 3704-3714.

[60] Boatright, K. M.; Deis, C.; Denault, J. B.; Sutherlin, D. P.; Salvesen, G. S. Activation of caspases-8 and -10 by FLIP(L). *Biochem. J.* **2004,** *382*, 651-657.

[61] Cottet, S.; Dupraz, P.; Hamburger, F.; Dolci, W.; Jaquet, M.; Thorens, B. cFLIP protein prevents tumor necrosis factor-alpha-mediated induction of caspase-8-dependent apoptosis in insulin-secreting betaTc-Tet cells. *Diabetes.* **2002,** *51*, 1805-1814.

[62] Fang, L. W.; Tai, T. S.; Yu, W. N.; Liao, F.; Lai, M. Z. Phosphatidylinositide 3-kinase priming couples c-FLIP to T cell activation. *J. Biol. Chem.* **2004,** *279*, 13-18 Epub 2003 Oct 2024.

[63] Chaudhary, P. M.; Eby, M. T.; Jasmin, A.; Kumar, A.; Liu, L.; Hood, L. Activation of the NF-kappaB pathway by caspase 8 and its homologs. *Oncogene.* **2000,** *19*, 4451-4460.

[64] Kataoka, T.; Budd, R. C.; Holler, N.; Thome, M.; Martinon, F.; Irmler, M.; Burns, K.; Hahne, M.; Kennedy, N.; Kovacsovics, M.; Tschopp, J. The caspase-8 inhibitor FLIP

promotes activation of NF-kappaB and Erk signaling pathways. *Curr. Biol.* **2000,** *10*, 640-648.

[65] Dohrman, A.; Kataoka, T.; Cuenin, S.; Russell, J. Q.; Tschopp, J.; Budd, R. C. Cellular FLIP (long form) regulates CD8+ T cell activation through caspase-8-dependent NF-kappa B activation. *J. Immunol.* **2005,** *174*, 5270-5278.

[66] Golks, A.; Brenner, D.; Krammer, P. H.; Lavrik, I. N. The c-FLIP-NH2 terminus (p22-FLIP) induces NF-kappaB activation. *J. Exp. Med.* **2006,** *203*, 1295-1305.

[67] Chang, L.; Kamata, H.; Solinas, G.; Luo, J. L.; Maeda, S.; Venuprasad, K.; Liu, Y. C.; Karin, M. The E3 ubiquitin ligase itch couples JNK activation to TNFalpha-induced cell death by inducing c-FLIP(L) turnover. *Cell.* **2006,** *124*, 601-613.

[68] Day, T. W.; Najafi, F.; Wu, C. H.; Safa, A. R. Cellular FLICE-like inhibitory protein (c-FLIP): A novel target for Taxol-induced apoptosis. *Biochem. Pharmacol.* **2006,** *71*, 1551-1561 Epub 2006 Mar 1531.

[69] Kim, Y. Y.; Park, B. J.; Seo, G. J.; Lim, J. Y.; Lee, S. M.; Kimm, K. C.; Park, C.; Kim, J.; Park, S. I. Long form of cellular FLICE-inhibitory protein interacts with Daxx and prevents Fas-induced JNK activation. *Biochem. Biophys. Res. Commun.* **2003,** *312*, 426-433.

[70] Nakajima, A.; Komazawa-Sakon, S.; Takekawa, M.; Sasazuki, T.; Yeh, W. C.; Yagita, H.; Okumura, K.; Nakano, H. An antiapoptotic protein, c-FLIPL, directly binds to MKK7 and inhibits the JNK pathway. *Embo J.* **2006,** *25*, 5549-5559 Epub 2006 Nov 5516.

[71] Yang, B. F.; Xiao, C.; Roa, W. H.; Krammer, P. H.; Hao, C. Calcium/calmodulin-dependent protein kinase II regulation of c-FLIP expression and phosphorylation in modulation of Fas-mediated signaling in malignant glioma cells. *J. Biol. Chem.* **2003,** *278*, 7043-7050 Epub 2002 Dec 7019.

[72] Higuchi, H.; Yoon, J. H.; Grambihler, A.; Werneburg, N.; Bronk, S. F.; Gores, G. J. Bile acids stimulate cFLIP phosphorylation enhancing TRAIL-mediated apoptosis. *J. Biol. Chem.* **2003,** *278*, 454-461 Epub 2002 Oct 2028.

[73] Misra, R. S.; Russell, J. Q.; Koenig, A.; Hinshaw-Makepeace, J. A.; Wen, R.; Wang, D.; Huo, H.; Littman, D. R.; Ferch, U.; Ruland, J.; Thome, M.; Budd, R. C. Caspase-8 and c-FLIPL Associate in Lipid Rafts with NF-{kappa}B Adaptors during T Cell Activation. *J. Biol. Chem.* **2007,** *282*, 19365-19374 Epub 12007 Apr 19326.

[74] Budd, R. C.; Yeh, W. C.; Tschopp, J. cFLIP regulation of lymphocyte activation and development. *Nat. Rev. Immunol.* **2006,** *6*, 196-204.

[75] Naito, M.; Katayama, R.; Ishioka, T.; Suga, A.; Takubo, K.; Nanjo, M.; Hashimoto, C.; Taira, M.; Takada, S.; Takada, R.; Kitagawa, M.; Matsuzawa, S.; Reed, J. C.; Tsuruo, T. Cellular FLIP inhibits beta-catenin ubiquitylation and enhances Wnt signaling. *Mol. Cell. Biol.* **2004,** *24*, 8418-8427.

[76] Wang, W.; Wang, S.; Song, X.; Sima, N.; Xu, X.; Luo, A.; Chen, G.; Deng, D.; Xu, Q.; Meng, L.; Lu, Y.; Ma, D. The relationship between c-FLIP expression and human papillomavirus E2 gene disruption in cervical carcinogenesis. *Gynecol. Oncol.* **2007,** *105*, 571-577 Epub 2007 Apr 2012.

[77] Gao, S.; Wang, H.; Lee, P.; Melamed, J.; Li, C. X.; Zhang, F.; Wu, H.; Zhou, L.; Wang, Z. Androgen receptor and prostate apoptosis response factor-4 target the c-FLIP gene to determine survival and apoptosis in the prostate gland. *J. Mol. Endocrinol.* **2006,** *36*, 463-483.

[78] Valnet-Rabier, M. B.; Challier, B.; Thiebault, S.; Angonin, R.; Margueritte, G.; Mougin, C.; Kantelip, B.; Deconinck, E.; Cahn, J. Y.; Fest, T. c-Flip protein expression in Burkitt's lymphomas is associated with a poor clinical outcome. *Br. J. Haematol.* **2005,** *128*, 767-773.

[79] Dolcet, X.; Llobet, D.; Pallares, J.; Rue, M.; Comella, J. X.; Matias-Guiu, X. FLIP is frequently expressed in endometrial carcinoma and has a role in resistance to TRAIL-induced apoptosis. *Lab. Invest.* **2005,** *85*, 885-894.

[80] Chen, H. X.; Liu, Y. J.; Zhou, X. D.; Luo, R. Y. Expression of cellular FLICE/caspase-8 inhibitory protein is associated with malignant potential in endometrial carcinoma. *Int. J. Gynecol. Cancer.* **2005,** *15*, 663-670.

[81] Ishioka, T.; Katayama, R.; Kikuchi, R.; Nishimoto, M.; Takada, S.; Takada, R.; Matsuzawa, S.; Reed, J. C.; Tsuruo, T.; Naito, M. Impairment of the ubiquitin-proteasome system by cellular FLIP. *Genes Cells.* **2007,** *12*, 735-744.

[82] Salon, C.; Eymin, B.; Micheau, O.; Chaperot, L.; Plumas, J.; Brambilla, C.; Brambilla, E.; Gazzeri, S. E2F1 induces apoptosis and sensitizes human lung adenocarcinoma cells to death-receptor-mediated apoptosis through specific downregulation of c-FLIP(short). *Cell Death Differ.* **2006,** *13*, 260-272.

[83] Zhou, X. D.; Yu, J. P.; Chen, H. X.; Yu, H. G.; Luo, H. S. Expression of cellular FLICE-inhibitory protein and its association with p53 mutation in colon cancer. *World J. Gastroenterol.* **2005,** *11*, 2482-2485.

[84] Bartke, T.; Siegmund, D.; Peters, N.; Reichwein, M.; Henkler, F.; Scheurich, P.; Wajant, H. p53 upregulates cFLIP, inhibits transcription of NF-kappaB-regulated genes and induces caspase-8-independent cell death in DLD-1 cells. *Oncogene.* **2001,** *20*, 571-580.

[85] Chandrasekaran, Y.; McKee, C. M.; Ye, Y.; Richburg, J. H. Influence of TRP53 status on FAS membrane localization, CFLAR (c-FLIP) ubiquitinylation, and sensitivity of GC-2spd (ts) cells to undergo FAS-mediated apoptosis. *Biol. Reprod.* **2006,** *74*, 560-568 Epub 2005 Nov 2023.

[86] Järvinen, K.; Hotti. A.; Santos, L.; Nummela, P.; Hölttä, E. Caspase-8, c-FLIP, and caspase-9 in c-Myc-induced apoptosis of fibroblasts. *Exp. Cell. Res.* **2011**, 317, 2602-2615.

[87] Ricci, M. S.; Jin, Z.; Dews, M.; Yu, D.; Thomas-Tikhonenko, A.; Dicker, D. T.; El-Deiry, W. S. Direct repression of FLIP expression by c-myc is a major determinant of TRAIL sensitivity. *Mol. Cell. Biol.* **2004,** *24*, 8541-8555.

[88] Li, W.; Zhang, X.; Olumi, A. F. MG-132 sensitizes TRAIL-resistant prostate cancer cells by activating c-Fos/c-Jun heterodimers and repressing c-FLIP(L). *Cancer Res.* **2007,** *67*, 2247-2255.

[89] Panner, A.; James, C. D.; Berger, M. S.; Pieper, R. O. mTOR controls FLIPS translation and TRAIL sensitivity in glioblastoma multiforme cells. *Mol. Cell. Biol.* **2005,** *25*, 8809-8823.

[90] Panner, A.; Nakamura, J. L.; Parsa, A. T.; Rodriguez-Viciana, P.; Berger, M. S.; Stokoe, D.; Pieper, R. O. mTOR-independent translational control of the extrinsic cell death pathway by RalA. *Mol. Cell. Biol.* **2006,** *26*, 7345-7357 Epub 2006 Aug 7347.

[91] Panner, A.; Parsa, A. T.; Pieper, R. O. Translational regulation of TRAIL sensitivity. *Cell Cycle.* **2006,** *5*, 147-150 Epub 2006 Jan 2016.

[92] Wolthuis, R. M.; Bos, J. L. Ras caught in another affair: the exchange factors for Ral. *Curr. Opin. Genet. Dev.* **1999,** *9*, 112-117.

[93] Jullien-Flores, V.; Dorseuil, O.; Romero, F.; Letourneur, F.; Saragosti, S.; Berger, R.; Tavitian, A.; Gacon, G.; Camonis, J. H. Bridging Ral GTPase to Rho pathways. RLIP76, a Ral effector with CDC42/Rac GTPase-activating protein activity. *J. Biol. Chem.* **1995,** *270*, 22473-22477.

[94] Zhang, S.; Shen, H. M.; Ong, C. N. Down-regulation of c-FLIP contributes to the sensitization effect of 3,3'-diindolylmethane on TRAIL-induced apoptosis in cancer cells. *Mol. Cancer Ther.* **2005,** *4*, 1972-1981.

[95] Palacios, C.; Yerbes, R.; Lopez-Rivas, A. Flavopiridol Induces Cellular FLICE-Inhibitory Protein Degradation by the Proteasome and Promotes TRAIL-Induced Early Signaling and Apoptosis in Breast Tumor Cells. *Cancer Res.* **2006,** *66*, 8858-8869.

[96] Kim, Y.; Suh, N.; Sporn, M.; Reed, J. C. An inducible pathway for degradation of FLIP protein sensitizes tumor cells to TRAIL-induced apoptosis. *J. Biol. Chem.* **2002,** *277*, 22320-22329.

[97] Zou, W.; Liu, X.; Yue, P.; Khuri, F. R.; Sun, S. Y. PPARgamma ligands enhance TRAIL-induced apoptosis through DR5 upregulation and c-FLIP downregulation in human lung cancer cells. *Cancer Biol. Ther.* **2007,** *6*, 99-106.

[98] Panner, A.; Crane, C.A.; Weng, C.; Feletti, A.; Fang, S.; Parsa, A.T.; Pieper, R.O. Ubiquitin-specific protease 8 links the PTEN-Akt-AIP4 pathway to the control of FLIPS stability and TRAIL sensitivity in glioblastoma multiforme. *Cancer Res.* **2010**, *70*, 5046-5053.

[99] Kabore, A. F.; Sun, J.; Hu, X.; McCrea, K.; Johnston, J. B.; Gibson, S. B. The TRAIL apoptotic pathway mediates proteasome inhibitor induced apoptosis in primary chronic lymphocytic leukemia cells. *Apoptosis.* **2006,** *11*, 1175-1193.

[100] Sayers, T. J.; Brooks, A. D.; Koh, C. Y.; Ma, W.; Seki, N.; Raziuddin, A.; Blazar, B. R.; Zhang, X.; Elliott, P. J.; Murphy, W. J. The proteasome inhibitor PS-341 sensitizes neoplastic cells to TRAIL-mediated apoptosis by reducing levels of c-FLIP. *Blood.* **2003,** *102*, 303-310.

[101] Abedini, M. R.; Qiu, Q.; Yan, X.; Tsang, B. K. Possible role of FLICE-like inhibitory protein (FLIP) in chemoresistant ovarian cancer cells *in vitro*. *Oncogene.* **2004,** *23*, 6997-7004.

[102] Wilson, T. R.; McLaughlin, K. M.; McEwan, M.; Sakai, H.; Rogers, K. M.; Redmond, K. M.; Johnston, P. G.; Longley, D. B. c-FLIP: a key regulator of colorectal cancer cell death. *Cancer Res.* **2007,** *67*, 5754-5762.

[103] Rogers, K. M.; Thomas, M.; Galligan, L.; Wilson, T. R.; Allen, W. L.; Sakai, H.; Johnston, P. G.; Longley, D. B. Cellular FLICE-inhibitory protein regulates chemotherapy-induced apoptosis in breast cancer cells. *Mol. Cancer Ther.* **2007,** *6*, 1544-1551.

[104] Dutton, A.; Young, L. S.; Murray, P. G. The role of cellular FLICE inhibitory protein (c-FLIP) in the pathogenesis and treatment of cancer. *Expert. Opin. Ther. Targets.* **2006,** *10*, 27-35.

[105] Day T.W.; Safa A.R. RNA interference in cancer: targeting the anti-apoptotic protein c-FLIP for drug discovery. *Mini. Rev. Med. Chem.* **2009,** 9, 741-748.

[106] Piggott, L.; Omidvar, N.; Martí Pérez, S.; Eberl, M.; Clarkson, R.W. Suppression of apoptosis inhibitor c-FLIP selectively eliminates breast cancer stem cell activity in response to the anti-cancer agent, TRAIL. *Breast Cancer Res.* **2011** Sep 14, *13*, R88

[107] Shivapurkar, N.; Reddy, J.; Matta, H.; Sathyanarayana, U. G.; Huang, C. X.; Toyooka, S.; Minna, J. D.; Chaudhary, P. M.; Gazdar, A. F. Loss of expression of death-inducing signaling complex (DISC) components in lung cancer cell lines and the influence of MYC amplification. *Oncogene.* **2002,** *21*, 8510-8514.

[108] Song, J. H.; Song, D. K.; Herlyn, M.; Petruk, K. C.; Hao, C. Cisplatin down-regulation of cellular Fas-associated death domain-like interleukin-1beta-converting enzyme-like

inhibitory proteins to restore tumor necrosis factor-related apoptosis-inducing ligand-induced apoptosis in human melanoma cells. *Clin. Cancer Res.* **2003,** *9*, 4255-4266.

[109] Kelly, M. M.; Hoel, B. D.; Voelkel-Johnson, C. Doxorubicin pretreatment sensitizes prostate cancer cell lines to TRAIL induced apoptosis which correlates with the loss of c-FLIP expression. *Cancer Biol. Ther.* **2002,** *1*, 520-527.

[110] Sun, C. L.; Chao, C. C. Cross-resistance to death ligand-induced apoptosis in cisplatin-selected HeLa cells associated with overexpression of DDB2 and subsequent induction of cFLIP. *Mol. Pharmacol.* **2005,** *67*, 1307-1314 Epub 2005 Jan 1311.

[111] Zhang, L.; Zhang, X.; Barrisford, G. W.; Olumi, A. F. Lexatumumab (TRAIL-receptor 2 mAb) induces expression of DR5 and promotes apoptosis in primary and metastatic renal cell carcinoma in a mouse orthotopic model. *Cancer Lett.* **2007,** *251*, 146-157.

[112] Zhao, X.; Qiu, W.; Kung, J.; Zhao, X.; Peng, X.; Yegappan, M.; Yen-Lieberman, B.; Hsi, E. D. Bortezomib induces caspase-dependent apoptosis in Hodgkin lymphoma cell lines and is associated with reduced c-FLIP expression: A gene expression profiling study with implications for potential combination therapies. *Leuk. Res.* **2007,** *18*, 18.

[113] Liu, X.; Yue, P.; Chen, S.; Hu, L.; Lonial, S.; Khuri, F. R.; Sun, S. Y. The proteasome inhibitor PS-341 (bortezomib) up-regulates DR5 expression leading to induction of apoptosis and enhancement of TRAIL-induced apoptosis despite up-regulation of c-FLIP and survivin expression in human NSCLC cells. *Cancer Res.* **2007,** *67*, 4981-4988.

[114] Hideshima, T.; Chauhan, D.; Richardson, P.; Mitsiades, C.; Mitsiades, N.; Hayashi, T.; Munshi, N.; Dang, L.; Castro, A.; Palombella, V.; Adams, J.; Anderson, K. C. NF-kappa B as a therapeutic target in multiple myeloma. *J. Biol. Chem.* **2002,** *277*, 16639-16647.

[115] Okamoto, K.; Fujisawa, J.; Reth, M.; Yonehara, S. Human T-cell leukemia virus type-I oncoprotein Tax inhibits Fas-mediated apoptosis by inducing cellular FLIP through activation of NF-kappaB. *Genes Cells.* **2006,** *11*, 177-191.

[116] Hyer, M. L.; Croxton, R.; Krajewska, M.; Krajewski, S.; Kress, C. L.; Lu, M.; Suh, N.; Sporn, M. B.; Cryns, V. L.; Zapata, J. M.; Reed, J. C. Synthetic triterpenoids cooperate with tumor necrosis factor-related apoptosis-inducing ligand to induce apoptosis of breast cancer cells. *Cancer Res.* **2005,** *65*, 4799-4808.

[117] Syed, V.; Mukherjee, K.; Godoy-Tundidor, S.; Ho, S. M. Progesterone induces Apoptosis in TRAIL-resistant ovarian cancer cells by circumventing c-FLIP(L) overexpression. *J. Cell. Biochem.* **2007,** *28*, 28.

[118] Komatsu, N.; Kawamata, N.; Takeuchi, S.; Yin, D.; Chien, W.; Miller, C. W.; Koeffler, H. P. SAHA, a HDAC inhibitor, has profound anti-growth activity against non-small cell lung cancer cells. *Oncol. Rep.* **2006,** *15*, 187-191.

[119] Minucci, S.; Pelicci, P. G. Histone deacetylase inhibitors and the promise of epigenetic (and more) treatments for cancer. *Nat. Rev. Cancer.* **2006,** *6*, 38-51.

[120] Liu, T.; Kuljaca, S.; Tee, A.; Marshall, G. M. Histone deacetylase inhibitors: multifunctional anticancer agents. *Cancer Treat. Rev.* **2006,** *32*, 157-165.

[121] Al-Yacoub, N.; Fecker, L.F.; Möbs, M.; Plötz, M.; Braun, F.K.; Sterry, W.; Eberle, J. Apoptosis induction by SAHA in cutaneous T-cell lymphoma cells is related to downregulation of c-FLIP and enhanced TRAIL signaling. *J. Invest. Dermatol.* **2012** May 3. doi: 10.1038/jid.2012.125. [Epub ahead of print].

[122] Yerbes, R.; López-Rivas, A.; Itch/AIP4-independent proteasomal degradation of cFLIP induced by the histone deacetylase inhibitor SAHA sensitizes breast tumour cells to TRAIL. *Invest. New Drugs.* **2012,** *30*, 541-547.

[123] Mawji, I.A.; Simpson, C.D.; Gronda, M.; Williams, M.A.; Hurren, R.; Henderson C.J.; Datti, A.; Wrana, J.L.; Schimmer, A.D. A chemical screen identifies anisomycin as an anoikis sensitizer that functions by decreasing FLIP protein synthesis. *Cancer Res.* **2007**, *67*, 8307-8315.

[124] Wood, T.E.; Dalili, S.; Simpson, C.D.; Sukhai, M.A.; Hurren, R.; Anyiwe, K.; Mao, X.; Suarez, Saiz F.; Gronda, M.; Eberhard, Y.; MacLean, N.; Ketela, T.; Reed, J. C.; Moffat, J.; Minden, M. D.; Batey, R. A.; Schimmer, A. D. Selective inhibition of histone deacetylases sensitizes malignant cells to death receptor ligands. *Mol. Cancer Ther.* **2010**, 9, 246-456.

[125] Bijangi-Vishehsaraei K.; Saadatzadeh M.R.; Huang, S.; Murphy, M.P.; Safa, A.R. 4-(4-Chloro-2-methylphenoxy)-N-hydroxybutanamide (CMH) targets mRNA of the c-FLIP variants and induces apoptosis in MCF-7 human breast cancer cells. *Mol. Cell. Biochem.* **2010,** *342*, 133-142.

[126] Kerr, E.; Holohan, C; McLaughlin K. M.; Majkut, J.; Dolan, S.; Redmond, K.; Riley, J.; McLaughlin, K.; Stasik, I.; Crudden, M.; Van Schaeybroeck S.; Fenning C.; O'Connor R.; Kiely, P.; Sgobba, M.; Haigh, D.; Johnston P. G.; Longley, D. B. Identification of an acetylation-dependent Ku70/FLIP complex that regulates FLIP expression and HDAC inhibitor-induced apoptosis. *Cell Death Differ.* **2012,** *19*, 1317-1327.

[127] Bleumink, M.; Köhler, R.; Giaisi, M.; Proksch, P.; Krammer, P.H.; Li-Weber, M. Rocaglamide breaks TRAIL resistance in HTLV-1-associated adult T-cell leukemia/lymphoma by translational suppression of c-FLIP expression. *Cell Death Differ.* **2011**, *18*, 362-370.

[128] Subramaniam, K.; Hirpara, JL.; Tucker-Kellogg, L.; Tucker-Kellogg, G.; Pervaiz, S. FLIP: A flop for execution signals. *Cancer Lett.* **2012** Jul 7. [Epub ahead of print].

Send Orders of Reprints at bspsaif@emirates.net.ae

Advances in Cancer Drug Targets, Vol. 1, 2013, 146-171

CHAPTER 5

Pin1: A Promising Novel Diagnostic and Therapeutic Target that Acts on Numerous Cancer-Driving Pathways

Greg Finn*, Man-Li Luo*, Xiao Zhen Zhou* and Kun Ping Lu*

Cancer Biology Program, Division of Hematology/Oncology, Department of Medicine, Beth Israel Deaconess Medical Center, Harvard Medical School, 3 Blankfan Circle, CLS 0408, Boston, MA 02115, USA

Abstract: Proline-directed phosphorylation is a common and central regulatory mechanism in cell proliferation and oncogenic transformation. In fact, numerous oncogenes and tumor suppressors themselves are directly regulated by proline-directed phosphorylation and/or can trigger signaling pathways involving proline-directed phosphorylation. Our recent identification of the phosphorylation dependent prolyl isomerase Pin1 has uncovered a novel signaling mechanism controlling protein function after phosphorylation *via* conformational changes. Importantly, Pin1 deregulation plays a pivotal role in the development of some diseases, providing a new therapeutic option, most notably for cancers. Pin1 is prevalently overexpressed and its levels correlate with poor clinical outcome in human cancers. Significantly, Pin1 is required for activation of multiple oncogenic pathways by acting on numeroous oncogenes and tumor suppressors. Moreover, Pin1 knockdown or knockout inhibits cancer cell growth and prevents cell transformation and tumorigenesis induced either by oncogenes or tumor suppressors *in vitro* and *in vivo*. Pin1-mediated post-phosphorylation isomerisation represents a unique regulatory mechanism in cell signalling whose upregulation during tumorigenesis promotes the pro-proliferative capacity of tumour cells. Accumulating evidences indicate that Pin1 may represent a novel tumour marker and potential therapeutic target. Therefore, there is an urgent need to develop Pin1-specific inhibitors because they may have the desired property to suppress numerous oncogenic pathways, which are often activated simultaneously in cancers, especially in those aggressive and drug-resistant ones.

Keywords: Proline-directed phosphorylation, cancer-driving pathways, cell transformation, tumorigenesis, Pin1, oncogenesis, *cis*-conformation, *trans*-conformation.

INTRODUCTION

Recent advances in the understanding of molecular mechanisms of oncogenesis

***Address correspondence to Kun Ping Lu, Greg Finn and Xiao Zhen Zhou:** Cancer Biology Program, Division of Hematology/Oncology, Department of Medicine, Beth Israel Deaconess Medical Center, Harvard Medical School, 77 Avenue Louis Pasteur, NRB 1030, Boston, MA 02115, USA; Tel: 617-735-2016; Fax, 617-735-2050; E-mail: klu@bidmc.harvard.edu; gfinn@bidmc.harvard.edu; xzhou@bidmc.harvard.edu have led to the development of an increasing number of exciting new drugs that selectively target specific oncogenic pathways [1]. However, since multiple interacting and/or redundant pathways are often activated simultaneously in many individual tumors, a major challenge remains how to control these multiple pathways at the same time.

A common and central regulatory mechanism in cell proliferation and transformation is proline-directed phosphorylation on certain Ser/Thr-Pro (pSer/Thr-Pro) motifs. In fact, numerous oncogenes and tumor suppressors themselves are directly regulated by Pro-directed phosphorylation and/or can trigger signaling pathways involving Pro-directed phosphorylation [2]. The unique stereochemistry of Pro means that it can adopt two distinct *cis* or *trans* conformations. However, the biological significance of these conformational switches was unappreciated for a long time and has not yet been explored for cancer treatments [3, 4].

A major advance in this area was the recent discovery of a unique prolyl isomerase, Pin1 that catalyzes *cis/trans* isomerization of specific pSer/Thr-Pro motifs in a subset of proteins to regulate cell signaling [4]. Importantly, Pin1 has emerged as a novel molecular timer to help drive certain cellular processes synergistically to one direction [5]. Moreover, Pin1 deregulation plays a pivotal role in the development of some diseases, providing a potentially new therapeutic option, most notably for cancers [2-6].

We and others have shown that Pin1 is prevalently overexpressed in human cancers and that high Pin1 levels correlate with poor clinical outcome in many cancers [2, 4]. In contrast, the Pin1 polymorphism that reduces Pin1 expression is associated with reduced cancer risk in humans. Significantly, Pin1 activates a huge and increasing number of oncogenes/growth enhancers and also inactivates an increasing number of tumor suppressors/growth inhibitors [6]. Furthermore, whereas Pin1 overexpression causes cell transformation and tumorigenesis [7], Pin1 knockdown inhibits cancer cell growth in cell cultures and mice [8]. Moreover, Pin1-null mice are highly resistant to tumorigenesis induced either by oncogenes such as activated Ras or HER2/Neu or tumor suppressors such as p53 [4, 9]. Thus, Pin1 inhibitors might have the desired property to suppress numerous oncogenic pathways simultaneously.

OVERVIEW & STRUCTURAL BASIS FOR Pin1 MODE OF ACTION

Pin1 belongs to a family of conserved proteins known as peptidyl-prolyl isomerases (PPIase) of which there are at least three major families namely, cyclophillins, FK506 binding proteins and parvulins. Pin1 is a parvulin type PPIase whose enzyme activity arises from the fact that proline has a unique five-carbonyl ring structure existing as two distinct conformers, cis and trans. In peptides, proline interconversion occurs spontaneously at a very slow rate, hence the need for PPIases. Furthermore, when a proline is positioned at the +1 position to an adjacent phosphorylated serine or threonine, the cis to trans conversion is even more thermodynamically hindered and rendered inaccessible to conventional PPIases such as cyclophillins and FKBPs [10]. This is where the action of Pin1 is distinguished from other PPIases as it remains the only PPIase thus far identified which functions in a phosphorylation specific manner. Pin1 has a modular domain architecture consisting of an N terminal WW domain, a flexible linker and a C terminal PPIase domain. Pin1 targets its substrates by means of the WW domain that binds to pSer/Thr-Proline motifs in substrate proteins [11-13]. The catalytic isomerase activity of Pin1 arises from the PPIase domain. The two domain structure of Pin1 allows for added control as the WW domain will only bind to phosphorylated Ser/Thr-pro motifs in target proteins which have been shown to be critical regulatory sites of function in many proteins [14]. Recent X-ray and NMR structural analyses not only confirmed this basic principle, but also revealed how Pin1 binds its substrates to regulate their conformation. Direct analysis of Pin1 activity on its substrate by means of NMR has illustrated the dynamics of Pin1 PPIase activity on the APP intracellular domain [15]. Specifically, the Thr668-Pro motif in APP exists in trans conformer prior to phosphorylation, and the cis conformation is favored after phosphorylation due to local structural constraints, indicating that Pin1 catalyzes the interconversion between both conformations. Of note, the Pin1 WW domain exhibits almost the same affinity for cis and trans pThr668-Pro in APP [15]. These results indicate that WW binding to cis or trans or both conformations of a pSer/Thr-Pro motif is sequence-specific, as the Pin1 WW domain binds to tau and CTD phosphopeptides in trans [16, 17]. NMR analysis of the interaction of Pin1 with Cdc25 phosphopeptide substrate also reveals dynamic changes in the side-chain flexibility in several regions including a hydrophobic cluster proximal to catalytic-site residues, residues within the catalytic loop, and residues forming the hydrophobic interface between the WW and PPIase domains [18, 19]. These elaborate studies have revealed the mechanism of Pin1 action on a subset of substrates, however further development of this knowledge is required to fully understand how Pin1 regulates some phospho-S/T-Pro bonds but not others. We believe that future developments in structural analysis techniques such as NMR and visualisation technologies such as Fret and Flim will add to our knowledge of the mechanism of action of not only Pin1 but other PPIases. One important future development will be the demonstration of PPIase activity and conformational regulation on substrates *in vivo.*

DISCOVERY AND CELL CYCLE FUNCTION

The Pin1 gene was originally identified in 1996 in a combined genetic and biochemical screen searching for proteins involved in mitotic regulation in yeast and was shown to be the first PPIase that is essential for cell division in yeast [14]. The original discovery of Pin1, lead to the discovery that Pin1 was a regulator of cell cycle transition primarily through mitosis. Subsequent studies in mammalian cells and higher organisms uncovered more varied and complex activities of this enzyme [20]. In particular, primary analysis of mice homozygous for deletion of Pin1 revealed phenotypes similar to those found for cyclin D1 deletion, namely that they displayed a range of cell-proliferative abnormalities, including decreased body weight and testicular and retinal atrophies [21]. Furthermore, in Pin1 null adult females, the breast epithelial compartment failed to undergo the massive proliferative changes associated with pregnancy [21]. Moreover, Pin1 directly bound to phosphorylated cyclin D1, increased cyclin D1 retention in the nucleus and stabilized cyclin D1 protein. These results indicated that Pin1 positively regulates cyclin D1. Further studies also demonstrated regulation of cyclin D1 in cells and tissues from cancer and normal subjects validating the role for Pin1 in cyclin D1 regulation [22]. Pin1 has been shown to be a key regulator of timely cell cycle transition by acting on multiple substrates. For example, Pin1 binds to Cdc25C during mitosis and catalyzes conformational changes in Cdc25C to regulate its catalytic activity directly or indirectly *via* regulation of its dephosphorylation [17, 23]. Pin1 is also a regulator of the anaphase-promoting complex(APC) early mitotic inhibitor 1(Emi1), which is required to induce S- and M-phase entries by stimulating the accumulation of cyclin A and cyclin B through APC inhibition [24]. Pin1 acts on phosphorylated Emi1, leading to Emi1 stabilization by preventing its association with SCF (beta-Trcp) during G2 phase of the cell cycle. In addition, Pin1 binds the pThr-Pro motif within the Wee-box which is phosphorylated by Cdc2 during M phase that functions to inactivate Wee1B, which is essential for the normal kinase activity of Wee1B during interphase [25]. The Pin1-dependent activation of Emi1 or inhibition of Wee1 may allow Emi1 and Wee1 to be controlled in such a fashion to allow co-ordination of cell cycle progression. Given that activated Cdc2 phosphorylates a large number of proteins which are also targeted by Pin1 and that Pin1 deletion leads to mitotic catastrophe, suggests Pin1 might help harmonize mitotic signaling cues following phosphorylation to provide a means for temporal regulation of signaling to proceed in a synchronous manner [26]. Recently, a role for Pin1 in mitotic chromosome condensation was demonstrated where the interaction of Pin1 with chromatin was enhanced in G2/M phase and this was accompanied by increased phosphorylated topoisomerase II alpha detected on chromosomes [27].

In addition a role for Pin1 in controlling cell cycle regulation was demonstrated by analysis of Pin1 null mouse embryonic fibroblasts (MEF) cells by at least two groups who showed that Pin1 null MEFs were slower in re-entry to the cell cycle following serum starvation [28, 29]. It therefore appears that Pin1 not only controls mitotic events but also coordinates G0/1 to S progression, further validated by the findings that Pin1 regulates Ki67, Cyclin E and c-MYC [30, 31]. Subsequent analysis of Pin1 null mice and cells has revealed novel roles for Pin1 apparently independent of its role in cell cycle regulation, specifically Pin1 has been found to play a role in both neurodegeneration and immune function reviewed in detail elsewhere [3, 32, 33].

PIN1 AND CANCER

The primary indications that Pin1 was involved in cancer came from the findings where Pin1 was found to be overexpressed in human cancer tissues [22, 34]. Subsequent studies have confirmed that the levels of Pin1 are indeed increased in cancerous cell lines and tissues of varied tissue origins [35, 36]. This has been confirmed and expanded by comparing Pin1 expression in 60 different human tumor types and their corresponding normal tissues. Pin1 overexpression is observed in most common cancers including prostate, breast, lung and colon cancer. Moreover, Pin1 overexpression in prostate cancer positively correlates with a higher probability of and a shorter period to tumor recurrence following radical prostatectomy [37, 38]. Pin1 overexpression has been shown to have some prognostic value in other cancers including colon and lung cancer. Meanwhile, the Pin1 polymorphisms that reduce Pin1 expression are associated with reduced cancer risk in humans [39-41]. Comparison of Pin1 expression with other tumor markers in human cancer tissues has uncovered the role of Pin1 in oncogenesis where, Pin1 expression is closely correlated with cyclin D1 levels, which is intrinsically involved in oncogenesis [42-44]. Subsequent studies using *in vitro* models, animal models and human tumor samples have demonstrated an essential role of Pin1 in regulating cyclin D1 function and consequently, oncogenesis. Given its role in regulating cell cycle coupled to its overexpression in certain cancers suggests that Pin1 may have a role as a novel therapeutic target and/or tumor marker. This was recently demonstrated in a study correlating Pin1 expression levels from 580 prostate cancer (PCa) patients to clinical outcome following radical prostatectomy [38]. Interestingly, this study showed that Pin1 expression is significantly overexpressed in PCa cells and in comparison to know pathological PCa markers of clinical outcome, Pin1 was a better indicator of not only recurrence but also of recurrent disease manifested as distant metastasis, suggesting that analysis of Pin1 status in PCa patients maybe of value in the clinic.

Mechanistically, Pin1 can increase cyclin D1 gene expression by multiple mechanisms, including activating c-Jun/c-Fos, β-catenin/TCF and NF-κB transcription factors [22, 34, 45, 46]. Furthermore, Pin1 can directly bind cyclin D1 to increase its half life [21]. Pin1 is an E2F target gene due to three E2F sites in the Pin1 promoter [47]. The transcription of E2F is activated in response to Her2/Neu or Ras activation and this is suggestive of a positive feedback loop. Furthermore, overexpression of Pin1 not only confers transforming properties on mammary epithelial cells but also enhances the transformed phenotypes of Neu/Ras-transformed mammary epithelial cells [47]. In contrast, inhibition of

Pin1 suppresses Neu- and Ras-induced transformed phenotypes, which can be rescued by expression of a constitutively active cyclin D1 mutant that is refractory to the Pin1 inhibition. A separate study demonstrated that Pin1interacts with Raf-1 to facilitate a regulatory mechanism that contributes to the sensitive modulation of Ras signalling [48]. Subsequently, using mouse models of mammary oncogenesis it was found that Pin1 ablation was highly effective in preventing oncogenic Neu or Ras from inducing cyclin D1 and breast cancer in mice, although it neither affects transgene expression nor mammary gland development [9]. Activation of the Wnt/β-catenin signaling pathway is a major feature of several human cancers [9, 49]. Deregulation of this signaling pathway has been found in a subset of human malignancies that carry mutations in proteins participating in this pathway, such as APC(adenomatous polyposis coli), axin and β-catenin [50]. The end result of this aberrant activation is always the cytosolic stabilization of β-catenin, which enhances the transcription of a number of target genes, including the cyclin D1 and MYC, which can lead to oncogenesis [50]. In addition, Pin1 is found to be a novel regulator of ErbB2 that modulates the ubiquitin-mediated degradation of ErbB2 [51]. Although Her2/Neu overexpression is primarily a result of ErbB2 amplification, the overexpression of Pin1 in a majority of Her2-overexpressing breast cancer may contribute to maintain ErbB2 levels.

A differential display screen for genes regulated by Pin1 that compared inducible Pin1-overexpressing MCF-7 breast cancer cells and control cells identified 17 known genes. Interestingly, four genes whose expression was unregulated are targets of β-catenin and its transcriptional partner TCF namely cyclin D1, MYC, PPAR-delta and fibronectin, furthermore β-catenin levels were decreased in Pin1-knockout mouse tissues [34]. The role of Pin1 in cancer is further supported by the recent findings that Pin1 overexpression correlates with centrosome amplification in human cancer tissues and that Pin1 overexpression induces centrosome amplification, aneuploidy and tumorigenesis *in vitro* and *in vivo* [7]. These results indicate that certain oncogenes can increase Pin1 expression *via* E2F, which in turn activates multiple upstream oncogenic signaling pathways allowing progression of downstream cell cycle events such as centrosome amplification cell cycle progression.

On the contrary, a recent study has intimated that Pin1 deletion may function to promote genomic instability at least in rodent fibroblasts. This study demonstrated that Pin1 null fibroblasts from isogenic B6 mice were more prone to transformation by Ras and the stability of c-MYC and cyclin E was enhanced due the loss of Pin1 and the authors suggested that Pin1 may be a conditional tumor suppressor in the isogenic B6 mice [31]. However, this hypothesis has been challenged by the findings that in double Pin1/p53 deficient mice in the B6 background, the instance of malignant tumor formation is completely blocked although these mice show increased normal proliferation of thymocytes due to a defective differentiation pathway [52]. It will be interesting to validate this finding in the context of epithelial cells of human origin where oncogenes such as Ras and MYC are established as true initiators of tumor formation.

Pin1 has been shown to also have role in regulation of the steroid receptor coactivator AIB1/SRC3 [53]. In this study, Pin1 cooperated with AIB1 to enhance estrogen dependent transactivation in breast cancer cells. The authors suggested that Pin1 functions as a transcriptional coactivator of nuclear receptors by modulating SRC-3 coactivator protein-protein complex formation and ultimately by also promoting the turnover of the activated SRC-3 oncoprotein, presumably affecting promoter occupancy turnover [53]. In addition, Pin1 has also been shown to regulate the stability of the ER transcriptional repressor SMRT downstream of growth factor receptors such as HER2 [54]. On a similar but distinct theme, a recent study has also shown a direct regulatory role for Pin1 on ERα where phosphorylation of ERα in the AF1 domain promotes binding and isomerisation of ERα and increased transactivation. Importantly, this regulation of AF1 function occurred in response to not only estrogen but also the antagonist pharmaceutical, tamoxifen and growth factors indicating that the activity of Pin1 may be promoting drug resistance and estrogen independent activation of ERα under certain circumstances. These findings are intriguing as they illustrate the complex orchestration of an oncogenic signalling pathway by Pin1 dependent isomerisation at multiple levels and also due to the observation that overexpression and increased activation of Pin1 in multiple types of breast cancer including those where ERα is not thought to play a significant role [55].

A recent paper also shows a role for Pin1 in controlling the maximal transcriptional activity of the transcription factor Stat-3, where Pin1 was found to target phosphorylated Stat3 following cytokine stimulation to promote Stat3 transcriptional activity and target gene expression, as well as recruitment of transcription coactivator, p300 [56]. Consequently, the authors suggested that Pin1 was an indispensable co-factor for coordinated Stat3 activity and speculated as to the regulatory crosstalk between Pin1 over-expression and the constitutive activation of Stat3 in breast cancer.

A role for Pin1 in response to genotoxic stress and apoptosis has also been demonstrated by several reports [57]. Firstly, Pin1 has been shown to regulate several key proteins regulating genotoxicity responses, most notably p53 and p73 [58-61]. Pin1 binds to phosphorylated p53 and p73 and increases p53 protein stability by inhibiting its binding to MDM2 or p73 protein stability by promoting its binding to and acetylation by p300 in c-Abl dependent manner similar to the mechanism observed for Pin1 on Stat3. As a consequence, Pin1 appears to be essential for activation of the apoptotic response by endogenous p73. In addition, Pin1 can also enhance the DNA-binding activity and transcriptional activity of both p53 and p73 towards their target genes. Similarly, Pin1 can affect the stability of Che-1, an RNA polymerase II-binding protein that plays an important role in transcriptional activation of p53 and in the maintenance of the G(2)/M checkpoint [62]. Functionally, Pin1 appears to be required for maintaining DNA damage checkpoint controls, protecting from DNA damage-induced apoptosis during normal cell cycle transition, but also to accelerate apoptosis depending on the cellular cues encountered by cells. A recent study examined the contribution of Pin1 in tumorigenesis *in vivo* using a p53 derived mouse model [52]. As described above they found that mice deleted for both Pin1 and p53 results in thymic hyperplasia due to defective differentiation and that while p53-deficient mice spontaneously developed lymphomas, mainly of thymic origin, as well as generalized lymphoma infiltration into other organs, the deletion of Pin1 completely prevented the development of malignant tumors induced by p53 knockout [52]. Mutation of p53 occurs in 15 to 20% of all breast cancers, and hotspot mutations turn p53 from a tumor suppressor into an oncogene. Interestingly, Pin1 also promotes the gain of function of mutant p53 [63]. Pin1 enhances tumorigenesis in a Li-Fraumeni mouse model and cooperates with mutant p53(R172H) in Ras-dependent transformation. In breast cancer cells, Pin1 promotes mutant p53 dependent inhibition of the antimetastatic factor p63 and induction of a mutant p53 transcriptional program to increase aggressiveness. Combination of high Pin1 levels and p53 mutation is a predictor of poor prognosis in breast cancer patients.

In addition, Pin1 can regulate mitochondrial import of the 66 kDa isoform of the growth factor adapter Shc(p66Shc) in response to oxidative damage [64]. Activation of protein kinase C β by oxidative conditions induces phosphorylation of p66Shc and triggers mitochondrial accumulation of the protein after it is recognized by Pin1, suggesting that Pin1 could promote aging. Together with the findings that Pin1 can be inactivated by oxidative stress suggest that Pin1 plays a role in response to different stress signals especially during aging [64, 65]. However, Pin1 knockout in mice causes a range of premature aging phenotypes and prevents oncogenesis induced by p53 knockout (20). Consequently, it will be interesting to examine the role of Pin1 in response to cellular stresses using Pin1 null mice as this will allow for a better comparison of these conflicting results.

Hepatitis B virus (HBV) is the most common etiological agent in hepatocellular carcinoma (HCC). Among the four proteins that are encoded by the HBV genome, HBV x (HBx) is the most potentially oncogenic factor. The role of Pin1 in hepatocarcinogenesis, particularly in HBV-related HCC, was investigated in a recent study where it was found that Pin1 binds to phosphorylated HBx in HBV infected cells to elevate its protein levels and transcription activity, as well as synergistically potentate the ability of HBx to increase proliferation *in vitro*, and to stimulate tumor formation in mice using non-transformed hepatocytes, suggesting that Pin1 contributes to hepatocarcinogenesis induced by HBV [50, 66]. This is not the first time a PPIase has been found to interact with a viral protein as is the case for cyclophillin A and the HIV1, gag envelope protein, but it does appear to be the first report for Pin1 binding to a viral phospho-protein [67]. Consequently, we suggest that Pin1 plays a role in the oncogenic "rewiring" of cellular signalling pathways to promote pro-proliferative signals *via* cell cycle regulation and ultimately tumorigenesis.

REGULATION OF PIN1

A number of studies have demonstrated that Pin1 itself is regulated by post-translational regulatory mechanisms. Firstly, Pin1 is known to be phosphorylated at serine 16 in the WW domain that serves to inhibit its interaction with substrates where it is thought that Pin1 is retained in an inactive form in resting cells by S16 phosphorylation [12, 68, 69]. Also, it has been shown that Pin1 is phosphorylated at serine 65 by polo like kinase 1 (Plk1) a kinase also found to be overexpressed in several cancers [70]. Interestingly, the phosphorylation of Pin1 by Plk1 did not affect its isomerase activity but rather prevented its degradation by the proteasome [65, 70, 71]. Recently, Pin1 has been found to be phosphorylated at Ser71 by death-associated protein kinase 1 (DAPK1) [72]. Such phosphorylation fully inactivates Pin1 catalytic activity and inhibits its nuclear location and cellular functions, including the ability of Pin1 to induce centrosome amplification and cell transformation. Pin1 is also found to be phosphorylated on a Ser138 site by mixed-lineage kinase 3 (MLK3), leading to an increased catalytic activity and nuclear translocation [73]. In addition, oxidative inactivation of Pin1 has been demonstrated during the early stages of AD [65, 74]. Pin1 is also regulated at the transcriptional level as it is a direct target of E2F during cell cycle transition and as a consequence it is evident of a positive feed back loop, where Pin1 is regulated by Ras/Neu expression that itself drives E2F and consequentially the expression and stability of cyclin D1 is positively affected and in this way proliferation is promoted [47]. It remains to be seen if Pin1 is regulated in a disease specific manner however, there are some indications that this maybe the case in both cancer and asthma and more information will be required to fully determine the contribution of such mechanisms to disease and pathological progression.

PIN1: A UNIQUE CANCER TARGET ACTING ON NUMEROUS CANCER-DRIVING PATHWAYS

Examination of the data as a whole obtained for Pin1 thus far suggests that Pin1 may represent a new target worthy of investigation in a variety of diseases, most notably cancer. There are a number of compelling reasons that make Pin1 as a unique and attractive new anti-cancer target. First, human Pin1 is a readily purified, active enzyme that has high substrate specificity and well-defined active site structure [75]. Second, Pin1 uses its WW domain to target itself to the substrate, where its PPIase domain isomerizes specific phosphorylated Ser/Thr-Pro motifs to regulate protein function [4]. Since the affinity of the PPIase domain towards substrates is quite weak, a potent catalytic inhibitor would effectively abolish Pin1 function. Third, Pin1 activates numerous oncogenes/growth enhancers, including β-catenin [34], cyclin D1 [21], NF-κB [46], c-Jun [22], c-fos [45], Raf-1 [48], Stat3 [56], c-Myb [76], Neu/ErbB2 [51], Notch [77], AKT [78], AIB1 [53], Mcl-1 [79], Hbx [80], Tax [81] and v-Rel [82], and also inactivates a large number of tumor suppressors/growth inhibitors, including FOXOs [83], PML [84], Daxx [85], Bcl2 [86], RARα [87], SMRT [54], Smad [88], Pin2/TRF1 [89], Fbw7 [90], AMPK [91], and Rb [92], and p53 (based on Pin1/p53 double KO mice) [52] (Fig. **1**). Fourth, Pin1 is overexpressed in 60-70% of total human cancers with high levels being correlated with poor clinical outcome [2, 4],

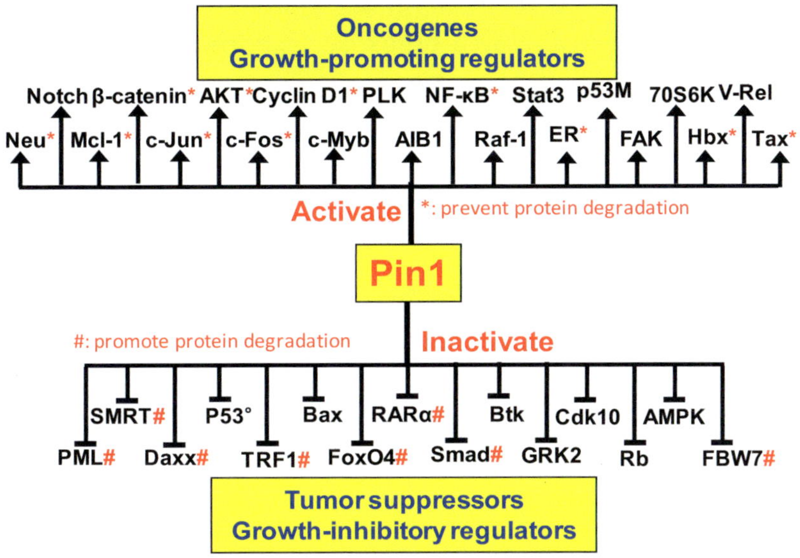

Figure 1: Pin1 is a promising diagnostic and therapeutic target that promotes tumorigenesis by activating numerous oncogenes and inactivating numerous tumor suppressors. (Modified from Lee, T. H., Pastorino, L. & Lu, K. P. Expet Rev Mol Med 13, e21(2011).

whereas low Pin1 expression is associated with reduced cancer risk. Fifth, Pin1 overexpression transforms normal cells, enhances transformed phenotype by oncogenes and causes tumorigenesis *in vitro* and *in vivo* [4, 7]. Sixth, Pin1 inhibition in cancer cells induces apoptosis or suppresses the transformed phenotype and Pin1 knockdown efficiently suppresses cancer cell growth *in vitro* and in mice [8]. Seventh, Pin1 knockout in mice prevents cancer development induced by overexpression of oncogenes such as Ras or Her2/Neu or knockout of tumor suppressors such as p53 [4, 9]. Of note, Pin1 knockout mice develop some age-dependent phenotypes, including retinal and neuronal degeneration, but only after more half of their life span without Pin1 [3, 4]. Together with the facts that Pin1-deficient mice develop normally to adulthood and that Pin1 knockdown has no effect on normal cell growth [8], these results suggest that short-term cancer treatments with Pin1 inhibitors might not have these age-related side effects, especially if the inhibitors cannot readily pass through the blood-brain barrier. Thus, Pin1 inhibitors might have the desired property to simultaneously inhibit numerous oncogenic pathways without general toxicity.

As results of these studies, there are several reports of Pin1 inhibitors discovered to date, which are completely different from the well known conventional PPIases inhibitors such as immunosuppressive drugs cyclosporine and FK506. Notably, Pin1 belongs to a parvulin family PPIases and is not inhibited by these conventional PPIase inhibitors [93]. The first inhibitors of Pin1 and its parvulin type PPIases was found to be juglone or 5-hydroxy-1,4-naphthoquinone, a naturally occurring aromatic compound [94]. The mode of action was studied by analyzing the inactivation kinetics and the nature of products of the reaction of *E. coli* parvulin and its Cys69Ala variant with juglone [94]. The inactivated parvulin was found to contain two juglone molecules covalently bound to active cysteines by Michael addition of the thiol groups to juglone [94]. Thus, partial unfolding of the active site of the parvulins was thought to be the cause of the loss of PPIase activity. Consequently, juglone inhibits enzyme activity but not substrate recognition *via* a functional WW domain. However, a subsequent investigation on juglone mechanism of action found that this compound inhibited RNA transcription directly by disrupting the formation of pre-initiation complexes by modifying sulfhydryl groups but did not have any significant effect on either initiation or elongation [95]. Importantly, both RNA polymerases I and III, but not T7 RNA polymerase, were inhibited by juglone. The primary target of juglone was suggested to be on RNA pol II as inhibition of RNA polymerase II was observed during factor-independent transcription of single-stranded DNA. Therefore, the growth inhibitory effects of juglone may be attributed to its effects on transcription rather than or in combination with inhibition of PPIase activity [95]. Of note, it is critical to keep in mind that juglone can affect many other cellular proteins by covalently inactivating active cysteines. Therefore, the specificity of juglone for Pin1 in the cell is highly questionable.

More recently, a study was undertaken to identify new parvulin inhibitors, to do so a screening of a chemical compound library was performed [96]. This method identified a set of compounds which inhibited PPIase activity of Pin1 and parvulin *in vitro* with low micro molar IC50s and inhibited the growth of several cancer lines as evaluated by MTT assay. Among the inhibitors, all shared a common aromatic ring structure similar to that observed for juglone. To demonstrate the specificity of these compounds the relative effects of the compounds on cell growth were examined on cells with opposing levels of Pin1, as examined by western blotting. Interestingly, several compounds appeared to show positive correlation to growth inhibition and Pin1 levels, this was further validated using mouse fibroblast cells from Pin1 WT and null mice [96]. However, no further developments regarding these drugs, were or have been demonstrated, such as preclinical mutagenesis/toxicity assays or solubility analysis but as a proof of principal it appears that these compounds act in a more specific manner than juglone.

In addition to small compound inhibitors, several groups have taken a biochemical approach to elucidation of the molecular surfaces required for efficient PPIase inhibition with the hope to extrapolate this data to structure based mining for chemical inhibitors. Specifically, peptidomimetic inhibitors have been designed and screened from synthesised non-natural amino containing peptide libraries [75, 97-99]. Using these approaches has not only uncovered several novel inhibitors of Pin1 but has also allowed a more definite description of the inhibitory mechanism required. Conformationally locked inhibitors have been described that were based on the preference of Pin1 for aromatic residues at the C terminus of its binding motif, these core Ser-cis-Pro and Ser-trans-pro alkenes were inert to isomerisation and therefore mimic cis and trans as they are “locked”. The conformational selectivity of the PPIase domain for cis and the WW domain for trans was demonstrated by both X-ray crystallography and NMR analysis [98, 99]. Inhibition of cell proliferation by these inhibitors was at the low to medium micromolar range of concentrations. In another study, reversible inhibitors were evaluated to determine the minimal structural requirement for Pin1 inhibition. In this case, tripeptides with pSer-Pro motifs were found to inhibit Pin1 and interestingly substitution of (D)-Ser instead of natural (L)-Ser rendered Pin1 substrates reversible inhibitors and the (D)-amino acid inhibitors were unexpectedly remarkably stable to phosphatase activity [99].

More recently, by screening a combinatorial peptide library, a series of nanomolar peptidic inhibitors of Pin1 were identified, with benzothienylalanine-d-phosphothreonine-homoproline-l-2-naphthylalanine being the most active at 1 nM of Kd [100, 101] . Nonproteinogenic amino acids, incorporated into 5-mer to 8-mer oligopeptides containing d-phosphothreonine as a central template, yielded selective inhibitors that blocked cell cycle progression in HeLa cells in a dose-dependent manner. This finding was further developed using co-crystal structure analysis of the inhibitors discovered from the screen described above and Pin1 [75]. These structures uncovered chemical elements that may further improve the affinity and pharmacological properties of future peptide-based Pin inhibitors. Finally, an intramolecular hydrogen bond observed in both peptide complexes was somewhat similar to that of the conformation described for FK506 and rapamycin, both being clinically important inhibitors of other peptidyl-prolyl cis-trans isomerases [75]. This comparative discovery suggested that a cyclic peptide polyketide bridge, like that found in FK506 and rapamycin, may significantly improve the binding affinity of structure-based Pin1 inhibitors. Notably, based on these studies, membrane permeable cyclic peptidyl inhibitors containing a consensus motif of d-phosphothreonine-homoproline-l-2-naphthylalanine with attachment of an octaarginine sequence were developed [102]. These Pin1 inhibitors inhibited breast cancer cell growth and increased the protein levels of PML and SMRT, two tumor suppressors that are Pin1 substrates, indicating that Pin1 inhibitors activates tumor suppressors [102].

Taken as a whole, these studies serve as a preamble for the discovery of Pin1 inhibitors based on rational design rather than combinatorial methodologies. More recently, a series of studies have reported potential new inhibitors of Pin1, which for the most part have been optimized from lead compounds based on their ability to inhibit Pin1's prolyl isomerase activity in the protease-coupled PPIase assay *in vitro*. For example, a series of phosphate containing small molecules have been discovered by structure-based design and have been optimized by phosphate-replacement with carboxylate groups, although these compounds displayed weaker activity than the phosphate containing inhibitors [103, 104]. Another report identified a series of Pin1 inhibitors based on a phenyl imidazole core that displayed sub-micromolar activity against prostate cancer cells *in vitro* [105]. The same group also reported a further series of related compounds which suffered from poor cell permeability, a common theme encountered by groups pursuing Pin1 inhibitors [106].

In addition, recent literature also reports dual Pin1:cyclophilin inhibitors [107], quinazoline-derived Pin1 inhibitors [108] and benzophenone analogues as Pin1 inhibitors [109]. As stated before, most if not all of these studies are based on either screening libraries of compounds or optimization of small molecule backbones based on *in vitro* inhibition of Pin1 activity or structural binding. The failure of most of these compounds to inhibit Pin1 in cellular models is a reflection of the current conundrum facing the field where selective *in vitro* inhibitors do not possess the require properties to perform inhibition in cells. Thus it suggests that a concerted effort to develop novel high throughput screening tools *in vitro* and *in vivo* is urgently needed.

CLOSING REMARKS

The identification of Pin1 as the first and thus far only phosphorylation dependent prolyl isomerase has opened the door on the highly regulated process of isomerisation during cell signalling. As more Pin1 substrates have been identified our understanding of the complexity between the balance of normal cell cycle control to the transition of uncontrolled cell growth and ultimately cancer becomes clearer, it has become evident that Pin1 activates numerous oncogenes and also inactivates a large number of tumor suppressors. However, all Pin1 inhibitors identified so far either lack the needed specificity and/or potency or fail to enter cells. Therefore, there is an urgent need to develop Pin1-specific inhibitors because they might have the unique property to simultaneously inhibit numerous oncogenic pathways that are needed to treat cancers, especially such aggressive and drug-resistant ones. One important recent innovation is the development of antibodies that can recognise either the cis or trans form of phosphorylated protein substrates of Pin1 such as Tau [110]. If this can be applied to other Pin1 substrates that are relevant to cancer and oncogenesis, one can imagine a scenario where Pin1 inhibitors can be monitored for efficacy *in vivo* in real time. This surely represents a worthy new avenue of investigation. It will be interesting to determine if other enzymes function in a similar way to Pin1 such that they function as molecular timers in signalling cascades which maybe deregulated in pathological disease. From a therapeutic view point, the identification and characterisation of compounds with specific activity for Pin1 *in vivo* will be the "acid test" for this molecules efficacy as a true molecular target in cancer.

ACKNOWLEDGEMENTS

We are grateful to L. Nicholson, T. Hunter, L. Cantley, B. Neel and to members of the Lu Lab for helpful and stimulating discussions and advice. Work done in the authors laboratory is supported by NIH grants R01CA167677, R03DA031663 to KP.L. and R01 CA122434 to X.Z.Z. We apologise to authors whose work isn't cited due to space limitations.

CONFLICT OF INTEREST

The author(s) confirm that this chapter content has no conflict of interest.

DISCLOSURE

The chapter submitted for the eBook Series entitled **"Advances in Cancer Drug Targets, Volume 1"** is an update of our article in **Current Cancer Drug Targets, Volume 8, Issue 3, 2008,** with additional text and references.

ABBREVIATIONS

Pin1	=	prolyl isomerase interacting with NIMA
FKBP	=	FK506 binding protein
Ser	=	Serine
Thr	=	Theronine
pSer/Thr-Pro	=	phosphorylated Ser-Pro or Thr-Pro
WW domain	=	Two conserved tryptophans domain

APP	=	Alzheimer' disease precursor protein
CTD	=	C terminal domain
NMR	=	Nuclear Magnetic resonance
APC	=	anaphase promoting complex
MEFs	=	Mouse embryonic fibroblasts
MYC	=	v-myc myelocytomatosis viral oncogene homolog
PCa	=	prostate cancer
E2F	=	E2F transcripton factor
NF-κB	=	Nuclear factor kappa B
AIB1/SRC3	=	Amplified in Breast cancer 1
Stat3	=	Signal transducer and activator of transcription
p300	=	p300 acetyltransferase
p53	=	p 53 transcription factor
p73	=	p73 transcription factor
MDM2	=	double minute 2
PLK1	=	Polo like kinase 1
HBV	=	Hepatitis B virus
Hbx	=	Hepatitis B protein x
AIB1	=	Amplified in breast cancer I
Mcl-1	=	Induced myeloid leukemia cell differentiation protein

Tax = human immunodeficiency virus type 1 Tat protein

v-Rel = The proto-oncogene Rel protein

FOXOs = Forkhead box proteins

PML = Promyelocytic leukemia protein

Daxx = death-domain-associated protein

Bcl2 = B-cell lymphoma 2

RARα = retinoic acid receptor α

SMRT = silencing mediator for retinoid or thyroid-hormone receptors

Smad = intracellular protein that transduces TGFβ signals

Pin2/TRF1 = Protein-interacting with NIMA 2/telomere-binding protein 1

Fbw7 = F-box protein 7

AMPK = AMP-Activated Protein Kinase

Rb = Retinoblastoma protein

REFERENCES

[1] Croce CM. Oncogenes and cancer. *The New England journal of medicine* **358**, 502-511 (2008).

[2] Lu KP. Prolyl isomerase Pin1 as a molecular target for cancer diagnostics and therapeutics. *Cancer cell* **4**, 175-180 (2003).

[3] Lu KP, Finn G, Lee TH, Nicholson LK. Prolyl cis-trans isomerization as a molecular timer. *Nature chemical biology* **3**, 619-629 (2007).

[4] Lu KP, Zhou XZ. The prolyl isomerase PIN1: a pivotal new twist in phosphorylation signalling and disease. *Nature reviews* **8**, 904-916 (2007).

[5] Liou YC, Zhou XZ, Lu KP. Prolyl isomerase Pin1 as a molecular switch to determine the fate of phosphoproteins. *Trends in biochemical sciences* **36**, 501-514 (2011).

[6] Lee TH, Pastorino L, Lu KP. Peptidyl-prolyl cis-trans isomerase Pin1 in ageing, cancer and Alzheimer disease. *Expert reviews in molecular medicine* **13**, e21 (2011).

[7] Suizu F, Ryo A, Wulf G, Lim J, Lu KP. Pin1 regulates centrosome duplication, and its overexpression induces centrosome amplification, chromosome instability, and oncogenesis. *Molecular and cellular biology* **26**, 1463-1479 (2006).

[8] Ryo A, Uemura H, Ishiguro H, Saitoh T, Yamaguchi A, Perrem K, Kubota Y, Lu KP, Aoki I. Stable suppression of tumorigenicity by Pin1-targeted RNA interference in prostate cancer. *Clin Cancer Res* **11**, 7523-7531 (2005).
[9] Wulf G, Garg P, Liou YC, Iglehart D, Lu KP. Modeling breast cancer *in vivo* and *ex vivo* reveals an essential role of Pin1 in tumorigenesis. *The EMBO journal* **23**, 3397-3407 (2004).
[10] Lu KP. Pinning down cell signaling, cancer and Alzheimer's disease. *Trends in biochemical sciences* **29**, 200-209 (2004).
[11] Wulf G, Finn G, Suizu F, Lu KP. Phosphorylation-specific prolyl isomerization: is there an underlying theme? *Nature cell biology* **7**, 435-441 (2005).
[12] Lu PJ, Zhou XZ, Liou YC, Noel JP, Lu KP. Critical role of WW domain phosphorylation in regulating phosphoserine binding activity and Pin1 function. *The Journal of biological chemistry* **277**, 2381-2384 (2002).
[13] Lu PJ, Zhou XZ, Shen M, Lu KP. Function of WW domains as phosphoserine- or phosphothreonine-binding modules. *Science (New York, NY* **283**, 1325-1328 (1999).
[14] Lu KP, Hanes SD, Hunter T. A human peptidyl-prolyl isomerase essential for regulation of mitosis. *Nature* **380**, 544-547 (1996).
[15] Pastorino L, Sun A, Lu PJ, Zhou XZ, Balastik M, Finn G, Wulf G, Lim J, Li SH, Li X, Xia W, Nicholson LK, Lu KP. The prolyl isomerase Pin1 regulates amyloid precursor protein processing and amyloid-beta production. *Nature* **440**, 528-534 (2006).
[16] Zhou XZ, Lu PJ, Wulf G, Lu KP. Phosphorylation-dependent prolyl isomerization: a novel signaling regulatory mechanism. *Cell Mol Life Sci* **56**, 788-806 (1999).
[17] Zhou XZ, Kops O, Werner A, Lu PJ, Shen M, Stoller G, Kullertz G, Stark M, Fischer G, Lu KP. Pin1-dependent prolyl isomerization regulates dephosphorylation of Cdc25C and tau proteins. *Molecular cell* **6**, 873-883 (2000).
[18] Landrieu I, Smet C, Wieruszeski JM, Sambo AV, Wintjens R, Buee L, Lippens G. Exploring the molecular function of PIN1 by nuclear magnetic resonance. *Current protein & peptide science* **7**, 179-194 (2006).
[19] Namanja AT, Peng T, Zintsmaster JS, Elson AC, Shakour MG, Peng JW. Substrate recognition reduces side-chain flexibility for conserved hydrophobic residues in human Pin1. *Structure* **15**, 313-327 (2007).
[20] Lu KP, Suizu F, Zhou XZ, Finn G, Lam P, Wulf G. Targeting carcinogenesis: a role for the prolyl isomerase Pin1? *Molecular carcinogenesis* **45**, 397-402 (2006).
[21] Liou YC, Ryo A, Huang HK, Lu PJ, Bronson R, Fujimori F, Uchida T, Hunter T, Lu KP. Loss of Pin1 function in the mouse causes phenotypes resembling cyclin D1-null phenotypes. *Proceedings of the National Academy of Sciences of the United States of America* **99**, 1335-1340 (2002).
[22] Wulf GM, Ryo A, Wulf GG, Lee SW, Niu T, Petkova V, Lu KP. Pin1 is overexpressed in breast cancer and cooperates with Ras signaling in increasing the transcriptional activity of c-Jun towards cyclin D1. *The EMBO journal* **20**, 3459-3472 (2001).
[23] Stukenberg PT, Kirschner MW. Pin1 acts catalytically to promote a conformational change in Cdc25. *Molecular cell* **7**, 1071-1083 (2001).
[24] Bernis C, Vigneron S, Burgess A, Labbe JC, Fesquet D, Castro A, Lorca T. Pin1 stabilizes Emi1 during G2 phase by preventing its association with SCF(betatrcp). *EMBO reports* **8**, 91-98 (2007).
[25] Okamoto K, Sagata N. Mechanism for inactivation of the mitotic inhibitory kinase Wee1 at M phase. *Proceedings of the National Academy of Sciences of the United States of America* **104**, 3753-3758 (2007).

[26] Shen M, Stukenberg PT, Kirschner MW, Lu KP. The essential mitotic peptidyl-prolyl isomerase Pin1 binds and regulates mitosis-specific phosphoproteins. *Genes & development* **12**, 706-720 (1998).

[27] Xu YX, Manley JL. The prolyl isomerase Pin1 functions in mitotic chromosome condensation. *Molecular cell* **26**, 287-300 (2007).

[28] Fujimori F, Takahashi K, Uchida C, Uchida T. Mice lacking Pin1 develop normally, but are defective in entering cell cycle from G(0) arrest. *Biochemical and biophysical research communications* **265**, 658-663 (1999).

[29] You H, Zheng H, Murray SA, Yu Q, Uchida T, Fan D, Xiao ZX. IGF-1 induces Pin1 expression in promoting cell cycle S-phase entry. *Journal of cellular biochemistry* **84**, 211-216 (2002).

[30] Yeh E, Cunningham M, Arnold H, Chasse D, Monteith T, Ivaldi G, Hahn WC, Stukenberg PT, Shenolikar S, Uchida T, Counter CM, Nevins JR, Means AR, Sears R. A signalling pathway controlling c-Myc degradation that impacts oncogenic transformation of human cells. *Nature cell biology* **6**, 308-318 (2004).

[31] Yeh ES, Lew BO, Means AR. The loss of PIN1 deregulates cyclin E and sensitizes mouse embryo fibroblasts to genomic instability. *The Journal of biological chemistry* **281**, 241-251 (2006).

[32] Lu KP. Phosphorylation-dependent prolyl isomerization: a novel cell cycle regulatory mechanism. *Progress in cell cycle research* **4**, 83-96 (2000).

[33] Anderson P. Pin1: a proline isomerase that makes you wheeze? *Nature immunology* **6**, 1211-1212 (2005).

[34] Ryo A, Nakamura M, Wulf G, Liou YC, Lu KP. Pin1 regulates turnover and subcellular localization of beta-catenin by inhibiting its interaction with APC. *Nature cell biology* **3**, 793-801 (2001).

[35] Bao L, Kimzey A, Sauter G, Sowadski JM, Lu KP, Wang DG. Prevalent overexpression of prolyl isomerase Pin1 in human cancers. *The American journal of pathology* **164**, 1727-1737 (2004).

[36] Ryo A, Liou YC, Lu KP, Wulf G. Prolyl isomerase Pin1: a catalyst for oncogenesis and a potential therapeutic target in cancer. *Journal of cell science* **116**, 773-783 (2003).

[37] Ayala G, Wang D, Wulf G, Frolov A, Li R, Sowadski J, Wheeler TM, Lu KP, Bao L. The prolyl isomerase Pin1 is a novel prognostic marker in human prostate cancer. *Cancer research* **63**, 6244-6251 (2003).

[38] Sasaki T, Ryo A, Uemura H, Ishiguro H, Inayama Y, Yamanaka S, Kubota Y, Nagashima Y, Harada M, Aoki I. An immunohistochemical scoring system of prolyl isomerase Pin1 for predicting relapse of prostate carcinoma after radical prostatectomy. *Pathology, research and practice* **202**, 357-364 (2006).

[39] Han CH, Lu J, Wei Q, Bondy ML, Brewster AM, Yu TK, Buchholz TA, Arun BK, Wang LE. The functional promoter polymorphism (-842G>C) in the PIN1 gene is associated with decreased risk of breast cancer in non-Hispanic white women 55 years and younger. *Breast cancer research and treatment* **122**, 243-249 (2010).

[40] Lu J, Hu Z, Wei S, Wang LE, Liu Z, El-Naggar AK, Sturgis EM, Wei Q. A novel functional variant (-842G>C) in the PIN1 promoter contributes to decreased risk of squamous cell carcinoma of the head and neck by diminishing the promoter activity. *Carcinogenesis* **30**, 1717-1721 (2009).

[41] Lu J, Yang L, Zhao H, Liu B, Li Y, Wu H, Li Q, Zeng B, Wang Y, Ji W, Zhou Y. The polymorphism and haplotypes of PIN1 gene are associated with the risk of lung cancer in Southern and Eastern Chinese populations. *Hum Mutat* **32**, 1299-1308 (2011).

[42] Fukuchi M, Fukai Y, Kimura H, Sohda M, Miyazaki T, Nakajima M, Masuda N, Tsukada K, Kato H, Kuwano H. Prolyl isomerase Pin1 expression predicts prognosis in patients with esophageal squamous cell carcinoma and correlates with cyclinD1 expression. *International journal of oncology* **29**, 329-334 (2006).

[43] Miyashita H, Mori S, Motegi K, Fukumoto M, Uchida T. Pin1 is overexpressed in oral squamous cell carcinoma and its levels correlate with cyclin D1 overexpression. *Oncology reports* **10**, 455-461 (2003).

[44] Miyashita H, Uchida T, Mori S, Echigo S, Motegi K. Expression status of Pin1 and cyclins in oral squamous cell carcinoma: Pin1 correlates with Cyclin D1 mRNA expression and clinical significance of cyclins. *Oncology reports* **10**, 1045-1048 (2003).

[45] Monje P, Hernandez-Losa J, Lyons RJ, Castellone MD, Gutkind JS. Regulation of the transcriptional activity of c-Fos by ERK. A novel role for the prolyl isomerase PIN1. *The Journal of biological chemistry* **280**, 35081-35084 (2005).

[46] Ryo A, Suizu F, Yoshida Y, Perrem K, Liou YC, Wulf G, Rottapel R, Yamaoka S, Lu KP. Regulation of NF-kappaB signaling by Pin1-dependent prolyl isomerization and ubiquitin-mediated proteolysis of p65/RelA. *Molecular cell* **12**, 1413-1426 (2003).

[47] Ryo A, Liou YC, Wulf G, Nakamura M, Lee SW, Lu KP. PIN1 is an E2F target gene essential for Neu/Ras-induced transformation of mammary epithelial cells. *Molecular and cellular biology* **22**, 5281-5295 (2002).

[48] Dougherty MK, Muller J, Ritt DA, Zhou M, Zhou XZ, Copeland TD, Conrads TP, Veenstra TD, Lu KP, Morrison DK. Regulation of Raf-1 by direct feedback phosphorylation. *Molecular cell* **17**, 215-224 (2005).

[49] Tzahor E. Wnt/beta-catenin signaling and cardiogenesis: timing does matter. *Developmental cell* **13**, 10-13 (2007).

[50] Pang R, Yuen J, Yuen MF, Lai CL, Lee TK, Man K, Poon RT, Fan ST, Wong CM, Ng IO, Kwong YL, Tse E. PIN1 overexpression and beta-catenin gene mutations are distinct oncogenic events in human hepatocellular carcinoma. *Oncogene* **23**, 4182-4186 (2004).

[51] Lam PB, Burga LN, Wu BP, Hofstatter EW, Lu KP, Wulf GM. Prolyl isomerase Pin1 is highly expressed in Her2-positive breast cancer and regulates erbB2 protein stability. *Molecular cancer* **7**, 91 (2008).

[52] Takahashi K, Akiyama H, Shimazaki K, Uchida C, Akiyama-Okunuki H, Tomita M, Fukumoto M, Uchida T. Ablation of a peptidyl prolyl isomerase Pin1 from p53-null mice accelerated thymic hyperplasia by increasing the level of the intracellular form of Notch1. *Oncogene* **26**, 3835-3845 (2007).

[53] Yi P, Wu RC, Sandquist J, Wong J, Tsai SY, Tsai MJ, Means AR, O'Malley BW. Peptidyl-prolyl isomerase 1 (Pin1) serves as a coactivator of steroid receptor by regulating the activity of phosphorylated steroid receptor coactivator 3 (SRC-3/AIB1). *Molecular and cellular biology* **25**, 9687-9699 (2005).

[54] Stanya KJ, Liu Y, Means AR, Kao HY. Cdk2 and Pin1 negatively regulate the transcriptional corepressor SMRT. *The Journal of cell biology* **183**, 49-61 (2008).

[55] Rajbhandari P, Finn G, Solodin NM, Singarapu KK, Sahu SC, Markley JL, Kadunc KJ, Ellison-Zelski SJ, Kariagina A, Haslam SZ, Lu KP, Alarid ET. Regulation of estrogen receptor alpha N-terminus conformation and function by peptidyl prolyl isomerase Pin1. *Molecular and cellular biology* **32**, 445-457 (2012).

[56] Lufei C, Koh TH, Uchida T, Cao X. Pin1 is required for the Ser727 phosphorylation-dependent Stat3 activity. *Oncogene* **26**, 7656-7664 (2007).

[57] Mantovani F, Piazza S, Gostissa M, Strano S, Zacchi P, Mantovani R, Blandino G, Del Sal G. Pin1 links the activities of c-Abl and p300 in regulating p73 function. *Molecular cell* **14**, 625-636 (2004).

[58] Zacchi P, Gostissa M, Uchida T, Salvagno C, Avolio F, Volinia S, Ronai Z, Blandino G, Schneider C, Del Sal G. The prolyl isomerase Pin1 reveals a mechanism to control p53 functions after genotoxic insults. *Nature* **419**, 853-857 (2002).

[59] Wulf GM, Liou YC, Ryo A, Lee SW, Lu KP. Role of Pin1 in the regulation of p53 stability and p21 transactivation, and cell cycle checkpoints in response to DNA damage. *The Journal of biological chemistry* **277**, 47976-47979 (2002).

[60] Zheng H, You H, Zhou XZ, Murray SA, Uchida T, Wulf G, Gu L, Tang X, Lu KP, Xiao ZX. The prolyl isomerase Pin1 is a regulator of p53 in genotoxic response. *Nature* **419**, 849-853 (2002).

[61] antovani F, Gostissa M, Collavin L, Del Sal G. KeePin' the p53 family in good shape. *Cell cycle (Georgetown, Tex* **3**, 905-911 (2004).

[62] De Nicola F, Bruno T, Iezzi S, Di Padova M, Floridi A, Passananti C, Del Sal G, Fanciulli M. The prolyl isomerase Pin1 affects Che-1 stability in response to apoptotic DNA damage. *The Journal of biological chemistry* **282**, 19685-19691 (2007).

[63] Girardini JE, Napoli M, Piazza S, Rustighi A, Marotta C, Radaelli E, Capaci V, Jordan L, Quinlan P, Thompson A, Mano M, Rosato A, Crook T, Scanziani E, Means AR, Lozano G, Schneider C, Del Sal G. A Pin1/mutant p53 axis promotes aggressiveness in breast cancer. *Cancer cell* **20**, 79-91 (2010).

[64] Pinton P, Rimessi A, Marchi S, Orsini F, Migliaccio E, Giorgio M, Contursi C, Minucci S, Mantovani F, Wieckowski MR, Del Sal G, Pelicci PG, Rizzuto R. Protein kinase C beta and prolyl isomerase 1 regulate mitochondrial effects of the life-span determinant p66Shc. *Science (New York, NY* **315**, 659-663 (2007).

[65] Sultana R, Boyd-Kimball D, Poon HF, Cai J, Pierce WM, Klein JB, Markesbery WR, Zhou XZ, Lu KP, Butterfield DA. Oxidative modification and down-regulation of Pin1 in Alzheimer's disease hippocampus: A redox proteomics analysis. *Neurobiology of aging* **27**, 918-925 (2006).

[66] Pang R, Lee TK, Poon RT, Fan ST, Wong KB, Kwong YL, Tse E. Pin1 interacts with a specific serine-proline motif of hepatitis B virus X-protein to enhance hepatocarcinogenesis. *Gastroenterology* **132**, 1088-1103 (2007).

[67] Zhao Y, Chen Y, Schutkowski M, Fischer G, Ke H. Cyclophilin A complexed with a fragment of HIV-1 gag protein: insights into HIV-1 infectious activity. *Structure* **5**, 139-146 (1997).

[68] Jacobs DM, Saxena K, Vogtherr M, Bernado P, Pons M, Fiebig KM. Peptide binding induces large scale changes in inter-domain mobility in human Pin1. *The Journal of biological chemistry* **278**, 26174-26182 (2003).

[69] Cho YS, Park SY, Kim DJ, Lee SH, Woo KM, Lee KA, Lee YJ, Cho YY, Shim JH. TPA-induced cell transformation provokes a complex formation between Pin1 and 90 kDa ribosomal protein S6 kinase 2. *Molecular and cellular biochemistry*, (2012).

[70] Eckerdt F, Yuan J, Saxena K, Martin B, Kappel S, Lindenau C, Kramer A, Naumann S, Daum S, Fischer G, Dikic I, Kaufmann M, Strebhardt K. Polo-like kinase 1-mediated phosphorylation stabilizes Pin1 by inhibiting its ubiquitination in human cells. *The Journal of biological chemistry* **280**, 36575-36583 (2005).

[71] Butterfield DA, Poon HF, St Clair D, Keller JN, Pierce WM, Klein JB, Markesbery WR. Redox proteomics identification of oxidatively modified hippocampal proteins in mild cognitive impairment: insights into the development of Alzheimer's disease. *Neurobiology of disease* **22**, 223-232 (2006).

[72] Lee TH, Chen CH, Suizu F, Huang P, Schiene-Fischer C, Daum S, Zhang YJ, Goate A, Chen RH, Zhou XZ, Lu KP. Death-associated protein kinase 1 phosphorylates Pin1 and inhibits its prolyl isomerase activity and cellular function. *Molecular cell* **42**, 147-159 (2011).

[73] Rangasamy V, Mishra R, Sondarva G, Das S, Lee TH, Bakowska JC, Tzivion G, Malter JS, Rana B, Lu KP, Kanthasamy A, Rana A. Mixed-lineage kinase 3 phosphorylates prolyl-isomerase Pin1 to regulate its nuclear translocation and cellular function. *Proceedings of the National Academy of Sciences of the United States of America*, (2012).

[74] Butterfield DA, Abdul HM, Opii W, Newman SF, Joshi G, Ansari MA, Sultana R. Pin1 in Alzheimer's disease. *Journal of neurochemistry* **98**, 1697-1706 (2006).

[75] Zhang Y, Daum S, Wildemann D, Zhou XZ, Verdecia MA, Bowman ME, Lucke C, Hunter T, Lu KP, Fischer G, Noel JP. Structural basis for high-affinity peptide inhibition of human Pin1. *ACS chemical biology* **2**, 320-328 (2007).

[76] Pani E, Menigatti M, Schubert S, Hess D, Gerrits B, Klempnauer KH, Ferrari S. Pin1 interacts with c-Myb in a phosphorylation-dependent manner and regulates its transactivation activity. *Biochimica et biophysica acta* **1783**, 1121-1128 (2008).

[77] Rustighi A, Tiberi L, Soldano A, Napoli M, Nuciforo P, Rosato A, Kaplan F, Capobianco A, Pece S, Di Fiore PP, Del Sal G. The prolyl-isomerase Pin1 is a Notch1 target that enhances Notch1 activation in cancer. *Nature cell biology* **11**, 133-142 (2009).

[78] Liao Y, Wei Y, Zhou X, Yang JY, Dai C, Chen YJ, Agarwal NK, Sarbassov D, Shi D, Yu D, Hung MC. Peptidyl-prolyl cis/trans isomerase Pin1 is critical for the regulation of PKB/Akt stability and activation phosphorylation. *Oncogene* **28**, 2436-2445 (2009).

[79] Ding Q, Huo L, Yang JY, Xia W, Wei Y, Liao Y, Chang CJ, Yang Y, Lai CC, Lee DF, Yen CJ, Chen YJ, Hsu JM, Kuo HP, Lin CY, Tsai FJ, Li LY, Tsai CH, Hung MC. Down-regulation of myeloid cell leukemia-1 through inhibiting Erk/Pin 1 pathway by sorafenib facilitates chemosensitization in breast cancer. *Cancer research* **68**, 6109-6117 (2008).

[80] Pang RW, Lee TK, Man K, Poon RT, Fan ST, Kwong YL, Tse E. PIN1 expression contributes to hepatic carcinogenesis. *The Journal of pathology* **210**, 19-25 (2006).

[81] Peloponese JM, Jr., Yasunaga J, Kinjo T, Watashi K, Jeang KT. Peptidylproline cis-trans-isomerase Pin1 interacts with human T-cell leukemia virus type 1 tax and modulates its activation of NF-kappaB. *Journal of virology* **83**, 3238-3248 (2009).

[82] Fan G, Fan Y, Gupta N, Matsuura I, Liu F, Zhou XZ, Lu KP, Gelinas C. Peptidyl-prolyl isomerase Pin1 markedly enhances the oncogenic activity of the rel proteins in the nuclear factor-kappaB family. *Cancer research* **69**, 4589-4597 (2009).

[83] Brenkman AB, de Keizer PL, van den Broek NJ, van der Groep P, van Diest PJ, van der Horst A, Smits AM, Burgering BM. The peptidyl-isomerase Pin1 regulates p27kip1 expression through inhibition of Forkhead box O tumor suppressors. *Cancer research* **68**, 7597-7605 (2008).

[84] Reineke EL, Lam M, Liu Q, Liu Y, Stanya KJ, Chang KS, Means AR, Kao HY. Degradation of the tumor suppressor PML by Pin1 contributes to the cancer phenotype of breast cancer MDA-MB-231 cells. *Molecular and cellular biology* **28**, 997-1006 (2008).

[85] Ryo A, Hirai A, Nishi M, Liou YC, Perrem K, Lin SC, Hirano H, Lee SW, Aoki I. A suppressive role of the prolyl isomerase Pin1 in cellular apoptosis mediated by the death-associated protein Daxx. *The Journal of biological chemistry* **282**, 36671-36681 (2007).

[86] Basu A, Das M, Qanungo S, Fan XJ, DuBois G, Haldar S. Proteasomal degradation of human peptidyl prolyl isomerase pin1-pointing phospho Bcl2 toward dephosphorylation. *Neoplasia (New York, NY* **4**, 218-227 (2002).

[87] Gianni M, Boldetti A, Guarnaccia V, Rambaldi A, Parrella E, Raska I, Jr., Rochette-Egly C, Del Sal G, Rustighi A, Terao M, Garattini E. Inhibition of the peptidyl-prolyl-isomerase Pin1 enhances the responses of acute myeloid leukemia cells to retinoic acid *via* stabilization of RARalpha and PML-RARalpha. *Cancer research* **69**, 1016-1026 (2009).

[88] Nakano A, Koinuma D, Miyazawa K, Uchida T, Saitoh M, Kawabata M, Hanai J, Akiyama H, Abe M, Miyazono K, Matsumoto T, Imamura T. Pin1 down-regulates transforming growth factor-beta (TGF-beta) signaling by inducing degradation of Smad proteins. *The Journal of biological chemistry* **284**, 6109-6115 (2009).

[89] Lee TH, Tun-Kyi A, Shi R, Lim J, Soohoo C, Finn G, Balastik M, Pastorino L, Wulf G, Zhou XZ, Lu KP. Essential role of Pin1 in the regulation of TRF1 stability and telomere maintenance. *Nature cell biology* **11**, 97-105 (2009).

[90] Min SH, Lau AW, Lee TH, Inuzuka H, Wei S, Huang P, Shaik S, Lee DY, Finn G, Balastik M, Chen CH, Luo ML, Tron AE, DeCaprio JA, Zhou XZ, Wei W, Lu KP. Negative Regulation of the Stability and Tumor Suppressor Function of Fbw7 by the Pin1 Prolyl Isomerase. *Molecular cell*, (In press).

[91] Khanal P, Kim G, Yun HJ, Cho HG, Choi HS. The prolyl isomerase Pin1 interacts with and downregulates the activity of AMPK leading to induction of tumorigenicity of hepatocarcinoma cells. *Molecular carcinogenesis*, (2012).

[92] Rizzolio F, Lucchetti C, Caligiuri I, Marchesi I, Caputo M, Klein-Szanto AJ, Bagella L, Castronovo M, Giordano A. Retinoblastoma tumor-suppressor protein phosphorylation and inactivation depend on direct interaction with Pin1. *Cell death and differentiation*, (2012).

[93] Wang XJ, Etzkorn FA. Peptidyl-prolyl isomerase inhibitors. *Biopolymers* **84**, 125-146 (2006).

[94] Hennig L, Christner C, Kipping M, Schelbert B, Rucknagel KP, Grabley S, Kullertz G, Fischer G. Selective inactivation of parvulin-like peptidyl-prolyl cis/trans isomerases by juglone. *Biochemistry* **37**, 5953-5960 (1998).

[95] Chao SH, Greenleaf AL, Price DH. Juglone, an inhibitor of the peptidyl-prolyl isomerase Pin1, also directly blocks transcription. *Nucleic acids research* **29**, 767-773 (2001).

[96] Uchida T, Takamiya M, Takahashi M, Miyashita H, Ikeda H, Terada T, Matsuo Y, Shirouzu M, Yokoyama S, Fujimori F, Hunter T. Pin1 and Par14 peptidyl prolyl isomerase inhibitors block cell proliferation. *Chemistry & biology* **10**, 15-24 (2003).

[97] Wang XJ, Hart SA, Xu B, Mason MD, Goodell JR, Etzkorn FA. Serine-cis-proline and serine-trans-proline isosteres: stereoselective synthesis of (Z)- and (E)-alkene mimics by Still-Wittig and Ireland-Claisen rearrangements. *The Journal of organic chemistry* **68**, 2343-2349 (2003).

[98] Wang XJ, Xu B, Mullins AB, Neiler FK, Etzkorn FA. Conformationally locked isostere of phosphoSer-cis-Pro inhibits Pin1 23-fold better than phosphoSer-trans-Pro isostere. *Journal of the American Chemical Society* **126**, 15533-15542 (2004).

[99] Zhang Y, Fussel S, Reimer U, Schutkowski M, Fischer G. Substrate-based design of reversible Pin1 inhibitors. *Biochemistry* **41**, 11868-11877 (2002).

[100] Wildemann D, Erdmann F, Alvarez BH, Stoller G, Zhou XZ, Fanghanel J, Schutkowski M, Lu KP, Fischer G. Nanomolar inhibitors of the peptidyl prolyl cis/trans isomerase Pin1 from combinatorial peptide libraries. *Journal of medicinal chemistry* **49**, 2147-2150 (2006).

[101] Wildemann D, Hernandez Alvarez B, Stoller G, Zhou XZ, Lu KP, Erdmann F, Ferrari D, Fischer G. An essential role for Pin1 in Xenopus laevis embryonic development revealed by specific inhibitors. *Biological chemistry* **388**, 1103-1111 (2007).

[102] Liu T, Liu Y, Kao HY, Pei D. Membrane permeable cyclic peptidyl inhibitors against human Peptidylprolyl Isomerase Pin1. *Journal of medicinal chemistry* **53**, 2494-2501 (2010).

[103] Guo C, Hou X, Dong L, Dagostino E, Greasley S, Ferre R, Marakovits J, Johnson MC, Matthews D, Mroczkowski B, Parge H, Vanarsdale T, Popoff I, Piraino J, Margosiak S, Thomson J, Los G, Murray BW. Structure-based design of novel human Pin1 inhibitors (I). *Bioorganic & medicinal chemistry letters* **19**, 5613-5616 (2009).

[104] Dong L, Marakovits J, Hou X, Guo C, Greasley S, Dagostino E, Ferre R, Johnson MC, Kraynov E, Thomson J, Pathak V, Murray BW. Structure-based design of novel human Pin1 inhibitors (II). *Bioorganic & medicinal chemistry letters* **20**, 2210-2214 (2010).

[105] Potter A, Oldfield V, Nunns C, Fromont C, Ray S, Northfield CJ, Bryant CJ, Scrace SF, Robinson D, Matossova N, Baker L, Dokurno P, Surgenor AE, Davis B, Richardson CM, Murray JB, Moore JD. Discovery of cell-active phenyl-imidazole Pin1 inhibitors by structure-guided fragment evolution. *Bioorganic & medicinal chemistry letters* **20**, 6483-6488 (2010).

[106] Potter AJ, Ray S, Gueritz L, Nunns CL, Bryant CJ, Scrace SF, Matassova N, Baker L, Dokurno P, Robinson DA, Surgenor AE, Davis B, Murray JB, Richardson CM, Moore JD. Structure-guided design of alpha-amino acid-derived Pin1 inhibitors. *Bioorganic & medicinal chemistry letters* **20**, 586-590 (2010).

[107] Mori T, Hidaka M, Lin YC, Yoshizawa I, Okabe T, Egashira S, Kojima H, Nagano T, Koketsu M, Takamiya M, Uchida T. A dual inhibitor against prolyl isomerase Pin1 and cyclophilin discovered by a novel real-time fluorescence detection method. *Biochemical and biophysical research communications* **406**, 439-443 (2011).

[108] Zhu L, Jin J, Liu C, Zhang C, Sun Y, Guo Y, Fu D, Chen X, Xu B. Synthesis and biological evaluation of novel quinazoline-derived human Pin1 inhibitors. *Bioorganic & medicinal chemistry* **19**, 2797-2807 (2011).

[109] Liu C, Jin J, Chen L, Zhou J, Chen X, Fu D, Song H, Xu B. Synthesis and biological evaluation of novel human Pin1 inhibitors with benzophenone skeleton. *Bioorganic & medicinal chemistry* **20**, 2992-2999 (2012).

[110] Nakamura K, Greenwood A, Binder L, Bigio EH, Denial S, Nicholson L, Zhou XZ, Lu KP. Proline isomer-specific antibodies reveal the early pathogenic tau conformation in Alzheimer's disease. *Cell* **149**, 232-244 (2012).

CHAPTER 6

Anticancer Immunotherapy in Combination with Proapoptotic Therapy - Possible Therapeutic Strategies for Enhancement of Anticancer Immune Reactivity in Autologous Immunocompetent Cells and After Allogeneic Stem Cell Transplantation

Håkon Reikvam[1,2], Elisabeth Ersvær[2], Guro Kristin Melve[3], Astrid Olsnes Kittang[1,2], Bjørn Tore Gjertsen[1,2] and Øystein Bruserud[1,2,*]

[1]Section for Hematology; Department of Medicine, Haukeland University Hospital; [2]Institute of Medicine, University of Bergen and [3]Department of Immunology and Transfusion Medicine, Haukeland University Hospital; Bergen, Norway

Abstract: Induction of immune responses against cancer-associated antigens is possible, but the optimal use of this strategy remains to be established and especially the combination of T cell therapy and new targeted therapeutic agents should be investigated. The design of future clinical studies has to consider several issues. Firstly, induction of anticancer T cell reactivity seems most effective in patients with low disease burden. Initial disease-reducing therapy including surgery, irradiation and conventional or new targeted chemotherapy should therefore be used, preferably through induction of immunogenic cancer cell death. Secondly, after the induction phase effector T cells will induce cancer cell apoptosis mainly through the intrinsic apoptosis-regulating pathway. The effect of this effector T cell function should be strengthened by administration of chemotherapy that mediates additional proapoptotic signalling through the external apoptosis-regulating pathway, inhibition of survival signalling or blocking of anti-apoptotic signalling. Thirdly, the status of the immune system has to be considered, including the postchemotherapy $CD4^+$ T cell defect, the balance between proinflammatory and immunosuppressive T cell subsets (*e.g.* regulatory T cells *versus* Th17 cells), and immunoregulatory mesenchymal cells that can be detected within tumors. Immunotherapy should probably be initiated early after disease-reducing therapy when the cancer cell burden is lowest and a focus should then be to alter the balance in favour of proinflammatory T cell subsets. All these issues need to be considered in the design of future clinical studies combining chemotherapy and immunotherapy.

Keywords: Cancer, T cells, Apoptosis, Immunotherapy, Chemotherapy, Allogeneic stem cell transplantation.

***Address correspondence to Øystein Bruserud:** Department of Medicine, Haukeland University Hospital, N-5021 Bergen, Norway; Tel +47 55975000; Fax +47 55972950 ; E-mail: oystein.bruserud@haukeland.no

Atta-ur-Rahman (Ed)

INTRODUCTION

Malignant cells often express cancer-associated antigens that can be recognized by T cells, and immunotherapy is therefore considered for the treatment of several human malignancies [1]. The possible immunotherapeutic strategies include various forms of cancer vaccines, *e.g.* peptide vaccines or dendritic cells pulsed with cancer cell lysates or transfected with cancer cell RNA [2-4]. These vaccines have often been tried as the only anticancer treatment. In this article we will review the results from recent studies suggesting that both previous chemotherapy and later targeted anticancer therapy may influence the final effect of immunotherapy. Taken together these observations support our suggestion that future immunotherapy in cancer should be used as an integrated part of treatment regimens including (i) initial chemotherapy (eventually combined with surgery or irradiation therapy) to achieve disease reduction and facilitate antigen presentation; and (ii) new targeted therapy that has proapoptotic effects on cancer cells and thereby will have additive or synergistic effects together with Natural Killer (NK) and T cell cytotoxity.

IMMUNOGENIC CANCER CELL DEATH

Scheffer *et al.* [5] described that apoptotic tumor cells, but not malignant cells in necrotic tumors, could provoke an antitumor immune response. This initial study thereby showed that the cell death mechanism is important for the immunogenicity of malignant cells. Furthermore, cytotoxic drugs often act by inducing apoptosis in the malignant cells, and in a recent experimental study Casares *et al.* [6] described that the apoptotic phenotype was important for induction of anticancer immunity. These authors compared the two DNA-binding and apoptosis-inducing drugs doxorubicin (an anthracyclin) and mitomycin in an experimental animal model and demonstrated that malignant cells could take different pathways to apoptosis. Killing by doxorubicin triggered an immune response, whereas the apoptotic cells killed by mitomycin did not. The authors demonstrated that colon-carcinoma cells (the CTC26 cell line) killed by doxorubicin were first taken up by dendritic cells that induced the proliferation of antitumor $CD8^{+}$ T cells. Direct injection of anthracyclin into the tumors caused immune-dependent regression. In contrast, neither dendritic cell uptake nor tumor regression was observed by using mitomycin. Thus, the anthracyclin-induced apoptosis and thereby development of cancer-specific immunity was critical for outcome. Studies in an alternative animal model also showed that the two anti-cancer drugs doxorubicin and melphalan did not reduce the effects of tumor antigen-specific vaccination, and this was true both when using peptide-pulsed dendritic cells as well as soluble antigen plus adjuvant [7]. A possible explanation is then that chemotherapy-induced immune responsiveness compensates for the immunosuppressive cytotoxic effect [8].

A recent study described that the cytotoxic drug cytarabine can induce differentiation in primary human AML cells with an increased surface expression of the costimulatory molecules CD80 and CD86 [9]. This observation further demonstrates that chemotherapy can enhance anticancer immune reactivity not only through modulation of cell trafficking and antigenic uptake but possibly also through induction of a more immunogenic but still viable cancer cell phenotype.

The results described above demonstrate that even though apoptotic tumor cells are more efficient than necrotic cells with regard to induction of immune responses [5], not all forms of apoptosis are equal in this respect [6]. The immunogenic, anthracyclin-induced apoptotic phenotype can be modulated by the caspase inhibition; the immunogenicity of the dying tumor cells is then suppressed but cell death is not inhibited [6]. On the other hand, combinatory therapy with recombinant calreticulin or pharmacological modulation of intracellular signaling may convert otherwise nonimmunogenic to immunogenic apoptosis [8]. An optimal combination of chemotherapy and immunotherapy will probably depend on the identification of cytotoxic drugs or drug combinations that show strong direct anticancer activity and at the same time induce cancer cell death through immunostimulatory apoptosis. There are several mechanisms by which chemotherapy can interfere with the induction of anti-cancer immune responses [6-18]; the experience from important animal models and the treatment of human malignancies is exemplified in Table **1**.

Table 1: Possible influence of chemotherapy on essential steps in anti-cancer immune responses.

Immunological Event	**Refs .**
Release of sufficient antigen for optimal presentation by professional antigen-presenting cells Apoptosis of cancer cells can be induced both by irradiation [5] or chemotherapy [6]. An experimental animal model demonstrated that vaccination with apoptotic cancer cells caused a strong local infiltration of T cells and professional antigen-presenting dendritic cells, and this was associated with protection against tumor outgrowth after later challenge [5]. In contrast, necrotic cancer cell vaccination caused local macrophage infiltration and no protection. This was observed for 3 different cell lines (colonic epithelial tumor, renal cell carcinoma, melanoma).	[5, 6]

Table 1: cont....

Antigen presentation resulting in the development of antitumor effector cells Animal models suggest that cross-arming of naive $CD8^+$ T cells to become effector cells following recognition of cross-presented tumor antigens in draining lymph nodes is thought to be a key event in development of cancer immunity [2]. This crosspresentation is dependent on $CD4^+$ T cell help or activation of dendritic cells through CD40 ligation [2]. Chemotherapy may cause selective $CD4^+$ T cell depletion (for a detailed discussion see [1]) or alter the differentiation/activation status of dendritic cells [7, 9]. The final chemotherapy is therefore difficult to predict.	[7, 9, 11, 12]
The immunostimulatory capacity of apoptotic cancer cells Irradiation and cytotoxic drugs can induce cancer cell apoptotis [5, 6], but *in vivo* chemotherapy in animals with established tumors animal studies have demonstrated that the ability of apoptotic cancer cells to induce an effective antitumor immune response depends on the apoptotic phenotype [6]. This immunostimulatory apoptotic phenotype is characterized by caspase activation in the cancer cell, it is in addition dependent on the ability of apoptotic cells to be phagocytosed by dendritic cells and thereafter initiate effector $CD8^+$ T cell development [6]. Dendritic cell activation alone is not sufficient and is also observed for nonstimulatory apoptotic phenotypes [6].	[5, 6]
T cell trafficking, chemotaxis of immunocompetent cells to the cancer cell microenvironment Solid tumors can be eridacated by antitumor $CD8^+$ T cell responses in certain animal models [12, 13]. The antitumor agent gemcitabine has a direct antitumor effect and at the same time augments the antigen-specific cellular antitumor immunity [3]. This augmentation is associated with increased tumor infiltration of $CD8^+$T cells [3]. Patients with advanced malignancies develop cachexia with altered immunoregulation; if chemotherapy improves the patients general condition (*e.g.* improved nutrition) this may reverse the immune defects associated with progressive disease/cachexia (for more detailed discussion see [4]). At least for acute leukemia patients receiving intensive chemotherapy this treatment can decrease the systemic serum levels of T cell chemotactic chemokines; this will increase local chemotactic gradients and may thereby fascilitate local recruitment of T cells to local cancer microenvironments [5].	[12-15]
Reduction of the malignant cell burden, sensitization to anti-cancer immune reactivity through pre-exposure to antineoplastic agents Tumor debulkment seems to increase the effect of anti-cancer immunotherapy, and this is clearly demonstrated by the increased antileukemic effect of allogeneic stem cell transplantation if the patients reach complete hematological remission before transplantation. *In vitro* studies of cancer cell lines (colon carcinoma, melanoma) have demonstrated that pretreatment with cytotoxic drugs before exposure to cytotoxic T cells [16, 17]. This effect is seen with different antineoplastic agents (5-fluorouracil, cisplatin, decarbacin, CPT-11), the molecular mechanisms behind this effect differ between the drugs, is mediated through the caspase pathway and in addition involve the perforin/granzyme pathway as well as Fas-initiated signaling [16, 17]. Partial sensitization of cancer cells for lysis by cytotoxic T cells.	[11, 16, 17]
Generation of immunological memory The experience from infectious diseases suggests that induction of long-tern antigen-specific memory depends on the clinical course of a disease [8]. Chronic antigenic exposure, that may be comparable to malignt disorders, was associated with the absence of antigen-independent persistence of T cell memory [8]. The interaction between chemotherapy and development of T cell memory is largely unknown.	[18]

INDUCTION OF ANTICANCER IMMUNE REACTIVITY: IMMUNOREGULATORY DENDRITIC CELLS ORCHESTRATE THE DEVELOPMENT OF ANTI-CANCER T CELL REACTIVITY

Animal models have demonstrated that development of anti-cancer immune reactivity depends on antigenic presentation by and activation of dendritic cells. These models have shown that dendritic cells are important for the presentation of tumor antigens; these specialized cells phagocytose apoptotic cells and crosspresent antigenic epitopes to $CD8^+$ T cells [12, 13]. Chemotherapy induces apoptosis in cancer cells, and the apoptotic cells then develop secondary necrosis [19, 20]. However, direct development of necrosis also seems possible [21]. Although apoptosis is important for presentation it does not necessarily induce the required maturation of the dendritic cells [22]. Rather the exposure to necrotic cells seems essential for the maturation and thereby presentation of the antigen in a context optimal for development of anti-tumor responsiveness and not tolerance induction [23]. Thus, exposure of the orchestrating dendritic cells to both antigen-donating/apoptotic and maturity-inducing/necrotic cells seems essential for the optimal development of anticancer immunity.

Development of apoptosis alone does not necessarily induce immunogenic cell death with antigenic uptake and presentation. Recent studies suggest that induction of an immunogenic apoptotic phenotype depends on the exposure of calreticulin [24]. In an experimental model anthracyclins induced rapid, preapoptotic translocation of calreticulin to the cell surface and thereby antigenic uptake, presentation and development of an antitumor immune response. The two other DNA-damaging drugs etoposide and mitomycin C did not induce calreticulin exposure and tumor immunity, but administration of recombinant calreticulin or combined pharmacological intervention to induce calreticulin exposure restored the immunogenicity of cell death elicited by these two drugs. Thus, apoptosis alone does not seem to be sufficient for induction of immunity, it has to be accompanied with calreticulin exposure. In contrast to apoptotic cells the plasma membrane shows an early destruction during necrosis, and optimal calreticulin exposure followed by phagocytosis by dendritic cells may then be difficult [25].

INDUCTION OF ANTI-CANCER T CELL REACTIVITY BY DENDRITIC CELL VACCINES

Dendritic cells have a crucial role in the induction of antigen-specific T cell responses, and dendritic cell-based therapy to enhance anti-cancer immune reactivity is now considered for several malignancies (for detailed information see the excellent review by Osada *et al.* [26]). Previous studies have investigated various methods for antigenic loading of normal dendritic cells, the role of dendritic cell maturation and various routes of immunization. Induction of anticancer reactivity has been demonstrated, but favorable clinical responses have been observed in only a few of these patients [26, 27]. However, the possible combination of immunostimulatory chemotherapy with dendritic cell-based therapy has not been investigated in humans, although the results from animal models (see above) suggest that the possibility to combine these two therapeutic approaches should be further explored.

Intradermal or subcutaneous injections have been used for dendritic cell vaccine administration and this may lead to better responses than intravenous administration [26-28]. These routes of administration rely on the capacity of injected dendritic cell to migrate to lymph nodes, and for this reason intranodal administration has also been tried [28]. This last approach may then disturb the structure of the lymph node. However, the hematopoietic malignancies may differ from other cancers with regard to the optimal route of administration. Both myeloid and lymphoid malignant cells can be induced to differentiate in the dendritic cell-direction and such cells may be used for vaccination instead of antigen-loaded normal dendritic cells [11, 26]. It is not known where these malignant dendritic cells then will home; they may home to lymph nodes like normal dendritic cells and/or home to disease-affected bone marrow or lymphoid organs like the original malignant cells. In case of migration to disease-affected organs repeated injection may then be used both to enhance immunity induction and to facilitate local chemotaxis and migration of effector T cells to the cancer cell microenvironments. Migration and chemotaxis by normal and malignant dendritic cell-vaccines should therefore be further explored before the optimal clinical use of dendritic cell vaccines (*e.g.* in combination with immunostimulatory chemotherapy) can be decided.

THE EFFECTOR PHASE OF ANTICANCER IMMUNITY

The Intrinsic Apoptosis-Inducing Pathway is Essential for Induction of Cancer Cell Apoptosis by Cytotoxic T Cells

T cells and Natural Killer (NK) cells use the same basic mechanisms for destroying their targets, although they are triggered by distinctive receptors [29]. The cells destroy their targets either by the granule-exocytosis pathway of cytotoxicity or by engaging cell surface death receptors (Fig. **1**). Cytotoxic granules are specialized secretory lysosomes and their content includes a family of serine proteases known as granzymes [29]. Perforin is another major component of the cytotoxic granules that is important for permeabilization of target cells to granzymes [30]. This molecule also seems important in tumor surveillance as perforin knock-out mice are more susceptible to tumorigenesis [31].

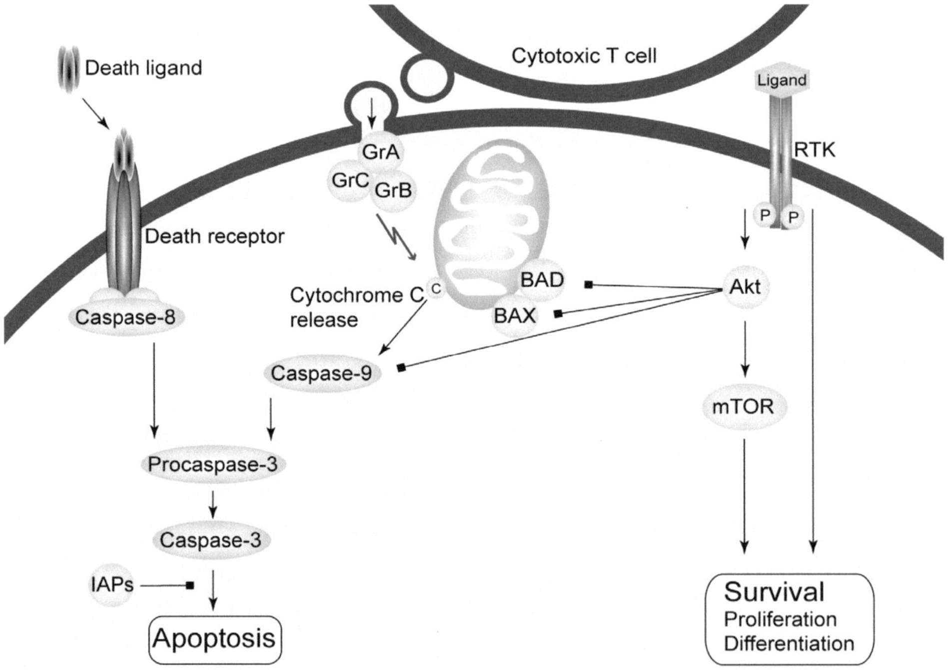

Figure 1: Cytotoxic T cell interactions with intracellular signaling pathways involved in the regulation of apoptosis and cell survival in cancer cells. (LEFT) Apoptosis can be induced through the extrinsic and intrinsic pathways. The extrinsic pathways involve extracellular death receptor ligands that bind to membrane receptors. Alternatively, intracellular events (*e.g.* cell damage caused by irradiation or chemotherapy, T cell cytotoxicity) can initiate apoptosis through the intrinsic pathway involving mitochondrial release of proapoptotic molecules like BCL2, BAX, cytochrome c (C) and inhibitors of

apoptosis (IAP). The T cell cytotoxicity with release of granzymes (GranA/B/C) mainly act on this pathway. However, there is a crosstalk between these pathways involving the bcl2/bax system upstream to their converging on caspase 3 (square symbols). (RIGHT) Many survival pathways converge on AKT (protein kinase B) and mTOR8 mammalian target of rapamycin), these pathways often involve membrane receptors with receptor tyrosine kinases (RTC). mTOR is also important for the regulation of energy metabolism in cancer cells.

Granzyme A activates the caspase-dependent pathway of apoptosis, and this process is dependent on perforin [29]. However, granzyme A also seems to induce apoptosis through caspase-independent and cytochrome c-independent mechanisms, although additional mitochondrial dysfunction also seems to contribute to this apoptotic phenotype (Table **2**). This granzyme may in addition have extracellular proinflammatory effects both through activation of procytokines (*e.g.* Interleukin-1β activation) or activation of neighboring macrophages to release cytokines [32].

Table 2: Possible alternatives for proapoptotic targeted therapy that increase the cancer cell susceptibility to T cell targeting immunotherapy.

Therapeutic Target for the Chemotherapy	**Refs.**
Enhanced proapoptotic signaling through the intrinsic regulatory pathway Heat shock protein 90 (HSP90) is a chaperon that stabilizes the structure of several client proteins [122], it is now considered for the treatment of several malignancies (for additional references see [120, 122]). Mitochondria can release several proapoptotic mediators including cytochrome c and inhibitors to IAPs (see below). Enhancement of anti-cancer T cell cytotoxicity can possibly be achieved through additional pharmacological targeting of the intrinsic pathway.	[120, 122] [51, 62]
Enhanced proapoptotic signaling through the extrinsic regulatory pathway Ligation of specific death receptors by the Tumor necrosis receptor related apoptosis-inducing ligand (TRAIL) will enhance the effect of anticancer therapy; the possible therapeutic use of recombinant human TRAIL is now considered [30, 40, 41]. TRAIL expression can be induced by histone deacetylase (HDAC) inhibitors [8]. Both chemo- and radiotherapy enhances TRAIL sensitivity [26, 44]. CD95/Fas-ligand activates the corresponding CD95/Fas death receptor [35], chemotherapy can sensitize cancer cells to T cell-mediated lysis [7]. The Inhibitors of apoptosis (IAP) gene family encodes molecules that can suppress apoptotic cell death [45], this is at least partly mediated through inhibition of caspases [46]. These molecules may be involved in carcinogenesis [48], and may therefor b considered as therapeutic target in cancer treatment. Peptide antagonists of IAPs are now developed [46, 47].	[26, 35, 38, 40, 41, 44] [17, 35] [45, 48]
Inhibition of survival pathways Cell membrane receptors for several growth and survival factors are linked to receptor tyrosine kinases that are phosphorylated and thereby activated by receptor ligation [44, 50, 51]. Receptor tyrosine kinase inhibitors inhibit this signal transduction; the drugs often inhibit several tyrosine kinases but the binding usually differ between various kinases and each drug thereby gets its own overall inhibitory profile.	[44, 50, 51]

Table 2: cont....

Inhibitory monoclonal antibodies can block receptor ligation and thereby initiation of signaling through growth factor receptors; this inhibition is often more specific than receptor tyrosine kinase inhibition [51]. These agents include inhibition of the epithelial growth factor receptor (trastuzumab) and vascular endothelial growth factor (VEGF) (bevacizumab) inhibition.	
Inhibition of nutrient supply and energy metabolism in the cancer cells Antiangiogenic therapy reduces the supply of oxygen and nutrients and will thereby alter cancer cell metabolism [50]; possible therapeutic approaches are inhibition of proangiogenic VEGF receptors (antibody blocking or tyrosine kinase inhibition), proangiogenic chemokine receptors and modulation of endothelial cell gene expression (HDAC inhibitors) (for a detailed discussion see reference [50]). Energy metabolism is often altered in malignant cells. mTOR (molecular target of rapamycin) is an important regulator of the energy metabolism, pharmacological inhibition of this mediator can alter the susceptibility of malignant cells to anticancer therapy [49]	[50] [49]

Granzyme B cleaves caspase-3 and some other caspases to unleash the caspase cascade (Fig. **1**), but several targets of this enzyme are in addition downstream caspase targets [29]. Another non-caspase target is BID (BH3-interacting domain death agonist) which, when cleaved, destroys the integrity of the mitochondrial outer membrane and thereby causes the release of proapoptotic cytochrome c as well as endogenous inhibitors of IAP (Inhibitor of Apoptosis Protein). This last effect thereby represents a mitochondrial amplification of the apoptosis pathway. Finally, granzyme B disrupts the mitochondrial transmembrane potential in a caspase- and BID-independent manner [33].

Other granzymes are also expressed in cytotoxic granules, and among these granzyme C can induce apoptosis with marked mitochondrial changes [29]. When comparing the apoptotic phenotypes of granzymes A, B and C several similarities are detected, including rapid loss of membrane integrity, surface Annexin-V expression, chromatin condensation, DNA damage and mitochondrial depolarization. However, the three granzyme-induced apoptotic phenotypes differ with regard to DNA as well as mitochondrial damage (*i.e.* bcl-2 inhibition, cytochrome c release, mitochondrial swelling). Taken together these observations show that cytotoxic cells induce apoptosis mainly through the intrinsic/intracellular pathways involving caspase activation, cytochrome c release as well as additional mechanisms involving mitochondrial damage. Therefore, a possible approach for enhancement of proapoptotic cytotoxic T cell effects in cancer cells would therefore be to combine the induction of T cell cytotoxicity with enhancement of additional proapoptotic signaling in cancer cells through (i) enhancement of signaling through the extrinsic pathways for apoptosis induction; (ii) pharmacological IAP (Inhibitors of apoptosis, see below) inhibition; and/or (iii) inhibition of signaling through survival pathways (Fig. **1**).

The External Death Receptor Pathways of Apoptotis Induction

The cell surface death receptors include the tumor necrosis factor receptor (TNFR) family [34-37]. Ligation of these death receptors causes apoptosis through activation of the caspase pathway (Fig. **1**) (Table **2**). CD95 (Fas) is one of the TNFR death receptors; its ligand is expressed on the killer cell surface and can thereby be a part of the cytotoxic cell reactivity [35, 37].

Another death receptor system is the TRAIL system (Tumor necrosis factor-related apoptosis-inducing ligand, otherwise known as Apo2Ligand/Apo2L). TRAIL induces apoptosis through interaction with the cell surface receptors TRAIL-R1 and TRAIL-R2, also known as death receptor 4 (DR4) and DR5 respectively. Both receptors contain death domains responsible for signal transduction leading to initial activation of caspase-8, thereafter activation of the effector caspase-3, -6 and -7 and finally apoptosis [34]. However, TRAIL can also bind to the two nonsignaling or decoy receptors TRAIL-R3 (DcR1) and TRAIL-R4 (DcR2). The importance of the TRAIL system in tumor surveillance is suggested by the increased frequency of spontaneous and experimental tumors in mice genetically deficient of TRAIL [34].

Several members of the death receptor family are expressed in malignant cells and can mediate anti-cancer effects, although the effects of ligation (*e.g.* CD40, TNFα) may differ and even receptor-induced antiapoptotic and growth-enhancing effects have been observed [36, 37]. Focused targeting by new therapeutic agents instead of the natural ligands may therefore become necessary to get a predictable proapoptotic signaling through these pathways.

Pharmacological Targeting of the External Death Receptor Pathway: A Possible Therapeutic Strategy to Increase Cancer Cell Susceptibility to T cell Cytotoxicity

Pharmacological targeting of the extrinsic death receptor pathway is now emerging as a possible approach in clinical anticancer therapy (Table **2**). One approach will then be to increase the expression of either death receptors or death receptor ligands by the malignant cells. A recent study described that histone deacetylase (HDAC) inhibitors could increase the expression of TRAIL in AML cells and thereby trigger leukemia-selective cell death [38]. This was observed with the three structurally different HDAC inhibitors valproic acid, suberoylanilide hydroxamic acid and MS275; all these drugs now being in clinical trials [39]. HDAC inhibitors can in addition activate both the extrinsic and intrinsic apoptosis pathway and alter the balance between pro- and antiapoptotic Bcl-2 family members in favor of apoptosis induction (for reference see [39]). Another class of new therapeutic agents is the proteasome inhibitors, these agents seem to inhibit NFκB activation and thereby induce the surface expression of the DR4 and DR5 death receptors [40]. DR5 seems to be more important than DR4 for induction of apoptosis [41], and for this reason future studies should possibly focus on this receptor.

An alternative approach would be to stimulate death receptors through administration of recombinant ligands or agonistic antibodies [41-43]. The possible use of recombinant human (rh) TRAIL is now considered, whereas severe systemic side effects of TNFα and the possibility of hepatotoxicity of rhFas-ligand suggest that systemic clinical use of these ligands is less likely [44]. However, TNFα is now approved for isolated limb perfusion in combination with chemotherapy in non-resectable high-grade sarcoma [43].

Inhibitors of apoptosis (IAP) are small proteins that suppress apoptosis through their ability to bind to and inactivate caspases that are critical for the initiation and execution phases of apoptosis [45]. IAP-inhibitors have been developed [46-48], and these agents may thereby represent a third alternative for induction of apoptosis through targeting of the death receptor pathways.

Finally, mammalian target of rapamycin (mTOR) is a kinase acting downstream to AKT, and is important for regulation of energy metabolism, cell proliferation and survival (see below). Rapamycin analogues are now in clinical trials, and preclinical data suggest an increased sensitivity to TRAIL-induced apoptosis when rhTRAIL is combined with rapamycin [41, 49].

Pharmacological Targeting of Survival Pathways: An Alternative Strategy to Increase Cancer Cell Susceptibility to T cell Cytotoxicity

Combination of apoptosis induction through the extrinsic pathway with inhibition of intracellular survival signaling is now suggested [41, 44]. Some of these receptors have mTOR as a downstream target, whereas other pathways/mediators are involved for other receptors (Fig. **1**). Signaling through these pathways may also affect the pathways of apoptosis induction, *e.g.* the Akt-induced inhibition of the intrinsic pathway *via* Bad, Bax and caspase 9 (Fig. **1**). A wide range of tyrosine kinase inhibitors have been characterized [50]; several of them are in clinical trials and the use of imatinib in the treatment of chronic myeloid leukemia and gastrointestinal stromal tumors is well established [51]. These agents can be used for inhibition of a wide range of growth factor receptors, their specificity profiles for different receptor kinases show a wide variation [50], and probably one has to consider the overall inhibitory profile of each individual drug when trying to identify the optimal inhibitor in different malignancies.

Another alternative for combined therapies could be to combine targeting of the extrinsic apoptosis pathway with targeting of survival pathways by inhibitory antibodies [52]. This is suggested by preclinical studies describing enhanced apoptosis of HER2 overexpressing cancer cell lines when combining rhTRAIL with the HER2-antagonistic tratuzumab antibody [49]. EGF-R inhibition can also sensitize human carcinoma cells to rhTRAIL-induced apoptosis by downregulating the antiapoptotic proteins AKT and Bcl-xl [44, 53].

IMMUNOSUPPRESSIVE EFFECTS OF CHEMOTHERAPY

The previous studies of immunostimulatory conventional chemotherapy were performed in animal models and with local injection of cytotoxic drugs into the tumor [5-7]. In clinical cancer therapy systemic administration is used and drug effects on the immune system therefore have to be considered [54-60]. In many cancers low-dose therapy is used either preoperatively to reduce tumor size or postoperatively to reduce the risk of later relapse. Chemotherapy may also be used in combination with radiotherapy. In these cases with low-dose therapy the effects on the immune system are limited; combination with immunotherapy should therefore be possible and may even enhance development of immunoreactivity (Table **1**).

However, it should be emphasized that certain drugs or drug combinations (*e.g.* fludarabine-containing regimen) have a stronger T cell suppressive effect than other drugs [54], and it will therefore be important to carefully develop chemotherapy regimens that induce immunostimulatory apoptosis in the malignant cells.

An important question will be whether it is possible to combine early immunotherapy with more intensive chemotherapy or high-dose therapy combined with autologous stem cell support. These patients develop a period of severe leukopenia, including severe lymphopenia and functional abnormalities of the cellular immune system, before hematologic and lymphoid reconstitution. These studies have demonstrated:

- Even during the period of severe chemotherapy-induced lymphopenia these patients have an operative T cell system. The functional characteristics of these circulating T cells in patients receiving intensive antileukemic therapy are summarized in Table **3** [55-58].

- Patients receiving peripheral blood mobilized stem cell support after high-dose therapy usually have a shorter period of severe leukopenia [57], but their T cell system during this period seems very similar to patients receiving conventional antileukemic therapy with only minor qualitative differences.

- After immune reconstitution there is often a CD4-lymphopenia that may last for several months [11, 59, 60], but this has only been investigated for patients with brain tumors, sarcomas and various hematological malignancies.

Table 3: The cellular immune system in cancer patients with severe chemotherapy-induced lymphopenia.

T cell subsets
- The CD4:CD8 ratio shows a wide variation but is often >1.0 [65].
- The majority of the circulating cells are T cell receptor $\alpha\beta^+$ [65].
T cell proliferative responsiveness
- Although a high frequency of clonogenic T cells persist after chemotherapy, the frequency is reduced [65].

Table 3: cont....

- A detectable proliferative response is often observed *in vitro* after stimulation through the TCR alone, but additional targeting of accessory pathways (*e.g.* anti-CD28 antibodies) will usually increase proliferation [56-58].
- Activated T cells can respond to a wide range of T cell growth factors, but the strongest responses are usually caused by IL2 and IL15 [14, 55-58, 61, 62].
T cell cytokine release
- The circulating clonogenic T cells release a wide range of cytokines, including tumor necrosis factor [14, 55].
- When investigating the whole T cell population a similar broad cytokine release profile is observed including (i) high levels of IFNγ and GM-CSF, (ii) intermediate levels of IL10 and IL13, and (iii) low but usually detectable levels of IL3 and IL4 [55].
Pharmacological targeting
Proliferative T cell responses are increased by the Protein Kinase C agonist Pep005 [55].

Taken together these studies clearly demonstrate that chemotherapy has immunosuppressive effects. However, for several reasons it would definitely be an advantage to start immunotherapy early after induction of immunostimulatory apoptosis in the cancer cell: (i) the cancer cell burden would then be relatively low and immunotherapy seems to be most effective in patients with a low disease burden and thereby a high T cell : cancer cell ratio [11]; (ii) it would thereby be possible to take advantage of the recently apoptosis-induced immune reactivity [11], and for example booster this chemotherapy-induced effect by additional immunotherapy. The results described in Table **2** suggest that early start of immunotherapy should be possible because circulating and functional T cells still exist even early after intensive chemotherapy during the period of severe lymphopenia.

Cancer diseases themselves will have systemic effects, the most extreme clinical manifestation being the picture of cachexia [14]. This picture will also include abnormalities in the immunoregulatory cytokine network. Thus, additional disease-induced immune defects have to be considered when immunotherapy is tried in such patients.

REGULATORY T CELLS, Th17 T CELLS AND MESENCHYMAL STROMAL/STEM CELLS - KEY REGULATORS OF ANTICANCER IMMUNE REACTIVITY

Treg cells are immunosuppressive cells [61]. In contrast, proinflammatory Th17 cells release the proinflammatory cytokine IL17 and differentiate from the

$CD161^+CD4^+$ T cell subset; one important function of IL17 seems to be coordination and regulation of local inflammation through upregulation of other proinflammatory cytokines and chemokines [61, 62]. Mesenchymal stromal cells are important immune regulators that interact with both these T cell subsets.

Treg Cells

One pathway for induction of immunological tolerance is through generation of regulatory T cells (Treg) that comprise approximately 5-15% of the peripheral $CD4^+$ T cells [62, 63]. In animal models these cells prevent autoimmune disorders, graft rejection and anticancer reactivity [62, 64]. Previous studies have demonstrated that the T cell depleting effects of anticancer chemotherapy is not a random effect [65, 66], and differences between cytotoxic agents in their elimination of Treg cells may therefore be important for the post-chemotherapy development of anti-cancer immune responses.

Several studies suggest that cytotoxic agents can alter the levels of Treg cells. In the majority of patients with chronic lymphocytic leukemia treatment with fludarabine-based regimen the activity of Treg cells is decreased or even abrogated and this is associated with a decreased frequency of these cells in peripheral blood [66]. Animal models have demonstrated that depletion of Treg cells is associated with generation of specific immune T cells in tumor-draining lymph nodes [67], whereas suppression of Treg cells by cyclophosphamide may allow immunotherapy of established tumors to be curative [68]. However, this cyclophospahmide effect may depend on the administration of the drug or the nature of the immunotherapy because no effect was observed of a single infusion of cyclophosphamide combined with nonspecific immunotherapy in humans with metastatic carcinoma [69]. The mTOR antagonist rapamycin that can be used both in immunosuppressive and anticancer therapy, increases the number of Treg cells [70], whereas docetaxel does not seem to have any effect [71]. Taken together these observations suggest that conventional as well as new targeted chemotherapy should not only be evaluated with regard to apoptosis induction and calreticulin expression by the apoptotic cancer cells, but also for their effects on Treg cells.

Th17 Cells - A Dynamic Proinflammatory Phenotype

As reviewed by Ersvaer *et al.* [61], the key regulators in human Th17 development are the transcription factor RORC2 and STAT3 [72]. In addition, IFNγ has a direct inhibitory effect but an indirect enhancing effect through increased IL-1β release [73, 74], STAT1 has inhibitory effects, [75], and the transcription factor aryl hydrocarbon receptor (AHR) [76] as well as prostaglandin E2 (PGE2) [77, 78] stimulate their development. The development of Th17 cells is inhibited by the cytokine Leukemia inhibitory factor (LIF) through activation of ERK signaling and upregulation of SOCS3 and mesenchymal stromal/stem cells can probably inhibit Th17 development by this mechanism [79]. LIF is also released by activated T cells; detectable release is then seen for most clonogenic T cells derived from normal donors as well as allogeneic stem cell recipients [80], and LIF may possibly serve as a negative feedback mechanism during inflammation.

Th17 cells typically express the surface molecules CCR4, CCR6, IL23-R and CD161 [81-83] and they release the signature cytokine IL17-A together with IL17-F, IL21, IL22, IL26 and CCL20 [81, 84, 85]. However, this is probably not a stable phenotype because: (i) *ex vivo* isolated murine Th17 cells can be converted into Thl/Th17 cells after exposure to IFN-γ and IL12 [86]; and (ii) both IL17-A and IL17-F can be only transiently produced during T cell stimulation [87]. These observations suggest that the Th17 phenotype does not represent an end-stage T helper cell subset. Human cancer cells may show constitutive release of a wide range of cytokines [88], but it is not known whether this cancer-associated modulations of local cytokine networks can alter the Th17 phenotype and thereby inhibit the anticancer immune reactivity.

The Th17: Treg Ratio After Intensive Chemotherapy

Conventional intensive chemotherapy is followed by a period of 2-4 weeks with a general bone marrow failure and severe lymphopenia [89]. As reviewed in detail previously [61, 90-92], rapid lymphoid reconstitution in patients receiving intensive anticancer chemotherapy is associated with increased leukemia-free survival. The mechanisms behind this effect are unknown, but may include increased efficiency of antileukemic immune reactivity during a period of low leukemia cell burden; or treatment-induced enhancement of immunostimulatory T cell networks (for additional references and a more detailed discussion see [61]).

As described above intensive chemotherapy is followed by a long-lasting defect in circulating $CD4^+$ cells. An important question is therefore whether intensive chemotherapy will alter the balance between proinflammatory and immunosuppressive T cell subsets. Previous studies suggest that at least certain cancer patients have increased levels of circulating immunosuppressive $CD4^+$ $CD25^{high}$ regulatory T cells, and these increased Treg levels may persist after chemotherapy [89, 93, 94]. On the other hand, the Th17 levels may not be altered even for patients receiving intensive chemotherapy for aggressive hematologic malignancies, *i.e.* acute myeloid leukemia (AML). The levels of circulating Th17 cells in patients with untreated AML have been investigated in two previous studies; these studies investigated different subsets of AML patients but they both described either increased or normal levels of circulating Th17 cells before treatment, during the period of severe chemotherapy-induced cytopenia and when patients achieved a complete hematological remission following intensive chemotherapy [89, 95]. Rapid lymphoid reconstitution with maintenance of normal Th17 levels may therefore counteract the immunosuppressive effects of Treg cells and thereby contribute to increased survival. Thus, it is justified to conclude that even though anticancer chemotherapy induces a general $CD4^+$ T cell defect this is not necessarily associated with a quantitative Th17 defect. However, future studies have to clarify whether this is true for cancer patients in general or differs between patients depending on the malignant disorder, disease stage and type of chemotherapy.

Mesenchymal Stromal/Stem Cells - Therapeutic Use *Versus* Therapeutic Targeting

Mesenchymal stromal cells have been established as important immunomodulatory cells [96, 97], and infusion of such cells is now tried as an immunosuppressive strategy [98, 99]. These cells are able to activate and expand Treg cells, but Treg cells are not necessary for their suppressive effects [100, 101]. Mesenchymal cells may also inhibit the development of Th17 cells possibly through the release of LIF with activation of ERK signaling and upregulation of SOCS3 [79, 102]. Infused mesenchymal cells are mainly trapped in the lungs and distant organs are affected through the release of soluble mediators [97-99, 103, 104]. These distant effects are the basis for using mesenchymal cell infusion as immunosuppression [98, 99]; the initial results suggest that this is a promising strategy for induction of immunological tolerance in GVHD as well as in autoimmune diseases and no acute infusional toxicity has been reported [105]. However, several aspects need to be clarified with regard to the use of such *ex vivo* expanded mesenchymal cells as a therapeutic strategy: (i) the optimal conditions for *ex vivo* expansion need to be established [106]; (ii) it has to be clarified whether autologous, haploidentical or third-party cells should be used; and (iii) efficiency markers to predict the clinical effects need to be identified. This strategy is now tried in the treatment of acute GVHD in allotransplanted patients [107], even though it is not known how such infusions will affect antileukemic T cell reactivity.

Mesenchymal immunoregulatory cells are also present within tumors and seem to be important for immunoediting as a part of the disease development. [108]. Experimental models suggest that T cell derived cytokines then activate mesenchymal cells to release chemotactic chemokines that attract T cells; direct T cell suppression is therefore mediated through the release of soluble mediators to their common microenvironment [109]. The mesenchymal cells then have dual effects: (i) dominating suppression is mediated through the T cell chemotaxis followed by local release of specific suppressive mediators; but (ii) the cell have additional immunostimulatory effects that become important if suppression is blocked [110]. Furthermore, a recent study described the presence of a specialized mesenchymal cell subset within pancreatic cancers, and these cells seem to initiate immunoediting with suppression of tumor-specific immune reactivity. Pharmacological targeting of such local/cancer-associated mesenchymal cells with blocking of their immunosuppressive activity may thus become a therapeutic strategy to initiate and enhance cancer-directed immune reactivity.

Finally, mesenchymal stem cells release a wide range of cytokines, including several growth factors that can be important both in the regulation of angiogenesis as well as cancer cell survival and proliferation [109]. These cells may even release soluble mediators in response to conventional chemotherapy that support cancer cell survival and induce chemoresistance [111]. Thus, therapeutic targeting of local mesenchymal cells should include inhibition of both the immunosuppressive effects and their growth factor release

ALLOGENEIC STEM CELL TRANSPLANTATION - AN ESTABLISHED COMBINATION OF PROAPOPTOTIC CHEMOTHERAPY AND IMMUNOTHERAPY

Allogeneic stem cell transplantation is the therapeutic strategy where the clinical importance of anti-cancer immune reactivity is best documented through graft *versus* host (GVH) and graft *versus* leukemia (GVL) reactivity [112]. The experience from allotransplantation can therefore be useful for the design of immunotherapy in the autologous setting. This treatment strategy consists of an initial conditioning chemotherapy and eventually irradiation therapy followed by the transplantation.

Allotransplantation in Leukemia - is Immunogenic Apoptosis Possible?

Allogeneic stem cell transplantation is mainly used for the treatment of hematological malignancies. The biological characteristics of immunogenic apoptosis were described above. Relatively few studies have addressed the question whether immunogenic apoptosis can be induced in malignant hematopoietic cells, but at least for AML cells an immunogenic apoptotic phenotype can be induced [25, 113, 114]. These studies showed that cytotoxic drugs can induce both calreticulin exposure, surface membrane expression of HSPs and release of soluble HSPs, and immunogenic apoptosis may thus be important for the posttransplant induction of leukemia-directed immune reactivity.

Reduction of the Cancer Cell Burden by Pretransplant Conditioning Therapy - Effects on Host Dendritic Cells and the Induction of Antileukemic Immune Reactivity

Pretransplant factors seem important for posttransplant immune reactivity [115], including the nature of the pretransplant conditioning therapy as well as the status of the cytokine network [116]. This can be illustrated by the effect G-CSF therapy in allotransplanted patients. A European study [117] demonstrated a negative outcome of posttransplant G-CSF therapy due to an increased risk of GVHD, whereas this was not detected in another study [118]. This difference can possibly be explained by pretransplant factors. Firstly, G-CSF has immunosuppressive effects [116], and the adverse effect of posttransplant G-CSF was not detected for patients receiving G-CSF mobilized PBSC allografts; these observations suggest that pretransplant G-CSF induced a suppression of graft immunocompetent cells. Secondly, the study without any G-CSF effect included a much lower number of patients receiving pretransplant total body irradiation (TBI), and a recent experimental study suggests that TBI upregulates G-CSF receptor expression by host dendritic cells and thereby initiate an anti-host immune response if G-CSF is administered early after conditioning when host dendritic cells are still present [119]. These observations thereby illustrate the importance of host dendritic cells for regulation of posttransplant immune responses, including antileukemic GVHD. Early therapeutic targeting of dendritic cells should therefore be considered not only in allotransplant recipients but possibly also after autotransplantation (*e.g.* start of cancer vaccination early after transplantation).

The Posttransplant Immune System - Pharmacological Agents with Immunosuppressive and Antileukemic Effects

Allotransplant recipients usually receive prophylactic immunosuppression against severe GVHD, and several new immunosuppressive agents also have anticancer effects, *e.g.* HSP90 and mTOR inhibitors [120-123]. A combined effect may therefore be possible with these new therapeutic agents, but only the mTOR inhibitor rapamycin is currently used as GVHD prophylaxis in allotransplanted patients [124].

Treg and Th17 Cells in Patients Receiving Allogeneic Stem Cell Transplantation

Treg cells seem to mediate anti-GVHD effects on cytolytic cellular effectors, proinflammatory mediators and proapoptotic soluble mediators [125, 126]. Recent animal studies suggest that Treg cells are important regulators of both GVH and GVL reactivity [126]. The observation that certain polymorphisms in the IL23 receptor and the IL17 genes are associated with an increased risk of GVHD suggest that Th17 cells are also important for development of GVH reactivity [128]. A small study also showed an association between later acute GVHD and the IL17 releasing capacity of circulating T cells derived during the early period of severe posttransplant cytopenia [129]. Finally, a third study described an increased frequency of acute GVHD in patients receiving a high number of Th17 in their stem cell grafts [130]; increased levels of Th17 cells were also observed at onset of acute GVHD but these levels normalized when patients responded to treatment. Taken together these studies strongly suggest that even though allografted patients also have a long-lasting $CD4^+$ T cell defect similar to patients receiving conventional intensive chemotherapy [90], the balance between Treg and Th17 cells seem to be important for the generation of antihost/antileukemic immune reactivity both in the autologous and allogeneic setting. Therapeutic targeting of these T cell subsets may therefore become possible to increase antileukemic immune reactivity and possibly separate the general GVH from the specific GVL reactivity.

What can we Learn from the Allotransplantation Experience About Combination of Chemotherapy and Immunotherapy?

Allogeneic stem cell transplantation represents a combination of pretransplant conditioning therapy (chemotherapy and eventually irradiation) and immunotherapy through GVH and GVL reactivity, and several general principles for anticancer immunotherapy are clearly illustrated by the experience from allogeneic stem cell transplantation. Firstly, immunotherapy is most effective in patients with a low cancer cell burden. Secondly, immunocompetent effector cells are able to eradicate residual cancer cells and thereby reduce the risk of relapse. Finally, even in patients with treatment-induced $CD4^+$ T cell defects effective anticancer immune reactivity can be seen; the induction of anticancer T cell reactivity seems to depend on the balance between proinflammatory and immunosuppressive T cell subsets rather than the general status of the immune system. However, other immunocompetent cells should also be considered in future studies, including antigen-presenting dendritic cells and immunoregulatory mesenchymal cells.

CONCLUDING REMARKS

In our opinion future anticancer therapy should try to combine different therapeutic approaches. T cell cytotoxicity should be regarded as a cancer-specific proapoptotic signal mediated mainly through the intrinsic pathway of apoptosis induction. This effect can probably be enhanced by an optimal combination with conventional proapoptotic chemotherapy and anticancer vaccination. However, new therapeutic strategies should also be considered for combination with immunotherapy, especially drugs that favor induction of apoptosis through the extrinsic pathway. We suggest that future clinical studies of immunotherapy should be based on the following guidelines that are summarized in Fig. **2**:

- An initial step to reduce the malignant cell burden is probably necessary because T cell targeting therapy seems most effective in patients with a limited cancer cell burden [11]. This could be surgery, irradiation or conventional chemotherapy. If possible one should use chemotherapy that induces immunogenic cell death and eventually in combination with vaccination.

- Immunotherapy should probably start early after tumor reduction when the cancer cell burden is at the lowest [11]. Although patients have a cellular immune defect early after chemotherapy, they still have circulating and functional T cells even after the most intensive treatment [55-58].

- Immunotherapy should be extended for a relatively long time, because chemotherapy-induced cellular immune defects may persist for several months in adult patients [11, 50, 59, 60].

- Several agents tried for proapoptotic targeted therapy are also considered as immunosuppressive agents [59, 131, 132]. These agents should therefore probably be administered after the initial development of an anticancer immune response, and treatment to further enhance the immune reactivity should then continue together with the proapoptotic targeted therapy.

This strategy is also supported by the experience from allogeneic stem cell transplantation in patients with hematologic malignancies, and by the fact that reduction of immunosuppression is used as a therapeutic strategy for patients with early posttransplant leukemia relapse [133]. The clinical effects of such combinatory regimen have to be carefully evaluated in properly designed clinical studies also involving detailed studies of the biological effects and possible side effects.

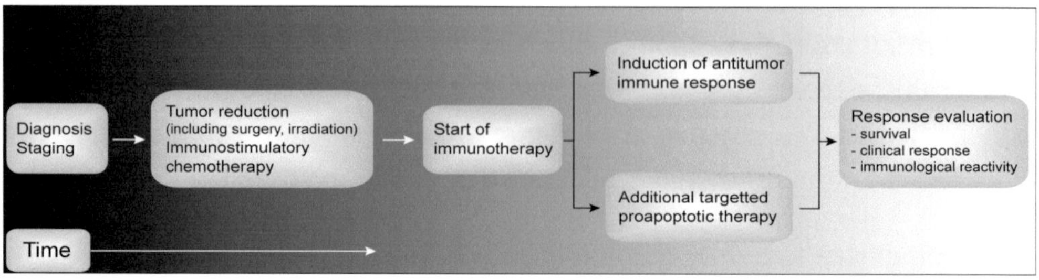

Figure 2: Design of future clinical studies combining conventional anticancer therapy, immunotherapy and new targeted anticancer therapy. The treatment should initially include conventional cancer-reducing therapy because studies of several malignancies suggest that anti-cancer immunoreactivity is most effective at a low cancer cell burden. If possible this step should include immunostimulatory chemotherapy. The next step should be start of immunotherapy to induce or enhance anticancer immune reactivity, this treatment should probably continue through an extended time period and its effect has to be evaluated before new targeted therapy is tried. Many of the new anticancer drugs have immunosuppressive effects; we suggest that the targeted therapy should start at least after a period of immunotherapy and preferable when increased anticancer immune reactivity is detected. When this total therapy is established; the effects have to be evaluated either as alteration in anticancer immune reactivity or preferably as difference in survival or clinical responses between randomized patients.

ACKNOWLEDGEMENTS

The study received financial support from the Norwegian Cancer Society and the Grieg Foundation.

CONFLICT OF INTEREST

The author(s) confirm that this chapter content has no conflict of interest.

DISCLOSURE

The chapter submitted for the eBook Series entitled **"Advances in Cancer Drug Targets, Volume 1"** is an update of our article in **Current Cancer Drug Targets, Volume 8, Issue 8, 2008,** with additional text and references.

ABBREVATIONS

AHR = Aryl hydrocarbon receptor

AML	=	Acute myeloid leukemia
Bax	=	Bcl2-associated X protein
Bcl-2	=	B-cell lymphoma 2
Bcl-xl	=	B-cell lymphoma – extra large
BID	=	BH3-interacting domain death agonist
CCL20	=	Chemokine (C-C motif) ligand 20
CCR4	=	Chemokine (C-C motif) receptor 4
CCR6	=	Chemokine (C-C motif) receptor 6
CD	=	Cluster of differentiation
DcR	=	Decoy receptor
DR	=	Death receptor
EBMT	=	European Group for Blood and Marrow Transplantation
EGF-R	=	Epidermal growth factor receptor
ERK	=	Extracellular signal-regulated kinases
G-CSF	=	Granulocyte-colony stimulating factor
GVHD	=	Graft *versus* host disease
GVL	=	Graft *versus* leukemia
HDAC inhibitor	=	Histone deacetylase inhibitor

HER2	=	Human Epidermal Growth Factor Receptor 2
HSP	=	Heat shock protein
IBMTR	=	International Bone Marrow Transplant Registry
IFNγ	=	Interferon gamma
IAP	=	Inhibitor of Apoptosis Protein
IL	=	Interleukin
LIF	=	Leukemia inhibitory factor
mTOR	=	Mammalian target of rapamycin
NFκB	=	Nuclear factor kappa B
NK cell	=	Natural Killer cell
PGE2	=	Prostaglandin E2
rh	=	Recombinant human
RORC2	=	Receptor-related orphan receptor C2
SOCS3	=	Suppressor of cytokine signalling 3
STAT	=	Signal transducer and activator of transcription
TBI	=	Total body irradiation
Th1	=	T helper 1 cell subset

Th17 = T helper 17 cell subset

TNFα = Tumor necrosis factor α

TNFR = Tumor necrosis factor receptor

TRAIL = Tumor necrosis factor-related apoptosis-inducing ligand

Treg cells = Regulatory T cells

REFERENCES

[1] Miles AK, Matharoo-Ball B, Li G, Ahmad M, Rees RC. The identification of human tumour antigens: Current status and future developments. Cancer Immunol Immunother 2006;55: 996-1003.

[2] Novellino L, Castelli C, Parmiani G. A listing of human tumor antigens recognized by T cells: March 2004 update. Cancer Immunol Immunother 2005;54: 187-207.

[3] Dalgleish AG, Whelan MA. Cancer vaccines as a therapeutic modality: The long trek. Cancer Immunol Immunother 2006;55: 1025-32.

[4] Yu M, Finn OJ. DNA vaccines for cancer too. Cancer Immunol Immunother 2006;55: 119-30.

[5] Scheffer SR, Nave H, Korangy F, Schlote K, Pabst R, Jaffee EM, Manns MP, Greten TF. Apoptotic, but not necrotic, tumor cell vaccines induce a potent immune response *in vivo*. Int J Cancer 2003;103: 205-11.

[6] Casares N, Pequignot MO, Tesniere A, Ghiringhelli F, Roux S, Chaput N, Schmitt E, Hamai A, Hervas-Stubbs S, Obeid M, Coutant F, Metivier D, Pichard E, Aucouturier P, Pierron G, Garrido C, Zitvogel L, Kroemer G. Caspase-dependent immunogenicity of doxorubicin-induced tumor cell death. J Exp Med 2005;202: 1691-701.

[7] Casati A, Zimmermann VS, Benigni F, Bertilaccio MT, Bellone M, Mondino A. The immunogenicity of dendritic cell-based vaccines is not hampered by doxorubicin and melphalan administration. J Immunol 2005;174: 3317-25.

[8] Clarke C, Smyth MJ. Calreticulin exposure increases cancer immunogenicity. Nat Biotechnol 2007;25: 192-3.

[9] Vereecque R, Saudemont A, Quesnel B. Cytosine arabinoside induces costimulatory molecule expression in acute myeloid leukemia cells. Leukemia 2004;18: 1223-30.

[10] Lake RA, Robinson BW. Immunotherapy and chemotherapy--a practical partnership. Nat Rev Cancer 2005;5: 397-405.

[11] Bruserud O, Wendelboe O. Biological treatment in acute myelogenous leukaemia: how should T-cell targeting immunotherapy be combined with intensive chemotherapy? Expert Opin Biol Ther 2001;1: 1005-16.

[12] Stumbles PA, Himbeck R, Frelinger JA, Collins EJ, Lake RA, Robinson BW. Cutting edge: tumor-specific CTL are constitutively cross-armed in draining lymph nodes and transiently disseminate to mediate tumor regression following systemic CD40 activatiol. J Immunol 2004;173: 5923-8.

[13] Nowak AK, Robinson BW, Lake RA. Synergy between chemotherapy and immunotherapy in the treatment of established murine solid tumors. Cancer Res 2003;63: 4490-6.

[14] Bruserud O, Glenjen N. A critical review of T cell targeting immunotherapy in pancreatic cancer: only a hypothesis or a real hope for the patients? Expert Opin Biol Ther 2002;2: 693-701.

[15] Olsnes AM, Motorin D, Ryningen A, Zaritskey AY, Bruserud O. T lymphocyte chemotactic chemokines in acute myelogenous leukemia (AML): local release by native human AML blasts and systemic levels of CXCL10 (IP-10), CCL5 (RANTES) and CCL17 (TARC). Cancer Immunol Immunother 2006;55: 830-40.

[16] Bergmann-Leitner ES, Abrams SI. Treatment of human colon carcinoma cell lines with anti-neoplastic agents enhances their lytic sensitivity to antigen-specific CD8+ cytotoxic T lymphocytes. Cancer Immunol Immunother 2001;50: 445-55.

[17] Yang S, Haluska FG. Treatment of melanoma with 5-fluorouracil or dacarbazine *in vitro* sensitizes cells to antigen-specific CTL lysis through perforin/granzyme- and Fas-mediated pathways. J Immunol 2004;172: 4599-608.

[18] Wherry EJ, Barber DL, Kaech SM, Blattman JN, Ahmed R. Antigen-independent memory CD8 T cells do not develop during chronic viral infection. Proc Natl Acad Sci USA 2004;101: 16004-9.

[19] Stapnes C, Doskeland AP, Hatfield K, Ersvaer E, Ryningen A, Lorens JB, Gjertsen BT, Bruserud O. The proteasome inhibitors bortezomib and PR-171 have antiproliferative and proapoptotic effects on primary human acute myeloid leukaemia cells. Br J Haematol 2007;136: 814-28.

[20] Ryningen A, Ersvaer E, Oyan AM, Kalland KH, Vintermyr OK, Gjertsen BT, Bruserud O. Stress-induced *in vitro* apoptosis of native human acute myelogenous leukemia (AML) cells shows a wide variation between patients and is associated with low BCL-2:Bax ratio and low levels of heat shock protein 70 and 90. Leuk Res 2006;30: 1531-40.

[21] Bruserud O, Ryningen A, Wergeland L, Glenjen NI, Gjertsen BT. Osteoblasts increase proliferation and release of pro-angiogenic interleukin 8 by native human acute myelogenous leukemia blasts. Haematologica 2004;89: 391-402.

[22] Steinman RM, Turley S, Mellman I, Inaba K. The induction of tolerance by dendritic cells that have captured apoptotic cells. J Exp Med 2000;191: 411-6.

[23] Sauter B, Albert ML, Francisco L, Larsson M, Somersan S, Bhardwaj N. Consequences of cell death: exposure to necrotic tumor cells, but not primary tissue cells or apoptotic cells, induces the maturation of immunostimulatory dendritic cells. J Exp Med 2000;191: 423-34.

[24] Obeid M, Tesniere A, Ghiringhelli F, Fimia GM, Apetoh L, Perfettini JL, Castedo M, Mignot G, Panaretakis T, Casares N, Metivier D, Larochette N, van Endert P, Ciccosanti F, Piacentini M, Zitvogel L, Kroemer G. Calreticulin exposure dictates the immunogenicity of cancer cell death. Nat Med 2007;13: 54-61.

[25] Chaput N, De Botton S, Obeid M, Apetoh L, Ghiringhelli F, Panaretakis T, Flament C, Zitvogel L, Kroemer G. Molecular determinants of immunogenic cell death: surface exposure of calreticulin makes the difference. J Mol Med 2007;85: 1069-76.

[26] Osada T, Clay TM, Woo CY, Morse MA, Lyerly HK. Dendritic cell-based immunotherapy. Int Rev Immunol 2006;25: 377-413.

[27] Kyte JA, Gaudernack G. Immuno-gene therapy of cancer with tumour-mRNA transfected dendritic cells. Cancer Immunol Immunother 2006;55: 1432-42.

[28] Houtenbos I, Westers TM, Ossenkoppele GJ, van de Loosdrecht AA. Leukemia-derived dendritic cells: towards clinical vaccination protocols in acute myeloid leukemia. Haematologica 2006;91: 348-55.

[29] Lieberman J. The ABCs of granule-mediated cytotoxicity: new weapons in the arsenal. Nat Rev Immunol 2003;3: 361-70.

[30] Catalfamo M, Henkart PA. Perforin and the granule exocytosis cytotoxicity pathway. Curr Opin Immunol 2003;15: 522-7.

[31] Smyth MJ, Thia KY, Street SE, MacGregor D, Godfrey DI, Trapani JA. Perforin-mediated cytotoxicity is critical for surveillance of spontaneous lymphoma. J Exp Med 2000;192: 755-60.

[32] Sower LE, Froelich CJ, Allegretto N, Rose PM, Hanna WD, Klimpel GR. Extracellular activities of human granzyme A. Monocyte activation by granzyme A *versus* alpha-thrombin. J Immunol 1996;156: 2585-90.

[33] Barry M, Heibein JA, Pinkoski MJ, Lee SF, Moyer RW, Green DR, Bleackley RC. Granzyme B short-circuits the need for caspase 8 activity during granule-mediated cytotoxic T-lymphocyte killing by directly cleaving Bid. Mol Cell Biol 2000;20: 3781-94.

[34] Wang S, El-Deiry WS. TRAIL and apoptosis induction by TNF-family death receptors. Oncogene 2003;22: 8628-33.

[35] Wajant H. CD95L/FasL and TRAIL in tumour surveillance and cancer therapy. Cancer Treat Res 2006;130: 141-65.

[36] Varfolomeev EE, Ashkenazi A. Tumor necrosis factor: an apoptosis JuNKie? Cell 2004;116: 491-7.

[37] Tamada K, Chen L. Renewed interest in cancer immunotherapy with the tumor necrosis factor superfamily molecules. Cancer Immunol Immunother 2006;55: 355-62.

[38] Nebbioso A, Clarke N, Voltz E, Germain E, Ambrosino C, Bontempo P, Alvarez R, Schiavone EM, Ferrara F, Bresciani F, Weisz A, de Lera AR, Gronemeyer H, Altucci L. Tumor-selective action of HDAC inhibitors involves TRAIL induction in acute myeloid leukemia cells. Nat Med 2005;11: 77-84.

[39] Bruserud O, Stapnes C, Ersvaer E, Gjertsen BT, Ryningen A. Histone deacetylase inhibitors in cancer treatment: a review of the clinical toxicity and the modulation of gene expression in cancer cell. Curr Pharm Biotechn 2007;8: 388-400.

[40] Nencioni A, Grunebach F, Patrone F, Ballestrero A, Brossart P. Proteasome inhibitors: antitumor effects and beyond. Leukemia 2007;21: 30-6.

[41] Duiker EW, Mom CH, de Jong S, Willemse PH, Gietema JA, van der Zee AG, de Vries EG. The clinical trail of TRAIL. Eur J Cancer 2006;42: 2233-40.

[42] Kelley RF, Totpal K, Lindstrom SH, Mathieu M, Billeci K, Deforge L, Pai R, Hymowitz SG, Ashkenazi A. Receptor-selective mutants of apoptosis-inducing ligand 2/tumor

necrosis factor-related apoptosis-inducing ligand reveal a greater contribution of death receptor (DR) 5 than DR4 to apoptosis signaling. J Biol Chem 2005;280: 2205-12.
[43] Ashkenazi A. Targeting death and decoy receptors of the tumour-necrosis factor superfamily. Nat Rev Cancer 2002;2: 420-30.
[44] Hougardy BM, Maduro JH, van der Zee AG, Willemse PH, de Jong S, de Vries EG. Clinical potential of inhibitors of survival pathways and activators of apoptotic pathways in treatment of cervical cancer: changing the apoptotic balance. Lancet Oncol 2005;6: 589-98.
[45] Salvesen GS, Duckett CS. IAP proteins: blocking the road to death's door. Nat Rev Mol Cell Biol 2002;3: 401-10.
[46] Vucic D, Franklin MC, Wallweber HJ, Das K, Eckelman BP, Shin H, Elliott LO, Kadkhodayan S, Deshayes K, Salvesen GS, Fairbrother WJ. Engineering ML-IAP to produce an extraordinarily potent caspase 9 inhibitor: implications for Smac-dependent anti-apoptotic activity of ML-IAP. Biochem J 2005;385: 11-20.
[47] Franklin MC, Kadkhodayan S, Ackerly H, Alexandru D, Distefano MD, Elliott LO, Flygare JA, Mausisa G, Okawa DC, Ong D, Vucic D, Deshayes K, Fairbrother WJ. Structure and function analysis of peptide antagonists of melanoma inhibitor of apoptosis (ML-IAP). Biochemistry 2003;42: 8223-31.
[48] Varfolomeev E, Wayson SM, Dixit VM, Fairbrother WJ, Vucic D. The inhibitor of apoptosis protein fusion c-IAP2.MALT1 stimulates NF-kappaB activation independently of TRAF1 AND TRAF2. J Biol Chem 2006;281: 29022-9.
[49] Panner A, James CD, Berger MS, Pieper RO. mTOR controls FLIPS translation and TRAIL sensitivity in glioblastoma multiforme cells. Mol Cell Biol 2005;25: 8809-23.
[50] Hatfield KJ, Olsnes AM, Gjertsen BT, Bruserud O. Antiangiogenic therapy in acute myelogenous leukemia: targeting of vascular endothelial growth factor and interleukin 8 as possible antileukemic strategies. Curr Cancer Drug Targets 2005;5: 229-48.
[51] Collins I, Workman P. New approaches to molecular cancer therapeutics. Nat Chem Biol 2006;2: 689-700.
[52] Cuello M, Ettenberg SA, Clark AS, Keane MM, Posner RH, Nau MM, Dennis PA, Lipkowitz S. Down-regulation of the erbB-2 receptor by trastuzumab (herceptin) enhances tumor necrosis factor-related apoptosis-inducing ligand-mediated apoptosis in breast and ovarian cancer cell lines that overexpress erbB-2. Cancer Res 2001;61: 4892-900.
[53] Park SY, Seol DW. Regulation of Akt by EGF-R inhibitors, a possible mechanism of EGF-R inhibitor-enhanced TRAIL-induced apoptosis. Biochem Biophys Res Commun 2002;295: 515-8.
[54] Ravandi F, O'Brien S. Immune defects in patients with chronic lymphocytic leukemia. Cancer Immunol Immunother 2006;55: 197-209.
[55] Ersvaer E, Hampson P, Hatfield K, Ulvestad E, Wendelbo O, Lord JM, Gjertsen BT, Bruserud O. T cells remaining after intensive chemotherapy for acute myelogenous leukemia show a broad cytokine release profile including high levels of interferon-gamma that can be further increased by a novel protein kinase C agonist PEP005. Cancer Immunol Immunother 2007;56: 913-25.
[56] Wendelbo O, Nesthus I, Sjo M, Paulsen K, Ernst P, Bruserud O. Functional characterization of T lymphocytes derived from patients with acute myelogenous leukemia and chemotherapy-induced leukopenia. Cancer Immunol Immunother 2004;53: 740-7.

[57] Wendelbo O, Nesthus I, Sjo M, Ernst P, Bruserud O. Cellular immune responses in multiple myeloma patients with treatment-induced cytopenia early after high-dose chemotherapy and autologous peripheral blood stem cell transplantation. Leuk Res 2004;28: 461-8.

[58] Wendelbo O, Glenjen N, Bruserud O. Interleukin-7 (IL-7) in patients receiving intensive chemotherapy for acute myelogenous leukemia: studies of systemic IL-7 Levels and IL-7 responsiveness of circulating T lymphocytes. J Interferon Cytokine Res 2002;22: 1057-65.

[59] Crooks GM, Weinberg K, Mackall C. Immune reconstitution: from stem cells to lymphocytes. Biol Blood Marrow Transplant 2006;12: 42-6.

[60] Mackall CL. T-cell immunodeficiency following cytotoxic antineoplastic therapy: a review. Stem Cells 2000;18: 10-8.

[61] Ersvaer E, Melve GK, Bruserud O. Future perspectives: should Th17 cells be considered as a possible therapeutic target in acute myeloid leukemia patients receiving allogeneic stem cell transplantation? Cancer Immunol Immunother 2011;60: 1669-81.

[62] Sakaguchi S. Naturally arising Foxp3-expressing CD25+CD4+ regulatory T cells in immunological tolerance to self and non-self. Nat Immunol 2005;6: 345-52.

[63] Gallegos AM, Bevan MJ. Central tolerance: good but imperfect. Immunol Rev 2006;209: 290-6.

[64] Shimizu J, Yamazaki S, Sakaguchi S. Induction of tumor immunity by removing CD25+CD4+ T cells: a common basis between tumor immunity and autoimmunity. J Immunol 1999;163: 5211-8.

[65] Bruserud O, Ulvestad E, Berentsen S, Bergheim J, Nesthus I. T-lymphocyte functions in acute leukaemia patients with severe chemotherapy-induced cytopenia: characterization of clonogenic T-cell proliferation. Scand J Immunol 1998;47: 54-62.

[66] Beyer M, Kochanek M, Darabi K, Popov A, Jensen M, Endl E, Knolle PA, Thomas RK, von Bergwelt-Baildon M, Debey S, Hallek M, Schultze JL. Reduced frequencies and suppressive function of CD4+CD25hi regulatory T cells in patients with chronic lymphocytic leukemia after therapy with fludarabine. Blood 2005;106: 2018-25.

[67] Tanaka H, Tanaka J, Kjaergaard J, Shu S. Depletion of CD4+ CD25+ regulatory cells augments the generation of specific immune T cells in tumor-draining lymph nodes. J Immunother 2002;25: 207-17.

[68] Ghiringhelli F, Larmonier N, Schmitt E, Parcellier A, Cathelin D, Garrido C, Chauffert B, Solary E, Bonnotte B, Martin F. CD4+CD25+ regulatory T cells suppress tumor immunity but are sensitive to cyclophosphamide which allows immunotherapy of established tumors to be curative. Eur J Immunol 2004;34: 336-44.

[69] Audia S, Nicolas A, Cathelin D, Larmonier N, Ferrand C, Foucher P, Fanton A, Bergoin E, Maynadie M, Arnould L, Bateman A, Lorcerie B, Solary E, Chauffert B, Bonnotte B. Increase of CD4+ CD25+ regulatory T cells in the peripheral blood of patients with metastatic carcinoma: a Phase I clinical trial using cyclophosphamide and immunotherapy to eliminate CD4+ CD25+ T lymphocytes. Clin Exp Immunol 2007;150: 523-30.

[70] Qu Y, Zhang B, Zhao L, Liu G, Ma H, Rao E, Zeng C, Zhao Y. The effect of immunosuppressive drug rapamycin on regulatory CD4+CD25+Foxp3+T cells in mice. Transpl Immunol 2007;17: 153-61.

[71] Garnett CT, Schlom J, Hodge JW. Combination of docetaxel and recombinant vaccine enhances T-cell responses and antitumor activity: effects of docetaxel on immune enhancement. Clin Cancer Res 2008;14: 3536-44.

[72] Ivanov, II, McKenzie BS, Zhou L, Tadokoro CE, Lepelley A, Lafaille JJ, Cua DJ, Littman DR. The orphan nuclear receptor RORgammat directs the differentiation program of proinflammatory IL-17+ T helper cells. Cell 2006;126: 1121-33.

[73] Masters SL, Mielke LA, Cornish AL, Sutton CE, O'Donnell J, Cengia LH, Roberts AW, Wicks IP, Mills KH, Croker BA. Regulation of interleukin-1beta by interferon-gamma is species specific, limited by suppressor of cytokine signalling 1 and influences interleukin-17 production. EMBO Rep 2010;11: 640-6.

[74] Lexberg MH, Taubner A, Albrecht I, Lepenies I, Richter A, Kamradt T, Radbruch A, Chang HD. IFN-gamma and IL-12 synergize to convert *in vivo* generated Th17 into Th1/Th17 cells. Eur J Immunol 2010;40: 3017-27.

[75] Ramgolam VS, Sha Y, Jin J, Zhang X, Markovic-Plese S. IFN-beta inhibits human Th17 cell differentiation. J Immunol 2009;183: 5418-27.

[76] Hirahara K, Ghoreschi K, Laurence A, Yang XP, Kanno Y, O'Shea JJ. Signal transduction pathways and transcriptional regulation in Th17 cell differentiation. Cytokine Growth Factor Rev 2010;21: 425-34.

[77] Chizzolini C, Chicheportiche R, Alvarez M, de Rham C, Roux-Lombard P, Ferrari-Lacraz S, Dayer JM. Prostaglandin E2 synergistically with interleukin-23 favors human Th17 expansion. Blood 2008;112: 3696-703.

[78] Boniface K, Bak-Jensen KS, Li Y, Blumenschein WM, McGeachy MJ, McClanahan TK, McKenzie BS, Kastelein RA, Cua DJ, de Waal Malefyt R. Prostaglandin E2 regulates Th17 cell differentiation and function through cyclic AMP and EP2/EP4 receptor signaling. J Exp Med 2009;206: 535-48.

[79] Cao W, Yang Y, Wang Z, Liu A, Fang L, Wu F, Hong J, Shi Y, Leung S, Dong C, Zhang JZ. Leukemia inhibitory factor inhibits T helper 17 cell differentiation and confers treatment effects of neural progenitor cell therapy in autoimmune disease. Immunity 2011;35: 273-84.

[80] Bruserud O, Hamann W, Pawelec G. Secretion of leukaemia inhibitory factor after allogeneic bone marrow transplantation: a study of CD4+ and CD8+ TCR alpha beta+ T-cell clones derived from four leukaemia patients. Eur J Haematol 1995;54: 106-10.

[81] Acosta-Rodriguez EV, Napolitani G, Lanzavecchia A, Sallusto F. Interleukins 1beta and 6 but not transforming growth factor-beta are essential for the differentiation of interleukin 17-producing human T helper cells. Nat Immunol 2007;8: 942-9.

[82] Cosmi L, De Palma R, Santarlasci V, Maggi L, Capone M, Frosali F, Rodolico G, Querci V, Abbate G, Angeli R, Berrino L, Fambrini M, Caproni M, Tonelli F, Lazzeri E, Parronchi P, Liotta F, Maggi E, Romagnani S, Annunziato F. Human interleukin 17-producing cells originate from a CD161+CD4+ T cell precursor. J Exp Med 2008;205: 1903-16.

[83] Maggi L, Santarlasci V, Capone M, Peired A, Frosali F, Crome SQ, Querci V, Fambrini M, Liotta F, Levings MK, Maggi E, Cosmi L, Romagnani S, Annunziato F. CD161 is a marker of all human IL-17-producing T-cell subsets and is induced by RORC. Eur J Immunol 2010;40: 2174-81.

[84] Annunziato F, Cosmi L, Santarlasci V, Maggi L, Liotta F, Mazzinghi B, Parente E, Fili L, Ferri S, Frosali F, Giudici F, Romagnani P, Parronchi P, Tonelli F, Maggi E, Romagnani S. Phenotypic and functional features of human Th17 cells. J Exp Med 2007;204: 1849-61.

[85] Wilson NJ, Boniface K, Chan JR, McKenzie BS, Blumenschein WM, Mattson JD, Basham B, Smith K, Chen T, Morel F, Lecron JC, Kastelein RA, Cua DJ, McClanahan TK, Bowman EP, de Waal Malefyt R. Development, cytokine profile and function of human interleukin 17-producing helper T cells. Nat Immunol 2007;8: 950-7.

[86] Lexberg MH, Taubner A, Albrecht I, Lepenies I, Richter A, Kamradt T, Radbruch A, Chang HD. IFN-gamma and IL-12 synergize to convert *in vivo* generated Th17 into Th1/Th17 cells. Eur J Immunol 2010;40: 3017-27.

[87] Kurschus FC, Croxford AL, Heinen AP, Wortge S, Ielo D, Waisman A. Genetic proof for the transient nature of the Th17 phenotype. Eur J Immunol 2010;40: 3336-46.

[88] Fredly H, Reikvam H, Gjertsen BT, Bruserud O. Disease-stabilizing treatment with all-trans retinoic acid and valproic acid in acute myeloid leukemia: serum hsp70 and hsp90 levels and serum cytokine profiles are determined by the disease, patient age, and anti-leukemic treatment. Amer J Hematol 2012;87: 368-76.

[89] Ersvaer E, Liseth K, Skavland J, Gjertsen BT, Bruserud O. Intensive chemotherapy for acute myeloid leukemia differentially affects circulating TC1, TH1, TH17 and TREG cells. BMC Immunol 2010;11: 38.

[90] Liseth K, Ersvaer E, Hervig T, Bruserud O. Combination of intensive chemotherapy and anticancer vaccines in the treatment of human malignancies: the hematological experience. J Biomedi Biotechnol 2010;2010: 692097.

[91] Porrata LF. Host immunity and survival. Leuk Lymphoma 2008;49: 843-4.

[92] Porrata LF, Markovic SN. Timely reconstitution of immune competence affects clinical outcome following autologous stem cell transplantation. Clin Exp Med 2004;4: 78-85.

[93] Szczepanski MJ, Szajnik M, Czystowska M, Mandapathil M, Strauss L, Welsh A, Foon KA, Whiteside TL, Boyiadzis M. Increased frequency and suppression by regulatory T cells in patients with acute myelogenous leukemia. Clini Cancer Res 2009;15: 3325-32.

[94] Wang X, Zheng J, Liu J, Yao J, He Y, Li X, Yu J, Yang J, Liu Z, Huang S. Increased population of CD4(+)CD25(high), regulatory T cells with their higher apoptotic and proliferating status in peripheral blood of acute myeloid leukemia patients. Eur J Haematol 2005;75: 468-76.

[95] Wu C, Wang S, Wang F, Chen Q, Peng S, Zhang Y, Qian J, Jin J, Xu H. Increased frequencies of T helper type 17 cells in the peripheral blood of patients with acute myeloid leukaemia. Clin Exp Immunol 2009;158: 199-204.

[96] Prockop DJ, Oh JY. Medical therapies with adult stem/progenitor cells (MSCs): A backward journey from dramatic results *in vivo* to the cellular and molecular explanations. J Cell Biochem 2012;113: 1460-9.

[97] Wernicke C, Grunewald T, Juenger H, Kuci S, Kuci Z, Koehl U, Mueller I, Doering M, Peters C, Lawitschka A, Kolb H-J, Bader P, Burdach S, von Luettichau I. Mesenchymal stromal cells for treatment of steroid-refractory GvHD: a review of the literature and two pediatric cases. Int Arch Med 2011;4: 27.

[98] Le Blanc K, Rasmusson I, Sundberg B, Gotherstrom C, Hassan M, Uzunel M, Ringden O. Treatment of severe acute graft-*versus*-host disease with third party haploidentical mesenchymal stem cells. Lancet 2004;363: 1439-41.

[99] Le Blanc K, Frassoni F, Ball L, Locatelli F, Roelofs H, Lewis I, Lanino E, Sundberg B, Bernardo ME, Remberger M, Dini G, Egeler RM, Bacigalupo A, Fibbe W, Ringden O. Mesenchymal stem cells for treatment of steroid-resistant, severe, acute graft-*versus*-host disease: a phase II study. Lancet 2008;371: 1579-86.

[100] Aggarwal S, Pittenger MF. Human mesenchymal stem cells modulate allogeneic immune cell responses. Blood 2005;105: 1815-22.

[101] Glennie S, Soeiro I, Dyson PJ, Lam EW, Dazzi F. Bone marrow mesenchymal stem cells induce division arrest anergy of activated T cells. Blood 2005;105: 2821-7.

[102] Egea V, von Baumgarten L, Schichor C, Berninger B, Popp T, Neth P, Goldbrunner R, Kienast Y, Winkler F, Jochum M, Ries C. TNF-alpha respecifies human mesenchymal stem cells to a neural fate and promotes migration toward experimental glioma. Cell Death Differ 2011;18: 853-63.

[103] Lee RH, Pulin AA, Seo MJ, Kota DJ, Ylostalo J, Larson BL, Semprun-Prieto L, Delafontaine P, Prockop DJ. Intravenous hMSCs improve myocardial infarction in mice because cells embolized in lung are activated to secrete the anti-inflammatory protein TSG-6. Cell Stem Cell 2009;5: 54-63.

[104] Block GJ, Ohkouchi S, Fung F, Frenkel J, Gregory C, Pochampally R, DiMattia G, Sullivan DE, Prockop DJ. Multipotent stromal cells are activated to reduce apoptosis in part by upregulation and secretion of stanniocalcin-1. Stem Cells 2009;27: 670-81.

[105] Prockop DJ, Brenner M, Fibbe WE, Horwitz E, Le Blanc K, Phinney DG, Simmons PJ, Sensebe L, Keating A. Defining the risks of mesenchymal stromal cell therapy. Cytotherapy 2010;12: 576-8.

[106] Roobrouck VD, Vanuytsel K, Verfaillie CM. Concise review: culture mediated changes in fate and/or potency of stem cells. Stem Cells 2011;29: 583-9.

[107] Ball LM, Bernardo ME, Roelofs H, Lankester A, Cometa A, Egeler RM, Locatelli F, Fibbe WE. Cotransplantation of *ex vivo* expanded mesenchymal stem cells accelerates lymphocyte recovery and may reduce the risk of graft failure in haploidentical hematopoietic stem-cell transplantation. Blood 2007;110: 2764-7.

[108] Kraman M, Bambrough PJ, Arnold JN, Roberts EW, Magiera L, Jones JO, Gopinathan A, Tuveson DA, Fearon DT. Suppression of antitumor immunity by stromal cells expressing fibroblast activation protein-alpha. Science 2010;330: 827-30.

[109] Shi Y, Su J, Roberts AI, Shou P, Rabson AB, Ren G. How mesenchymal stem cells interact with tissue immune responses. Trends Immunol 2012;33: 136-43.

[110] Ren C, Kumar S, Chanda D, Chen J, Mountz JD, Ponnazhagan S. Therapeutic potential of mesenchymal stem cells producing interferon-alpha in a mouse melanoma lung metastasis model. Stem Cells 2008;26: 2332-8.

[111] Roodhart JM, Daenen LG, Stigter EC, Prins HJ, Gerrits J, Houthuijzen JM, Gerritsen MG, Schipper HS, Backer MJ, van Amersfoort M, Vermaat JS, Moerer P, Ishihara K, Kalkhoven E, Beijnen JH, Derksen PW, Medema RH, Martens AC, Brenkman AB, Voest

EE. Mesenchymal stem cells induce resistance to chemotherapy through the release of platinum-induced fatty acids. Cancer Cell 2011;20: 370-83.

[112] Kersey JH. The role of allogeneic-cell transplantation in leukemia. N Engl J Med 2010;363: 2158-9.

[113] Fredly H, Ersvaer E, Gjertsen BT, Bruserud O. Immunogenic apoptosis in human acute myeloid leukemia (AML): primary human AML cells expose calreticulin and release heat shock protein (HSP) 70 and HSP90 during apoptosis. Oncol Rep 2011;25: 1549-56.

[114] Lasunskaia EB, Fridlianskaia, II, Guzhova IV, Bozhkov VM, Margulis BA. Accumulation of major stress protein 70kDa protects myeloid and lymphoid cells from death by apoptosis. Apoptosis 1997;2: 156-63.

[115] Reikvam H, Mosevoll KA, Melve GK, Gunther CC, Sjo M, Bentsen PT, Bruserud O. The Pretransplantation Serum Cytokine Profile in Allogeneic Stem Cell Recipients Differs from Healthy Individuals, and Various Profiles are Associated with Different Risks of Posttransplantation Complications. Biol Blood Marrow Transplant 2012;18: 190-9.

[116] Melve GK, Ersvssr E, Kittang AO, Bruserud O. The chemokine system in allogeneic stem-cell transplantation: a possible therapeutic target? Exp Rev Hematol 2011;4: 563-76.

[117] Ringden O, Labopin M, Gorin NC, Le Blanc K, Rocha V, Gluckman E, Reiffers J, Arcese W, Vossen JM, Jouet JP, Cordonnier C, Frassoni F. Treatment with granulocyte colony-stimulating factor after allogeneic bone marrow transplantation for acute leukemia increases the risk of graft-*versus*-host disease and death: a study from the Acute Leukemia Working Party of the European Group for Blood and Marrow Transplantation. J Clin Oncol 2004;22: 416-23.

[118] Khoury HJ, Loberiza FR, Jr., Ringden O, Barrett AJ, Bolwell BJ, Cahn JY, Champlin RE, Gale RP, Hale GA, Urbano-Ispizua A, Martino R, McCarthy PL, Tiberghien P, Verdonck LF, Horowitz MM. Impact of posttransplantation G-CSF on outcomes of allogeneic hematopoietic stem cell transplantation. Blood 2006;107: 1712-6.

[119] Morris ES, MacDonald KP, Kuns RD, Morris HM, Banovic T, Don AL, Rowe V, Wilson YA, Raffelt NC, Engwerda CR, Burman AC, Markey KA, Godfrey DI, Smyth MJ, Hill GR. Induction of natural killer T cell-dependent alloreactivity by administration of granulocyte colony-stimulating factor after bone marrow transplantation. Nat Med 2009;15: 436-41.

[120] Reikvam H, Hatfield KJ, Ersvaer E, Hovland R, Skavland J, Gjertsen BT, Petersen K, Bruserud O. Expression profile of heat shock proteins in acute myeloid leukaemia patients reveals a distinct signature strongly associated with FLT3 mutation status - consequences and potentials for pharmacological intervention. Br J Haematol 2012;156: 468-80.

[121] Reikvam H, Hatfield K, Ersvaer E, Ryningen A, Bruserud Ø. Pharmacological targeting of the PI3K-AKT/PKB-mTOR pathway alters local angioregulation in acute myelogenous leukemia. Haematologica 2010;95(s2): Abstract no 0634.

[122] Reikvam H, Ersvaer E, Bruserud O. Heat shock protein 90 - a potential target in the treatment of human acute myelogenous leukemia. Curr Cancer Drug Targets 2009;9: 761-76.

[123] Bruserud O, Ersvaer E, Olsnes A, Gjertsen BT. Anticancer immunotherapy in combination with proapoptotic therapy. Curr Cancer Drug Targets 2008;8: 666-75.

[124] Rodriguez R, Nakamura R, Palmer JM, Parker P, Shayani S, Nademanee A, Snyder D, Pullarkat V, Kogut N, Rosenthal J, Smith E, Karanes C, O'Donnell M, Krishnan AY, Senitzer D, Forman SJ. A phase II pilot study of tacrolimus/sirolimus GVHD prophylaxis for sibling donor hematopoietic stem cell transplantation using 3 conditioning regimens. Blood 2010;115: 1098-1105.

[125] Paczesny S, Hanauer D, Sun Y, Reddy P. New perspectives on the biology of acute GVHD. Bone Marrow Transplant. 2010;45: 1-11.

[126] Engelhardt BG, Crowe JE, Jr. Homing in on acute graft *vs.* host disease: tissue-specific T regulatory and Th17 cells. Curr Top Microbiol Immunol. 2010;341: 121-46.

[127] Kittan NA, Hildebrandt GC. The chemokine system: a possible therapeutic target in acute graft *versus* host disease. Curr Top Microbiol Immunol 2010;341: 97-120.

[128] Carvalho A, Cunha C, Di Ianni M, Pitzurra L, Aloisi T, Falzetti F, Carotti A, Bistoni F, Aversa F, Romani L. Prognostic significance of genetic variants in the IL-23/Th17 pathway for the outcome of T cell-depleted allogeneic stem cell transplantation. Bone Marrow Transplant 2010;45: 1645-52.

[129] Liseth K, Sjo M, Paulsen K, Bruserud O, Ersvaer E. Early pre-engraftment, functional, *in vitro* responsiveness of T lymphocytes in allotransplanted, acute leukemia patients: proliferation and release of a broad profile of cytokines, possibly predictive of graft-*versus*-host disease. Eur Cytokine Netw 2010;21: 40-9.

[130] Zhao XY, Xu LL, Lu SY, Huang XJ. IL-17-producing T cells contribute to acute graft-*versus*-host disease in patients undergoing unmanipulated blood and marrow transplantation. Eur J Immunol 2011;41: 514-26.

[131] Bruserud O, Tronstad KJ, McCormack E, Gjertsen BT. Is targeted chemotherapy an alternative to immunotherapy in chronic lymphocytic leukemia? Cancer Immunol Immunother 2006;55: 221-8.

[132] Bruserud O, McCormack E, Gjertsen BT. Immunotherapy in chronic lymphocytic leukemia. Cancer Immunol Immunother 2006;55: 185-7.

[133] Reikvam H, Kittang AO, Melve G, Mosevoll KA, Bentsen PT, Ersvær E, Gjertsen BT, Bruserud Ø. Targeted anti-leukemic therapy as disease-stabilizing treatment for leukemia relapse after allogeneic stem cell transplantation: Will it be possible to combine these strategies with retransplantation or donor lymphocyte infusions? Curr Cancer Drug Targets 2012; Epub ahead of print.

Send Orders of Reprints at bspsaif@emirates.net.ae
Advances in Cancer Drug Targets, Vol. 1, 2013, 207-237

CHAPTER 7

Melatonin and Breast Cancer: Selective Estrogen Enzyme Modulator Actions

Samuel Cos*, Alicia González, Virginia Alvarez-García, Carolina Alonso-González and Carlos Martínez-Campa

Department of Physiology and Pharmacology, School of Medicine, University of Cantabria, 39011 Santander, Spain

Abstract: Melatonin exerts oncostatic effects on different kinds of tumors, especially on hormone-dependent breast cancer. The general conclusion is that melatonin, *in vivo*, reduces the incidence and growth of chemically-induced mammary tumors in rodents, and, *in vitro*, inhibits the proliferation and invasiveness of human breast cancer cells. Both studies support the hypothesis that melatonin inhibits the growth of breast cancer by interacting with estrogen-signaling pathways through three different mechanisms: (a) indirect neuroendocrine effect which includes the melatonin down-regulation of the hypothalamic-pituitary-reproductive axis and the consequent reduction of circulating levels of gonadal estrogens, (b) direct melatonin actions at tumor cell level by interacting with the activation of the estrogen receptor, thus behaving as a selective estrogen receptor modulator (SERM), and (c) the regulation of the enzymes involved in the biosynthesis of estrogens in peripheral tissues, thus behaving as a selective estrogen enzyme modulator (SEEM). As melatonin reduces the activity and expression of aromatase, sulfatase and 17β-hydroxysteroid dehydrogenase and increases the activity and expression of estrogen sulfotransferase, it may protect mammary tissue from excessive estrogenic effects. Thus, a single molecule has both SERM and SEEM properties, one of the main objectives desired for the breast antitumoral drugs. Since the inhibition of enzymes involved in the biosynthesis of estrogens is currently one of the first therapeutic strategies used against the growth of breast cancer, melatonin modulation of different enzymes involved in the synthesis of steroid hormones make, collectively, this indolamine an interesting anticancer drug in the prevention and treatment of estrogen-dependent mammary tumors.

Keywords: Melatonin, estrogen, tumors, SERM, SEEM, carcinogenesis, oncostatic, indolamine, carcinoma, estradiol, 17β-hydroxysteroid dehydrogenase, androgens.

***Address correspondence to Samuel Cos:** Departamento de Fisiología y Farmacología, Facultad de Medicina, Universidad de Cantabria, Cardenal Herrera Oria s/n, 39011 Santander, Spain; Tel: 34 942 201988. Fax: 34 942 201903; E-mail: coss@unican.es.

Atta-ur-Rahman (Ed)

INTRODUCTION

Melatonin, the main hormone secreted by the pineal gland, has been involved in different physiological actions in a great variety of biological contexts [1]. The role of melatonin in the regulation of cancer cell growth has been widely studied during the last few decades [2-5]. There has been considerable study into the oncostatic actions of melatonin on different kinds of tumors and especially on estrogen-dependent breast cancer [5, 6]. It is well established that, *in vivo*, experimental manipulations activating the pineal gland, or the administration of melatonin, reduce both the incidence and growth rate of spontaneous or chemically induced mammary tumors in rodents, while pinealectomy or situations which implicate a reduction of melatonin production usually stimulate mammary carcinogenesis [2, 3, 7], whereas *in vitro* melatonin inhibits breast cancer cell proliferation and invasiveness [2-6].

Several mechanisms have been proposed to explain the oncostatic actions of melatonin in breast tumors: a) indirect effects derived from the interaction of melatonin with the neuroendocrine reproductive axis, leading to a down-regulation of some of the hormones influencing tumor growth, especially gonadal estrogens [1]; b) melatonin antiestrogenic actions directly on the epithelial mammary cells [8, 9]; c) antioxidant effects of melatonin [10]; d) melatonin regulatory effects in hemopoiesis and immunoenhancement, which is believed to be closely involved in several aspects of host defense and has the potential to be useful as an adjuvant tumor immunotherapeutic agent [11]; e) inhibitory effects of melatonin on telomerase activity in tumor cells [12]; or f) melatonin's suppression of fatty acid uptake and metabolism [13, 14].

In this review, we will firstly point out the importance of estrogens in the genesis and development of breast cancer and how the intratumoral metabolism and synthesis of estrogens, as a result of the interactions of various enzymes, are considered to play a very important role in the pathogenesis and development of hormone dependent breast carcinoma; secondly, we will underline how the interaction between estrogens and melatonin has long been described to explain the melatonin oncostatic actions and, finally, we will outline the possible mechanisms through which melatonin may inhibit the growth of breast cancer and how some of these mechanisms recently described involve interactions with the intratumoral metabolism and biosynthesis of estrogens, with melatonin behaving as a selective estrogen enzyme modulator (SEEM).

THE ROLE OF ESTROGENS IN BREAST CANCER

Breast cancer continues to be a major cause of death in European and American women. The incidence of breast cancer is rising throughout the world and is the most frequent cancer in women. There are more than 1,000,000 new cases of breast cancer in the world each year [15]. Breast cancer is a classic model of hormone dependent malignancy. More than 95% of new cases of breast cancer are initially hormone-dependent, either in pre- or postmenopausal women, and estradiol plays a main role in their genesis and progression. It is known that breast development at puberty and during sexual maturity is stimulated by 17β-estradiol, which is the predominant circulating ovarian steroid and the most biologically active hormone in breast tissue. However, there is also considerable evidence that estrogens are also mammary carcinogens [16-19]. The dependence on ovarian function of breast cancer was first recognized in 1896, when Beatson observed regression of advanced and metastatic breast cancer induced by bilateral ovariectomy in premenopausal women. From then on, considerable clinical and experimental studies link cumulative and sustained exposure to estrogens with an increased risk of developing breast cancer [20]. The importance of ovarian steroidogenesis in the genesis of breast cancer is highlighted by the facts that early menarche and late menopause are associated with greater breast cancer risk, whereas late menarche and early menopause result in a significant reduction of the same. However, what is not clear are the mechanisms through which estrogens cause cancer. Most hypotheses consider that estrogens binding to ERα stimulate cell proliferation, thus increasing the possibility of errors in DNA replication which would result in point mutations [21]. Furthermore, direct genotoxic effects of 17β-estradiol by itself and its metabolites could also explain the estrogen-induced carcinogenesis [17, 22].

In relation to the role of estrogens in the genesis and growth of mammary tumors, it is important to consider that two–thirds of breast cancer occur in postmenopausal women, where ovaries have ceased to be functional and circulating levels of estrogens are low. In premenopausal women 70% of estrogens come from the ovaries and 30% from the conversion of androgens (mainly dehydroepiandrosterone and dehydroepiandrosterone sulfate) to estrogens in peripheral tissues. After the cessation of the follicular function, in postmenopausal women, except for a small contribution from ovarian and/or adrenal testosterone and androstenedione, 100% of sex estrogens are synthesized in peripheral tissues, such as mesenquimal-cells of the adipose tissue and skin, osteoblasts, condrocites, vascular endothelium, aortic soft muscle and different areas of the brain such as hypothalamus (preoptic, anterior and mediobasal areas) and tonsil, from precursors of adrenal [23]. In this situation, plasma levels of estrogens are low, and, however, the concentration of estradiol in peripheral tissues such as the mammary gland is high, as a result of the *in situ* biosynthesis [24, 25]. Yue *et al.* reported that *in situ* synthesis of estrogen predominates over uptake from plasma as a means of maintaining breast tissues estradiol concentrations after menopause [25, 26]. Estrogen-dependent breast carcinoma in which *in situ* conversion from serum androgen to biologically active estrogens occurs without release into the extracellular space is considered "intracrine" tissue [26].

INTRACRINOLOGY OF ESTROGEN DEPENDENT HUMAN BREAST CARCINOMA

There is extensive information describing that mammary cancer tissue contains all the enzymes responsible for the local biosynthesis of estrogens. The most important precursors (steroids C19) for the local synthesis of estrogens are dehydroepyandrosterone (DHEA) and its sulphate (DHEAS), which come mainly from the adrenal cortex. Fig. **1** shows a general view of the basic enzymatic mechanisms involved in the formation and transformation of estrogens in human breast cancer. Two principal pathways are involved in the final steps of estrogens formation: the aromatase pathway, which transforms androgens into estrogens and the sulfatase pathway which converts estrogen sulfates into estrone and estradiol [27, 28]. The main enzymes involved in the regulation of local estrogen production are:

A) Aromatase is an enzymatic complex which consists of two components: aromatase cytochrome P-450 protein and, coupled to it, an ubiquitous flavoprotein, NADPH-cytochrome P-450 reductase [29]. The gene coding for the cytochrome P-450 protein is the largest of the cytochrome P-450 family. Because

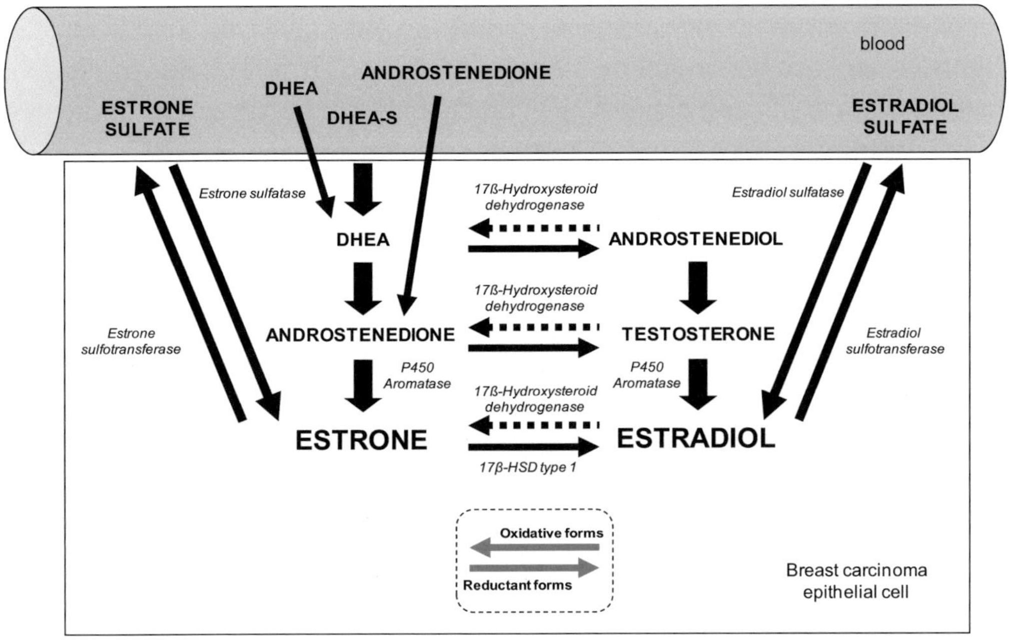

Figure 1: Enzymatic mechanisms involved in the local production of estrogens in human breast carcinoma tissues. (Abbreviations: DHEA, dehydroepiandrosterone; DHEA-S, dehydroepiandrosterone sulphate; *17β-HSD type 1,* 17β-hydroxysteroid dehidrogenase type 1).

its overall homology to other members of the P-450 superfamily is low, aromatase belongs to a separate gene family designated CYP19 [30]. The transcription of the aromatase gene is highly regulated and each tissue can regulate the amount of aromatase transcribed in a highly specific manner [29]. The catalytic process leading to the aromatization of androgens requires the sequential transfer of three pairs of electrons and consumes three moles of reduced NADPH in the synthesis of one mole of estrogen. The reaction is thought to involve three oxidative cycles at the C19 methyl group of the steroid substrate which are involved in the conversion of androstenedione to estrone or testosterone to estradiol. In the premenopausal state the major source of aromatase and of its substrates is the ovary. However, in the postmenopausal state, the ovary loses its complement of aromatase enzyme, although it does continue to secrete androstenedione. The adrenal subsumes the primary role of providing substrate for aromatase by directly secreting testosterone and androstenedione. The major source of the aromatase enzyme in postmenopausal women is peripheral tissues and particularly fat and muscle. In humans, the expression of aromatase has a broader tissue distribution and occurs in many organs, including ovary, placenta, hypothalamus, liver, muscle, adipose tissue and mammary tissue itself. It is well known that the P450 aromatase activity and expression is much higher in breast cancer tissue than in normal mammary tissue, and this is one of the reasons why the estrogen concentration in this type of tissue is very elevated [26, 31]. Two-thirds of breast cancer contain aromatase and synthesize biologically significant amounts of estrogens locally in the tumor. The level of aromatase mRNA expression is highest in the stromal compartment of breast tumors but it is also present in epithelial cells as well [30].

B) Sulfatase (STS) is an enzyme which hydrolyzes several sulphated steroids such as estrone sulphate, estradiol sulphate, dehydroepiandrosterone sulphate and cholesterol sulphate [31]. The estrogen sulfate can act as an estrogen reserve, which could be formed from the sulphated-estrogens by the estrogen sulfatase, present in the mammary gland in both normal and tumoral tissues. Estrone sulphate has a relatively long half-life in the peripheral blood and the levels of estrone sulphate are 5 to 10 times higher than those of unconjugated estrogens such as estrone, estradiol and estriol during the menstrual cycle and in postmenopausal women [27, 31]. In mammary tumors, the estrone production from the sulphated-estrone is ten-time higher than that obtained by the aromatase [31].

C) In breast cancer tissues the estrogen sulfotransferase (EST) is also present; it is a member of the superfamily of steroid-sulfotransferases which converts estrogens into their biologically inactive estrogen sulfates [31, 32]. The estrogen sulfotransferase is widely distributed in various normal human tissues, including the breast, and it is involved in protecting peripheral tissues from excessive estrogenic effects. However, in the breast carcinoma tissues the estrogen sulfotransferase activity and expression tend to be decreased [27, 31, 32].

D) 17β-hydroxysteroid dehydrogenase (17β-HSD) is a widely distributed enzyme in mammalian tissues which catalyzes an interconversion of estrogens or androgens. This enzyme catalyzes the reactions between 17-hydroxysteroids and 17-ketosteroids. At least twelve different isoforms of 17β-HSD have been cloned in humans [27, 28]. Some of these isoforms are reductant and are essential for the gonadal and extragonadal biosynthesis of estradiol and testosterone. The oxidative isoforms catalize the formation of steroids of low activity, thus exerting a protective role in different tissues, including the mammary gland, against the steroid actions. The final step of steroidogenesis is the conversion of the weak estrone to the potent biologically active estradiol by the action of a reductive 17β-hydroxysteroid dehydrogenase activity (17β-HSD1). The 17β-HSD1 converts the relatively inactive estrone, androstenedione and 5-androstenedione into the most potent estradiol, testosterone and 5-dihydrotestosterone and *vice versa* [27, 31, 32]. The presence of 17β-HSD1 has been probed in 50% of the mammary carcinoma in postmenopausal women and also in numerous breast tumor cellular lines, T47D and MCF-7 included [27, 28, 31].

In normal mammary tissue the local estrogen production is displaced towards the production of estrone (low activity) whereas in breast adenocarcinomas the formation of the active 17β-estradiol predominates. This is because, in normal tissue, the high concentrations of circulating inactive steroids, androstenedione and estrone sulfates, are the major precursor substrates of local estrogen production. Aromatase catalyzes androstenedione into estrone and sulfatase hydrolyzes the estrone sulfates to estrone. Estrone is subsequently converted to potent 17β-estradiol by 17β-HSD1. In normal tissue, the activity of 17β-HSD type 2 (17β-HSD2), which converts 17β-estradiol to estrone, and the EST, which inactives estrone and 17β-estradiol, are high and protect from excessive estrogenic effects. In the breast carcinoma tissue, sulfatase, aromatase and 17β-HSD1 tend to be overexpressed, while EST and 17β-HSD2 are frequently decreased, which may result in the accumulation of 17β-estradiol [32].

HORMONAL THERAPY IN BREAST CANCER

Because of the role of estrogens as mammary carcinogenic, one of the main objectives in the treatment of breast cancer has always been to neutralize the effects of estrogens on the breast. Ovariectomy, as mentioned above, was the first "antiestrogenic" therapy. Since then, the treatment of breast cancer has included localized treatment on the breast region (surgery and radiotherapy) and general treatment that centers around chemotherapy and hormonotherapy. The pharmacological strategies employed to selectively neutralize the effects of estrogens on the breast are: a) drugs that act through the estrogen receptor interfering with the effects of the endogenous estrogens; this group includes the so-called selective estrogen receptor modulators (SERMs), of which tamoxifen and its derivatives are the most representative examples that for many years have had a significantly beneficial effect both on freedom from symptoms of the disease and reduction in mortality; b) drugs that interfere with the synthesis of steroid hormones by inhibiting the enzymes controlling the interconversion from androgenic precursors: the SEEMs (selective estrogen enzyme modulators). At present, antiaromatases which include steroidal (formestane, exemestane, *etc.*) as well as non-steroidal (anastrozole, letrozole, *etc.*) compounds are extensively used in breast cancer treatment with positive benefits [33-35]. Recent data, in trials with breast cancer patients, have shown that the utilization of selective agents to regulate other enzymes involved in the biosynthesis and transformation of estrogens (estrogen sulfotransferases, sulfatases and 17β-hydroxysteroid deshidrogenases type 1), in combination, with antiaromatase drugs, may also have possible important therapeutic potential as an endocrine therapy for the total blockade of local estrogens in breast cancer and may provide new possibilities in the treatment of this disease [26, 27].

MELATONIN, THE MAIN PINEAL HORMONE

Fifty years ago, melatonin, the main biologically active substance secreted by the pineal gland, was isolated by Lerner and collaborators [36]. Melatonin synthesis from tryptophan is made in successive steps involving different enzymes. The rate-limiting step in this biosynthetic pathway is the activity of the enzyme arylalkylamine N-acetyltransferase (NAT), controlled by the light-dark cycle, which catalyzes the transformation of serotonin to N-acetylserotonin, the direct precursor of melatonin. The regulation of the NAT activity depends on the suprachiasmatic nucleus of hypothalamus which projects axons to the paraventricular nucleus of hypothalamus and from there to the thoracic spinal cord, where the axons synapses with preganglionic sympathetic neurons. These neurons project to the superior cervical ganglion, which sends postganglionic terminals to the pineal gland. The release of norepinephrine from these sympathetic terminals induces the activity of the NAT and drives the synthesis of melatonin. The neurons of the suprachiasmatic nucleus act as an endogenous oscillator with period lengths close to 24 h, which is synchronized by the light/dark signals perceived by the eyes and transmitted by the retino-hypothalamic tract. The light-dark cycle thus entrains the rhythm of melatonin synthesis. Circulating levels of melatonin are low during the day and show a large increase at night. The nocturnal rise of melatonin is abolished, or substantially decreased, in animals exposed to constant light whereas, in animals kept in constant darkness, melatonin is secreted following the endogenous rhythm driven by the suprachiasmatic nucleus of the hypothalamus [1, 37].

Some of the major biological actions of melatonin depend on its binding to specific receptors in the target tissues. Two melatonin receptors, termed MT-1 and MT-2, have been described in the central nervous system and in numerous peripheral tissues [37]. They are Gi-protein coupled membrane receptors which decrease intracellular concentration of cAMP [37]. Melatonin effects on other second messengers such as $[Ca^{++}]_I$, cGMP, diacylglycerol or protein kinase C have been described depending on the cell type studied [37]. Although controversial, some reports based on the lipophilic nature of melatonin have also suggested that this hormone is able to bind and activate nuclear receptor members of the family of retinoid orphan nuclear receptors (RZR/ROR_{α}) [38]. It has not, though, been possible to subsequently confirm this action mechanism. Alternative mechanisms of melatonin actions, not mediated by receptors, have been also proposed. Melatonin may act at intracellular sites, binding to cytosolic calmodulin and thus affecting the calcium signaling and modulating cytoskeletical structural proteins [39]. Finally, recent *in vivo* and *in vitro* studies have shown that melatonin is a potent direct scavenger of hydroxyl radicals and other oxygen centered free radicals, protecting cells against oxidative damage [10].

Different physiological actions, in a great variety of biological contexts, have been attributed to melatonin. In mammals, this indolamine is involved in the synchronization of circadian rhythms as well as in seasonal reproduction [1, 40]. A considerable number of reports have appeared describing the effects of melatonin on the immune system, which suggests that melatonin has immunomodulatory actions [11]. Melatonin has also been described as an efficient free radical scavenger with antioxidant properties [10].

MELATONIN AND ESTROGENS IN BREAST CANCER

The pineal gland is a neuroendocrine organ which, through the synthesis and secretion of melatonin, plays a main role in the regulation of reproductive physiology. Melatonin was formerly considered as a hormone controlling seasonal reproduction in wild animals through its effects on the hypothalamic-pituitary reproductive axis [1, 40]. In seasonally breeding mammals, melatonin controls the reproductive function through the activation of receptor sites within the hypothalamic-pituitary axis thus driving the levels of gonadal activity [41, 42]. Melatonin down-regulation of the ovarian estrogen secretion has been observed in a variety of mammals (the so-called long breeders) [1] whereas in others, such as sheep (short breeders), the control of reproduction depends on the melatonin-induced up-regulation of the synthesis of estrogens during the winter [43]. In humans the role of melatonin on the reproductive system is not completely clear and even controversial. An inverse relationship between serum melatonin and ovarian activity [44] and a certain role of melatonin in the modulation of the neuroendocrine-reproductive axis has been proposed [45]. Furthermore, direct stimulatory effects of melatonin on ovarian steroidogenesis have been demonstrated in human granulosa-luteal cells [46]. However, some other reports indicate no effect of melatonin on estrogen production by granulosa cells [47]. Together, these data suggest that melatonin modulates ovarian function although, in humans, this control on gonadal activity has not been solidly demonstrated. Based on the role of the pineal in inhibiting gonadal maduration and sex hormone secretion in mammals, Cohen and collaborators, in 1978 [48], proposed a possible relationship between the pineal function and the etiology of breast cancer and introduced, for the first time, the hypothesis that diminished function of the pineal gland may promote the development of breast cancer in human beings. They supported their hypothesis by indirect data such as a strong correlation between pineal calcification (interpreted as diminished pineal function) and the incidence of breast cancer and a low incidence of breast cancer in psychiatric patients taking chlorpromazine, which raises serum melatonin. The authors suggested that a decrease in pineal function, whatever its cause, decreases melatonin levels and induces a relative "hyperestrogenism", which underlies the development of breast cancer in human beings [48]. Since then, numerous studies have suggested an association between melatonin levels and cancer progression [4, 14, 49]. Tamarkin and collaborators [50] stated that the amplitude of the nightime peak of plasma melatonin is diminished in women with estrogen receptor-positive breast cancer *versus* those with estrogen receptor-negative disease or healthy, matched controls. Whether the decline in the nocturnal peak of plasma melatonin represents a long-term pineal failure or a change that occurs at the time of breast cancer development is not clear. An inverse correlation between nuclear grade and tumor melatonin concentration and a positive association between tumor melatonin and estrogen receptor status suggested that high tumor melatonin concentration may reflect the differentiation state and constitute a good prognostic marker [51]. Pineal melatonin secretion may be modified in quantity as well as in rhythmicity in breast cancer patients [52]. The relationship between pineal function and risk of breast cancer has also been proposed because of the low incidence of breast cancer among blind women [53] as well as the inverse association between breast cancer incidence and degree of visual impairment [54].

Melatonin represents an important nocturnal output component of the circadian system which exerts an important influence over many physiologic activities. Indirect evidence is emerging that disruption of circadian clock activity is associated with cancer in humans [55]. It has recently been described that the exposure to light at night and the endocrine disruption induced by light pollution increases the growth of DMBA-induced mammary adenocarcinomas in rats [56]. In healthy premenopausal women the exposure to bright white light at night has been also postulated to result from the enhancement of breast oncogenesis *via* disruption of the circadian oncostatic melatonin signal [49]. This kind of experiments encourage the study of melatonin-based treatments to reduce the risk of carcinogenesis.

Besides clinical and epidemiological studies, there is evidence from *in vivo* studies on animal models that supports the hypothesis that melatonin oncostatic actions on hormone-dependent mammary tumors are based on antiestrogenic actions. Most *in vivo* studies have used, as an animal model, the chemically induced (7,12-dimethylbenz(a)anthracene or N-nitrosomethylurea) mammary cancer in rats (see revisions [2, 3]) and the general conclusions are that the animals with enhanced pineal function or those treated with melatonin, in contrast to pinealectomized animals or to those animals with decreased melatonin levels, have: (a) an increase in tumor latency or time elapsing between the administration of the carcinogen and the appearance of palpable mammary tumors, (b) a lower tumor incidence, (c) a reduction in the number and size of the tumors, (d) a lower rate of tumor growth, (e) a more frequent incidence of tumor regression in previously induced tumors, (f) a decrease in serum estradiol and pituitary FSH and LH, and (g) a decrease in the estrogen receptor concentration at the tumor level [2, 3].

The growth of chemically-induced estrogen receptor-positive mammary tumors in ovariectomized rats treated daily with exogenous estradiol was significantly reduced when these animals were subjected to some of the experimental manipulations known as enhancers of pineal-dependent effects (anosmia, underfeeding or exposure to cold, associated with light deprivation) [2, 3]. These animals subjected to increased pineal function, which had lower tumor growth than control and pinealectomized animals, also showed a reduction in the concentration of the estrogen receptor at the tumor level. In this case, these antitumor effects could not be explained by a pineal-dependent decline in circulating estrogens, since serum estradiol concentrations were kept stable because of the exogenous administration of steroids and the lack of changes in the rate of metabolism of steroids. The results of these experiments and other similar ones suggested that melatonin may directly counteract the effects of estrogens at tumor level. The direct antiestrogenic effects of melatonin have been established from *in vitro* studies mainly with the estrogen-sensitive MCF-7 human breast cancer cell line. At mammary tumor cell level, melatonin interferes with the estrogen receptor and counteracts the effects of estrogens, thus behaving as a selective estrogen receptor modulator (SERM). In these estrogen-responsive MCF-7 cells, melatonin exerts a direct antiproliferative effect, including a decrease in cell number, DNA content and thymidine incorporation [57-59]. This effect is dependent on the presence of estrogen receptors in the cells. The fact that only human breast cancer cell lines that express estrogen receptors have been found to be responsive to the antimitogenic effects of melatonin, strengthen the hypothesis that melatonin's oncostatic actions are mediated through its effects at different levels of the estrogen signalling pathway [58]. The link between the antiproliferative effect of melatonin on MCF-7 cell growth and the estrogen-response pathway is further supported: (a) by the ability of melatonin to block, under different culture systems (monolayer and clonogenic soft agar) the mitogenic effect of estradiol [2, 9, 57]; (b) by the blockade mediated by melatonin of the estrogen-rescue of tamoxifen-inhibited cells in clonogenic agar and monolayer culture [9]; (c) by the ability of tamoxifen, a non-steroidal antiestrogen, to reduce the antiproliferative action of melatonin, which suggests that both tamoxifen and melatonin may be working through the same or related mechanisms [58]; (d) by melatonin's down-regulation of both ER_{α} protein and ER_{α} mRNA expression in a time- and dose-dependent manner in MCF-7 cells [8, 60]; (e) by the modulation mediated by melatonin of estrogen-regulated proteins, growth factors and protooncogenes (TGF_{α}, *c-myc*, pS2, progesterone receptor, *c-fox*, TGF_{β}) in human breast cancer cells [61, 62]; (f) by the enhanced growth suppression effects of melatonin in MT_1-transfected ER_{α}-positive cells in comparison to parental and vector-transfected MCF-7 cells but, however, MT_1-overexpression did not induce a melatonin-sensitive phenotype in ER_{α}-negative breast cancer cells [63]; (g) by the enhanced inhibition of ER_{α} mRNA expression induced by melatonin in MT_1-transfected MCF-7 cells [63]; and (h) by the ability of melatonin to counteract the estradiol-induced invasiveness of mammary tumor cells [64].

The oncostatic properties of melatonin based on its ability to interact with the estrogen receptors has been reviewed elsewhere [6, 7]. Therefore, in this review what is exclusively summarized is the recent information on the oncostatic properties of melatonin based on its ability to regulate the activity and expression of some enzymes involved in the biosynthesis of estrogens in peripheral tissues.

MELATONIN AS A SELECTIVE ESTROGEN ENZYME MODULATOR

Anti-Aromatase Actions of Melatonin

In all the experimental models (*in vivo* and *in vitro* studies) relating melatonin with tumor growth, estradiol reaches the tumor tissue from sources different from the mammary gland tissue (ovaries in *in vivo* models and estradiol added to the culture medium in *in vitro* models) [2, 3]. However, as we have previously commented, in the breast cancer of postmenopausal women, estrogens are synthesized in the mammary tissue by transformation from androgens precursors of adrenal origin or from biologically inactive estrogens.

Most of the *in vitro* studies which have demonstrated the direct effects of melatonin on the control of the enzymes involved in the biosynthesis and transformation of estrogens in breast cancer cells were carried out on the MCF-7 human breast cancer cell line, which was derived from a pleural effusion of a woman with metastatic carcinoma of the breast [65]. This cell line is a good breast cancer model because, in addition to melatonin receptors [63, 66], it contains Arom, STS, 17βHSD1 and EST enzymes [27, 28, 31], the enzymes involved in the intratumoral biosynthesis and transformation of estrogens.

As indicated above, one of the major pathways involved in the synthesis of estrogens in mammary tumor cells is the aromatization of androstenedione to estrone by aromatase. MCF-7 human breast cancer cells respond to the presence of androgens, like testosterone, in the culture medium increasing their proliferation. Physiological concentrations of melatonin are able to counteract the testosterone-induced cell proliferation dependent on the local biosynthesis of estrogens from testosterone by the aromatase activity of the cells [67]. In particular, melatonin reduces the aromatase activity of MCF-7 cells both at basal conditions and when aromatase activity is stimulated by cAMP or cortisol [67]. The greatest inhibition of the aromatase activity has been obtained with 1 nM melatonin, the same concentration that gives the highest antiproliferative and anti-invasive effects on MCF-7 cells [2, 57, 64]. In addition, it has been shown, by RT-PCR, that melatonin also down-regulates aromatase mRNA steady state levels in these cells (Fig. **2**) [67]. Transfection of the MT_1 melatonin receptor in MCF-7 cells significantly decreases aromatase activity of the cells and MT_1-transfected cells show a level of aromatase activity that is 50 % of vector-transfected MCF-7 cells [68]. The proliferation of estrogen-sensitive MCF-7 cells in an estradiol-free medium but in the presence of testosterone (an indirect measure of aromatase activity) is strongly inhibited by melatonin in those cells overexpressing the MT_1 receptor. This inhibitory effect of melatonin on cell growth is higher in MT_1 transfected cells than in vector transfected ones. In MT_1-transfected cells, aromatase activity is inhibited by melatonin. The same concentrations of melatonin do not significantly influence at the same level the aromatase activity of vector-transfected cells. MT_1 melatonin receptor transfection also induces a significant 55 % inhibition of aromatase steady-state mRNA expression in comparison to vector-transfected MCF-7 cells. In addition, in MT_1-transfected cells melatonin treatment is able to inhibit aromatase mRNA expression and 1 nM melatonin induces a higher and significant downregulation of aromatase mRNA expression than in vector-transfected cells [68]. These findings point to the importance of MT_1 melatonin receptor in mediating melatonin's oncostatic action in MCF-7 human breast cancer cells and confirm MT_1 melatonin receptor as a major mediator in the melatonin signaling pathway in breast cancer.

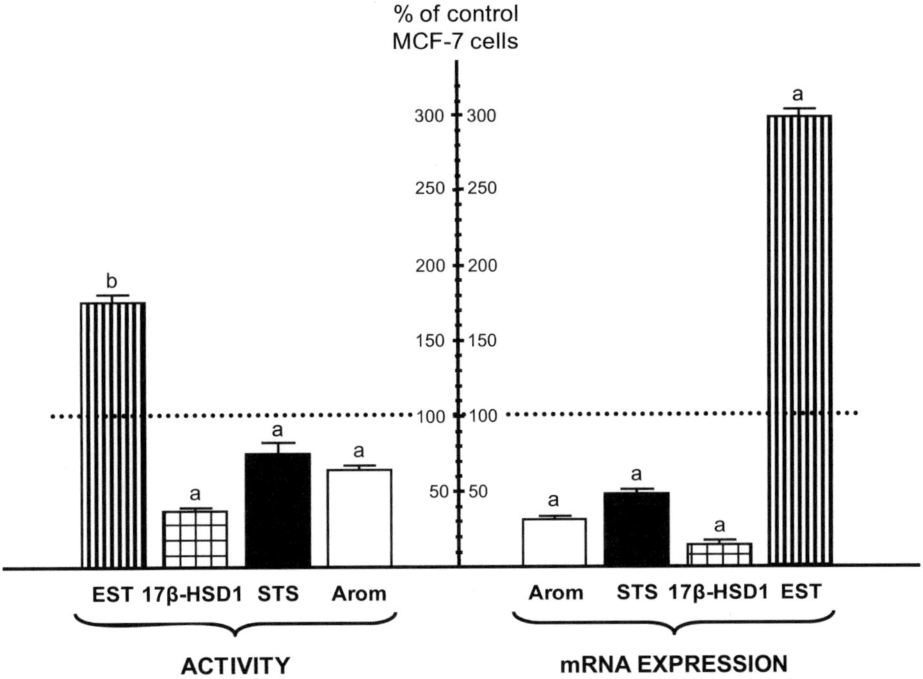

Figure 2: Effects of physiological concentration of melatonin (1 nM) on aromatase (Arom), sulfatase (STS), 17β-hydroxysteroid dehydrogenase type 1 (17β-HSD1) and estrogen sulfotransferase (EST) activity and mRNA expression in MCF-7 human breast cancer cells. Data are expressed as the percentage of the untreated-control group (mean ± S.E.M.). a, $p<0.001$ *vs.* unpretreated-control cells; b, $p<0.01$ *vs.* unpretreated-control cells. Modified from Cos *et al.* 2005 [67] and González *et al.* 2008 [89].

This modulator effect of melatonin on the enzyme which controls the conversion from androgenic precursors to estrogens has been also described *in vivo*, in rats bearing DMBA-induced mammary tumors [69]. The growth of these mammary tumors is estrogen-dependent and the ovariectomy significantly reduces the size and number of the tumors, while the administration of testosterone to ovariectomized animals is able to maintain the tumor growth at the control animals' level. The stimulatory effect of tumor development induced by testosterone, which depends on the local synthesis of estrogens from androgens, due to the aromatase action, is suppressed by the administration of melatonin (Fig. **3**) [69]. The growth-stimulatory effects of testosterone on the tumors depend exclusively on locally formed estrogens, since no changes in serum estradiol have been described in testosterone-treated rats. Tumors from animals treated with melatonin showed the lowest microsomal aromatase activity (Fig. **3**). This finding supports that melatonin could exert at least part of its antitumor effects on hormone-dependent mammary tumors by inhibiting the aromatase activity of the tumor tissue and then reducing the intratumoral conversion of androgens to estrogens [69].

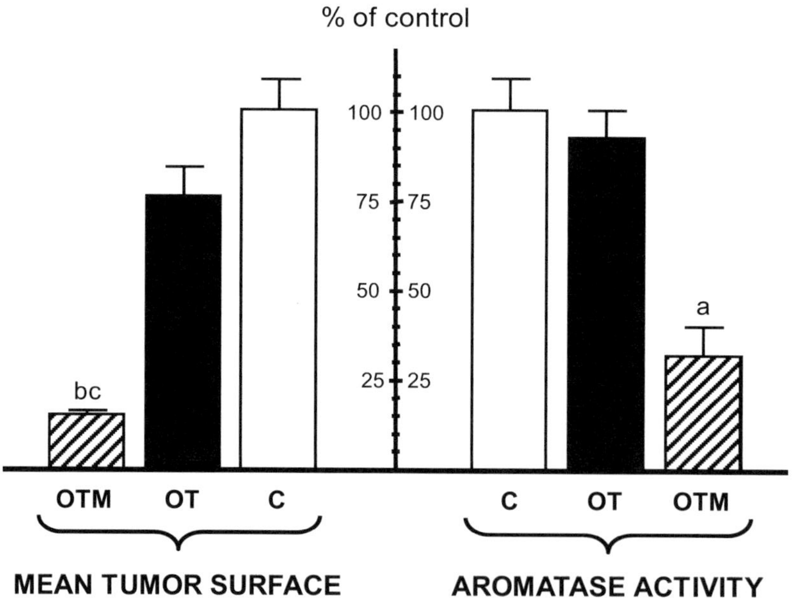

Figure 3: Changes in DMBA-induced tumor size and microsomal aromatase activity in rats 9 weeks after ovariectomy (O) and treatment with testosterone (T) and melatonin (M). Data are expressed as the percentage of the control (C) group (mean ± S.E.M.). a, $p<0.05$ *vs.* C; b, $p<0.001$ *vs.* C; c, $p<0.001$ *vs.* OT. Modified from Cos *et al.* 2006 [69].

Aminoglutethimide, the first non-steroidal aromatase inhibitor used clinically in mammary cancer, is a reversible competitive inhibitor which binds competitively to the heme moiety of aromatase. When melatonin has been used in combination with an aromatase inhibitor such as aminoglutethimide, an increase in the efficacy of the competitive inhibitor used in treating breast cancer has been reported [70]. A sequential regimen of melatonin (1 nM) followed 24 hrs later by aminoglutethimide (100 μM) induces a significantly higher decrease in MCF-7 cell aromatase activity to below the values obtained in unpretreated cells and a significant inhibition in the aromatase mRNA expression as compared to cells exposed to the same doses of aminoglutethimide, but without melatonin pretreatment. The aminoglutethimide inhibitory effect is more potent when MCF-7 cells are pre-exposed to melatonin [70]. Melatonin pretreatment increases the reduction of the aromatase activity of cells exposed to aminoglutethimide as a result of the decrease in the aromatase mRNA expression. Aminoglutethimide modulation on aromatase expression is suppressed by adenylate cyclase inhibitors, thus indicating that a cAMP-dependent mechanism might be involved [71]. Again cAMP has been suggested as one of the possible molecules linking melatonin, aminoglutethimide and aromatase activity and expression in human breast cancer cells.

The antiaromatase effect of melatonin has been shown not only in breast cancer cells. In C6 glioma cells, which express estrogen receptors and also have the ability to synthesize estrogens from androgens, melatonin also counteracts the growth stimulatory effects of testosterone, which is dependent on the local synthesis of estrogens from testosterone, reduces the aromatase activity of C6 cells and downregulates aromatase mRNA steady state levels [72]. By analogy to the implications of aromatase in other forms of estrogen-sensitive tumors, it is conceivable that the modulation of the aromatase by melatonin may play a role in the growth of glioblastomas.

It is now known that expression of the aromatase gene (CYP19) is regulated in a tissue-specific manner by the use of alternative promoters. In normal mammary glands the aromatase gene (CYP19) is under the control of promoter I.4 and is regulated by the combined action of a glucocorticoid and a member of the class I cytokine family (*e.g.*, interleukin-6, interleukin-11, oncostatin-M, leukemia inhibitory factor) [73]. The 5'-upstream region of promoter I.4 contains a glucocorticoid response element which can bind transcription factors of the 'signal transducer and activator of transcription' family. Cytokines, in the presence of glucocorticoids, regulate aromatase gene expression *via* the promoter

I.4. However, in mammary cancer cells, aromatase expression is primarily regulated by increased activity of the proximally located promoters II and I.3, which are regulated by cAMP and factors that regulate cAMP levels [74]. Prostaglandin E_2 (PGE_2) is an important regulator of aromatase gene expression *via* promoters II and I.3. [73, 75, 76]. The formation of PGE_2 occurs through the activity of the cyclooxygenases (COX), rate-limiting enzymes that catalyze the conversion of arachidonic acid to prostaglandins. There are two isoforms, COX-1 and COX-2. COX-1 is constitutively expressed in most tissues; both its activity and expression are also elevated in many breast tumors. COX-2 is present in breast cancer tissue but not in the normal breast tissue and can undergo rapid induction in response to a variety of stimuli, including mitogens, hormones, cytokines and growth factors. It has been proposed a model to explain the interrelationship between aromatase and COX enzymes. High levels of expression of COX genes and increased cyclooxygenases activity result in higher levels of PGE_2. Elevated PGE_2 levels increase intracellular cAMP and result in increased aromatase expression *via* activation of promoters I.3 and II [73, 75, 76]. Melatonin modulates aromatase enzyme in breast cancer cells through a down-regulatory action on the expression of both cyclooxygenase enzymes (COX-1 and, above all, COX-2) which decrease the levels of PGE_2. Lower levels of PGE_2 decrease intracellular levels of cAMP which in turn decrease the activation of promoters I.3 and II and result in reduced aromatase expression. Lower levels of aromatase lead to lower levels of estrogens, resulting in decreased growth and development of the breast tumor [77, 78].

Over the last decade many studies have been carried out to identify potential aromatase stimulator factors. Interleukin-6 has been one of the most potent factors detected. Cultured fibroblasts derived from normal or malignant breast tissue were also found to be a rich source of interleukin-6. Other cytokines and growth factors that can stimulate aromatase activity include tumor necrosis factor-α (TNF-α), oncostatin M, leukaemia inhibitory factor and insulin-like growth factor type I [79]. Since melatonin is able to regulate the cytokine production in both immunocompetent cells [11] and human breast cancer cells [80] the actions of melatonin on cytokine production in breast tumors may also be another link between melatonin and tumor estrogen synthesis.

Several lines of evidence highlight the contribution of the tumor microenvironment to its growth and maintenance. Adjacent adipose fibroblasts and vascular endothelial cells provide structural and biochemical support for tumor growth, mainly by increasing their estrogen biosynthesis in response to paracrine signals which are secreted by breast cancer cells [81, 82]. Malignant epithelial cells secrete cytokines (TNF-α, interleukin-11, interleukin-6) that inhibit the differentiation of surrounding fibroblasts into mature adipocytes, mediated by the selective inhibition of expression of peroxisome proliferator-activated receptor (PPARγ) and CCAAT/enhancer binding protein (C/EBP)α, and also stimulate aromatase expression in these undifferentiated adipose fibroblasts. This biological phenomenon is commonly known as the desmoplastic reaction or accumulation of undifferentiated fibroblasts with high aromatase activity around malignant epithelial cells. Tumor cells also secrete factors like prostaglandin E_2 that stimulate aromatase activity and expression in these undifferentiated fibroblasts and upregulate antiadipogenic cytokines. Melatonin reduces the formation of undifferentiated fibroblasts surrounding malignant epithelial cells by stimulating their differentiation to mature adipocytes and adipogenesis and by decreasing the aromatase activity of the fibroblasts through a downregulatory action on the expression of antiadipogenic cytokines, which decreases the levels of these cytokines (Fig. **4**). Lower levels of TNF-α, interleukin-6 and interleukin-11 allow the differentiation of fibroblasts and decrease the aromatase activity and expression, thereby reducing the number of cells contributing to estrogen production in the tumor adjacent tissue [80, 83, 84]. PPARγ and C/EBPα, the two main regulators of terminal adipogenesis, are up-regulated by melatonin in preadipocytes [80]. Melatonin also decreases the production of PGE_2 by malignant cells, which upregulates aromatase expression both in the tumor itself and in the surrounding adipose tissue and enhances the production of interleukin-11 by tumor cells. Then, lower levels of aromatase lead to lower levels of estrogens, resulting in decreased growth and development of breast tumor (Fig. **4**).

Endothelial cells surrounding tumor cells, may provide another source of estrogens since they also express aromatase [85, 86]. Melatonin also inhibits aromatase activity and expression in endothelial cells by down-regulating the expression of the endothelial specific aromatase promoter region I.7, one of the major promoter directing aromatase expression in endothelial cells [87].

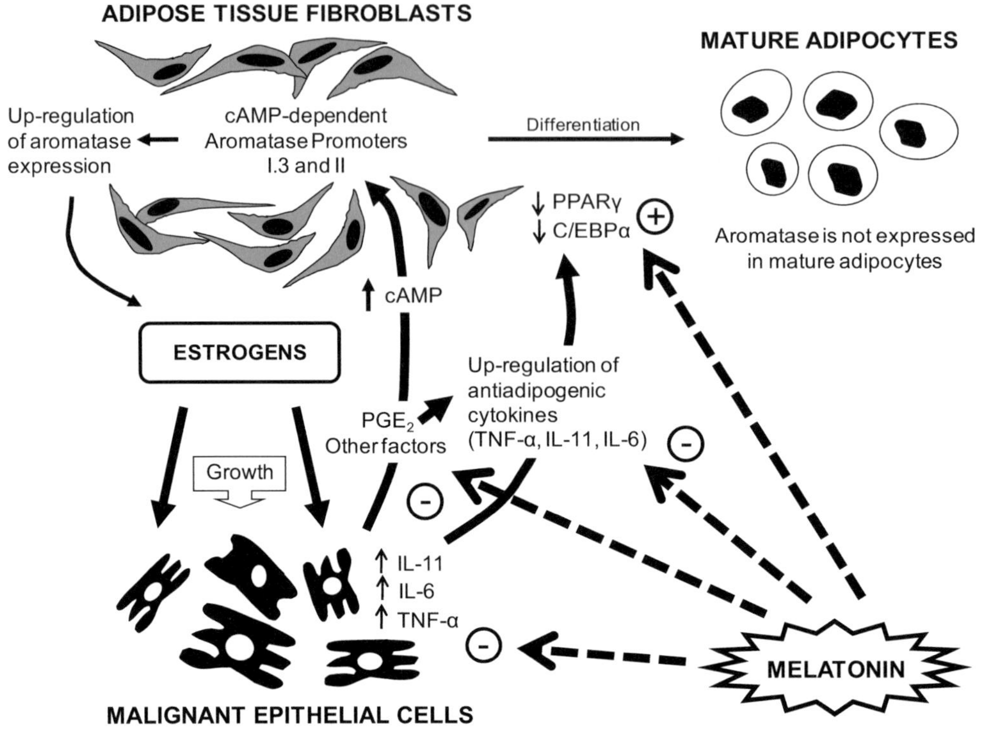

Figure 4: Epithelial-stromal interactions in breast tumors inhibits adipogenic differentiation and enhance estrogen formation by increasing the aromatase activity of the undifferentiated fibroblasts. All these actions are mediated by cytokines such as tumor necrosis factor-α (TNF-α), interleukin-6 (IL-6) and interleukin-11 (IL-11) produced by malignant epithelial cells. Melatonin reduces the formation of undifferentiated fibroblasts surrounding malignant epithelial cells by stimulating the differentiation of fibroblasts to mature adipocytes and adipogenesis and by decreasing the aromatase activity of the fibroblasts and adipocytes through a downregulatory action on the expression of antiadipogenic cytokines, which decrease the levels of these cytokines. Lower levels of TNF-α, IL-6 and IL-11 stimulate the differentiation of fibroblasts and decrease the aromatase activity and expression. Melatonin also decreases the production of PGE_2 by malignant cells, which upregulates aromatase expression both in the tumor itself and in the surrounding adipose tissue and enhances the production of interleukin-11 by tumor cells. Modified from Alvarez-García *et al.* 2012 [80].

Anti-Sulfatase Actions of Melatonin

Since estrone sulphate is quantitatively the most important precursor of estradiol [27] and the estrogen sulfatase activity is 40-500 times higher than aromatase activity in breast cancer tissues [28, 88], the interest of these enzymes as targets for anticancer drugs seems clear. In recent years, it has been demonstrated that some progestins (promegestone, nomegestrol acetate, medrogestone, dyhidrogesterone, norelgestromin), various synthetic steroids (tibolone and its metabolites) as well as other steroidal (sulfamates) and non-steroidal compounds are potent inhibitors of sulfatase [27, 28]. Melatonin at physiological (1 nM) concentrations also reduces the synthesis of biologically active estrogens in MCF-7 cells, through the inhibition of the conversion from biologically inactive forms of estrogens to bioactive unconjugated estrogens *via* sulfatase [89]. It has been demonstrated that the mRNA expression of the enzyme responsible for converting estrone-sulfate and estradiol-sulfate into estrone and estradiol respectively, is also significantly reduced by melatonin (Fig. **2**) [89].

This modulator effect of melatonin on the sulfatase has also been described *in vivo*, in rats bearing DMBA-induced mammary tumors. Since the growth of these mammary tumors is estrogen-dependent, the ovariectomy significantly reduces the size, while the administration of estrone sulphate to ovariectomized animals is able to maintain the tumor growth at the control animals'level. The stimulatory effect of tumor development induced by estrone sulfate which depends on the local synthesis of estrogens because of the action of the sulfatase enzyme on the biologically inactive estrogens, is suppressed by the administration of melatonin [90]. Mammary tumors from animals ovariectomized and treated with estrone sulfate have high sulfatase activity and sulfatase expression and melatonin counteracts the stimulatory effect of estrone sulfate on both sulfatase activity and expression. These findings support that melatonin could exert its antitumoral effects on hormone-dependent mammary tumors by down-regulating the sulfatase pathway of the tumoral tissue [90]. Synthetic antiestrogens, like tamoxifen and its derivates, seem to exert some of their effects on breast tumors by also blocking estrogen biosynthesis through inhibition of sulfatase activity and/or expression [27, 91]. In addition, melatonin also decreases the local production of estrogens in glioblastoma cells by decreasing the activity and expression of sulfatase [92].

17β-Hydroxysteroid Dehydrogenase Inhibitory Actions of Melatonin

The last step of steroidogenesis in peripheral tissues is the conversion of the weak estrone to the potent biologically active estradiol by the activity of 17β-HSD1 [27, 31] and it has been suggested that this enzyme might be a marker for hormone-dependent breast cancer [93]. It has been reported that the production of 17β-estradiol from estrone in MCF-7 cells decreases (2- to 3-fold) in the presence of 1 nM melatonin [89]. Furthermore, physiological or pharmacological doses of melatonin also decreased 17β-HSD1 expression, especially with physiological doses of the indoleamine (a 6-fold reduction of 17β-HSD1 expression with 1 nM melatonin) (Fig. **2**) [89]. Effects of melatonin on the steroidogenic activity of the testes, mediated by an inhibition of 17β-HSD activity and/or expression, have also been previously described in rat and hamster [94, 95]. A significant decrease in the activity of 17β-HSD was described in the testes of melatonin-treated rats maintained under normal light-dark schedules [94]. In isolated Leydig cells from active testes of adult hamsters kept in a long-day (14 h light, 10 h dark) photoperiod and from regressed testes of adult animals exposed to a short-day photoperiod during 16 weeks (6 h light, 18 h dark), melatonin significantly decreased the expression of P450 side chain cleavage, 3β-hydroxysteroid dehydrogenase and 17β-hydroxysteroid dehydrogenase [95]. Antiestrogens such as tamoxifen, 4-hydroxytamoxifen or ICI 164384 can also inhibit by competition the 17β-HSD1 effects in both rat mammary and human breast tumor tissues [27, 28]. In addition, melatonin also decreases the local production of estrogens in glioblastoma cells by decreasing the activity and expression of 17β-hydroxysteroid dehydrogenase [92].

Estrogen Sulfotranferase Stimulatory Actions of Melatonin

Since the sulfoestrogens are the biologically inactive forms of the estrogens, another possibility to control the tissular concentration of active estradiol is to stimulate the enzymes involved in the sulphate formation. In this concern, it is remarkable that melatonin, at physiological doses, can increase almost 2-times the estrogen sulfotransferase activity and up to 3-times the estrogen sulfotransferase expression in MCF-7 (Fig. **2**) [89].

Regulation of the Enzymes Related to the Local Production of Estrogens in Human Normal Breast Tissue and Breast Carcinoma Tissue by Melatonin

Most melatonin actions on enzymes involved in the intratumoral metabolism and biosynthesis of estrogens in breast tumors take account at physiological doses in the nanomolar range, the same concentration at which melatonin exerts the highest antiproliferative and anti-invasive effects [2, 64]. However, other mechanisms by which melatonin exert its oncostatic actions, such as by its antioxidant or immunoenhancement effects, have been described using very high pharmacological concentrations of melatonin [10, 11].

As pointed out above, in the normal breast tissue the local estrogen production is displaced towards the production of estrone, whereas in breast carcinoma tissues what predominates is the formation of the active 17β-estradiol, because in normal tissue, the high concentrations of circulating inactive steroids, androstenedione and estrone sulfates, are the major precursor substrates of local estrogen production (Fig. **5**).

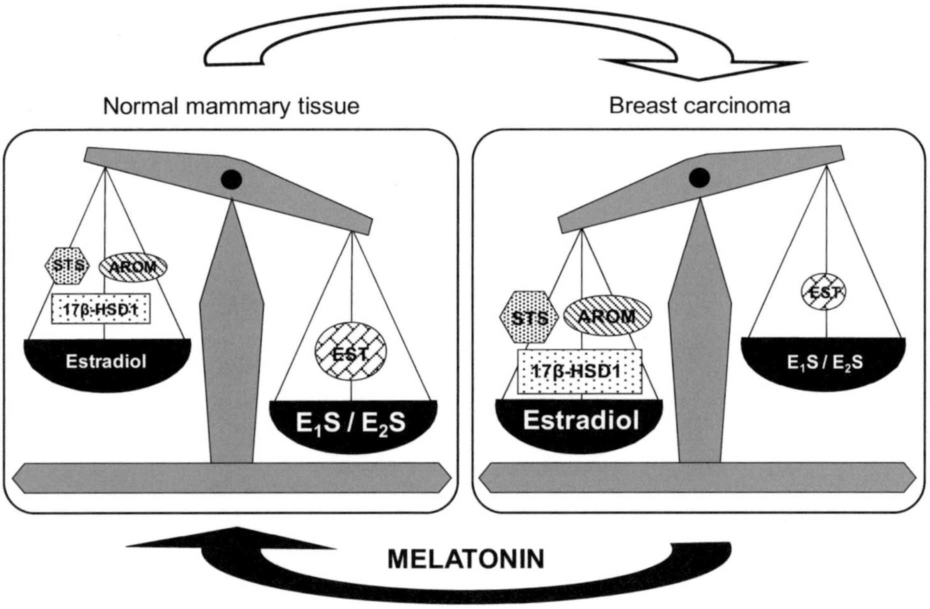

Figure 5: Expression of enzymes related to the local production of estrogens in human normal tissue and breast carcinoma tissue. In the breast carcinoma tissue STS, Arom and 17β-HSD1 tend to be overexpressed, while EST is decreased. Melatonin decreases the expression of aromatase, sulfatase and 17β-HSD1 and increases the estrogen sulfotransferase expression. Thus, melatonin tends to modify the expression of the enzymes involved in the local synthesis of estrogens, causing it to be similar to the expression of enzymes in the mammary normal tissue.

In the breast carcinoma tissue, aromatase, which catalyzes androstenedione into estrone, sulfatase, which hydrolyzes the estrone sulfates to estrone, and 17β-HSD1, which converts the estrone to the potent 17β-estradiol, tend to be overexpressed, while the expression of estrogen sulfotransferase, the enzyme that inactivates estrone and 17β-estradiol, is frequently decreased, which may result in the accumulation of

17β-estradiol in breast cancer tissues (Fig. **5**) [32]. However, since melatonin decreases the activity and expression of aromatase, sulfatase and 17β-HSD1 and increases the activity and expression of estrogen sulfotransferase (Fig. **6**), it may protect mammary tissue from excessive estrogenic effects and, as shown in Fig. **5**, it tends to modify the activity and expression of the enzymes involved in the local synthesis of estrogens turning them back to similar expression and activity of enzymes in the mammary normal tissue. Melatonin is able not only to interact with the estrogen-signaling pathway, but also to modulate the biosynthesis of estrogens directly at mammary tumor cell level.

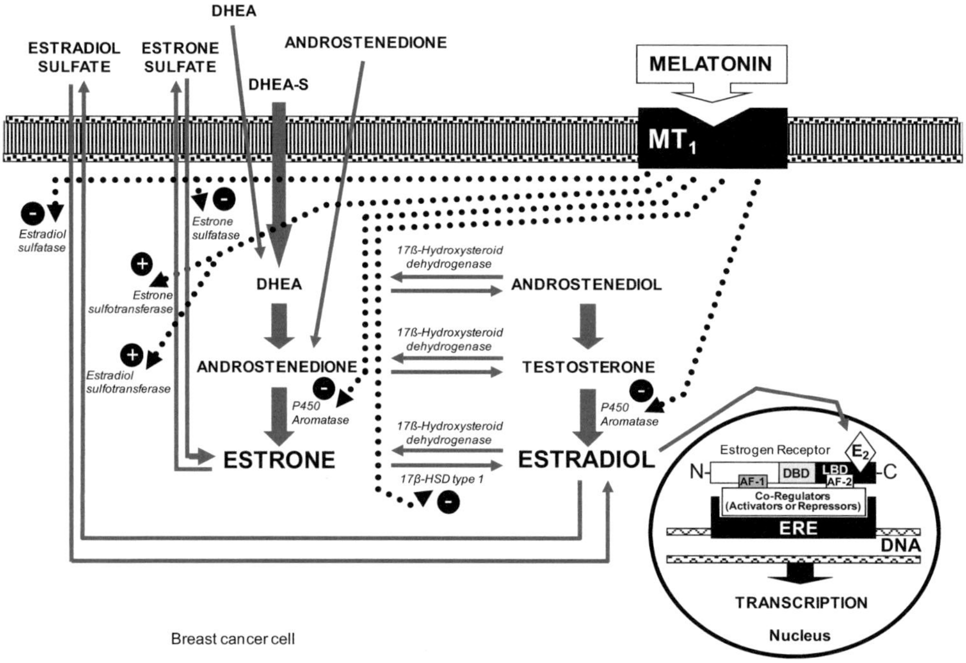

Figrue 6: Sites of action of melatonin as selective estrogen enzyme modulator in human breast cancer cells. (Abbreviations: DHEA, dehydroepiandrosterone; DHEA-S, dehydroepiandrosterone sulphate; *17β-HSD type 1,* 17β-hydroxysteroid dehydrogenase type 1).

Little is known about the factors regulating estrogen sulfatase, 17β-HSD1 and sulfotransferase expression in humans. However, it is now evident that cytokines, growth factors and PGE_2 have crucial roles in regulating estrogen synthesis in breast tumors. Interleukin-6 and tumor necrosis factor-α can stimulate the activities of all the enzymes involved in estrogen synthesis [79]. The activities of the aromatase, 17β-HSD1 and estrone sulfatase are all increased in a co-ordinated manner by the actions of cytokines such as interleukin-6 and tumor necrosis factor-α, and PGE_2. Macrophages and lymphocytes, which invade many breast tumors, are thought to be an important source of factors that can stimulate estrogen synthesis in malignant breast tissue. As pointed out above, since melatonin is able to modulate the cytokine production in immunocompetent cells [11] and human breast cancer cells [80], the actions of melatonin on cytokines and PGE_2 production in breast tumors may also be other mechanisms which might modulate the activity and expression of the enzymes involved in tumor estrogen synthesis.

CONCLUSIONS

Estrogens, besides being involved in the growth and differentiation of the normal mammary gland, contribute greatly to the genesis, growth and development of breast cancer and some of the mammary tumors require estrogens for continued growth. Melatonin, the main secretory product of the pineal gland, acts as a regulator of neoplastic cell growth, particularly on those tumors corresponding to the mammary gland, especially on estrogen-dependent mammary tumors. Melatonin reduces the estrogen-mediated development of breast cancer on the basis of two different mechanisms: indirect neuroendocrine mechanisms, such as the melatonin down-regulation of the neuroendocrine reproductive axis and the consequent reduction of estrogenic hormones responsible for the normal and pathological growth of the mammary gland, and, on the other hand, direct melatonin actions at the tumor cell level. Evidence from *in vivo* studies on animal models and *in vitro* studies on human breast cancer cell lines supports the hypothesis that melatonin oncostatic actions on hormone-dependent mammary tumors are mainly based on its antiestrogenic actions and they are due to melatonin interactions with the estrogen-signaling pathways on tumor cells. At the level of the mammary tumor cell, melatonin interacts with the estrogen-response pathway and counteracts the effects of estrogens, thus behaving as a selective estrogen receptor modulator. Recently, melatonin has been described as also being able to regulate the activity of some enzymes (aromatase, sulfatase, 17β-hydroxysteroid dehydrogenase, estrogen sulfotransferase) responsible for the local synthesis of estrogens, thus behaving as a selective estrogen enzyme modulator. Melatonin decreases the activity and expression of some enzymes like aromatase, sulfatase and 17β-hydroxysteroid dehydrogenase, whose function is increase local estrogens, and increases the activity and expression of the estrogen sulfotransferase, an enzyme whose role in the mammary tissue is to sulfonate estrogens to inactive estrogen sulfates (Fig. **5**). All these melatonin actions on sex steroid-producing enzymes in breast malignant epithelial cells, surrounding fibroblasts and endothelial cells may serve to protect mammary tissue from excessive estrogenic effects. Melatonin is a naturally occurring antiestrogen which shares properties with most of the synthetic drugs used to either interact with estrogens at the estrogen receptor level (SERMs), or to decrease the biosynthesis of estrogens at tumor level (SEEMs). Both properties of melatonin are focused to selectively neutralize the effects of estrogens on the breast, one of the main objectives of the antitumor pharmacological therapeutics. All these actions at different levels of the estrogen-signaling pathways, collectively, make melatonin an interesting anticancer drug in the prevention and treatment of estrogen-dependent mammary tumors and opens up new and interesting possibilities in clinical applications of melatonin in breast cancer.

ACKNOWLEDGEMENTS

This work was supported by grants from the Spanish MCYT (SAF2007-60659) and MICINN (SAF2010-19579).

CONFLICT OF INTEREST

The author(s) confirm that this chapter content has no conflict of interest.

DISCLOSURE

The chapter submitted for the eBook Series entitled **"Advances in Cancer Drug Targets, Volume 1"** is an update of our article in **Current Cancer Drug Targets, Volume 8, Issue 8, 2008,** with additional text and references.

REFERENCES

[1] Reiter RJ. The pineal and its hormones in the control of reproduction in mammals. *Endocr. Rev.* 1980, 1, 109-131.

[2] Cos S, Sánchez-Barceló EJ. Melatonin and mammary pathological growth. *Front. Neuroendocrinol.* 2000, 21, 133-170.

[3] Cos S, Sánchez-Barceló EJ. Melatonin, experimental basis for a possible application in breast cancer prevention and treatment. *Histol. Histopathol.* 2000, 15, 637-647.

[4] Blask DE, Sauer LA, Dauchy RT. Melatonin as a chronobiotic/ anticancer agent: cellular, biochemical and molecular mechanisms of action and their implications for circadian-based cancer therapy. *Curr. Topics Med. Chem.* 2002, 2, 113-132.

[5] Sánchez-Barceló EJ, Cos S, Fernández R, Mediavilla MD. Melatonin and mammary cancer: a short review. *Endocr. Relat. Cancer* 2003, 10, 153-159.
[6] Sánchez-Barceló EJ, Cos S, Mediavilla MD, Martínez-Campa CM, González A, Alonso-González C. Melatonin-estrogen interactions in breast cancer. *J. Pineal Res.* 2005, 38, 217-222.
[7] Cos S, González A, Martínez-Campa C, Mediavilla MD, Alonso-González C, Sánchez-Barceló EJ. Estrogen-signaling pathway: a link between breast cancer and melatonin oncostatic actions. *Cancer Detect. Prev.* 2006, 30, 118-128.
[8] Molis TM, Spriggs LL, Hill SM. Modulation of estrogen receptor mRNA expression by melatonin in MCF-7 human breast cancer cells. *Mol. Endocrinol.* 1994, 8, 1681-1690.
[9] Cos S, Blask DE, Lemus-Wilson A, Hill SM. Effects of melatonin on the cell cycle kinetics and estrogen rescue of MCF-7 human breast cancer cells in culture. *J. Pineal Res.* 1991, 10, 36-42.
[10] Allegra M, Reiter RJ, Tan DX, Gentile C, Tesoriere L, Livrea MA. The chemistry of melatonin's interaction with reactive species. *J. Pineal Res.* 2003, 34, 1-10.
[11] Fraschini F, Demartini G, Esposti D, Scaglione F. Melatonin involvement in immunity and cancer. *Biol. Signals Recept.* 1998, 7, 61-72.
[12] Leon-Blanco MM, Guerrero JM, Reiter RJ, Calvo JR, Pozo D. Melatonin inhibits telomerase activity in the MCF-7 tumor cell line both *in vivo* and *in vitro*. *J. Pineal Res.* 2003, 35, 204-211.
[13] Blask DE, Dauchy RT, Sauer LA, Krause JA, Brainard GC. Growth and fatty acid metabolism of human breast cancer (MCF-7) xenografts in nude rats: impact of constant light-induced nocturnal melatonin suppression. *Breast Cancer Res. Treat.* 2003, 79, 313-320.
[14] Blask DE, Dauchy RT, Sauer LA. Putting cancer to sleep at night. *Endocrine* 2005, 27, 179-188.
[15] Dumitrescu RG, Cotarla I. Understanding breast cancer risk – where do we stand in 2005?. *J. Cell Mol. Med.* 2005, 9, 208-221.
[16] Russo IH, Russo J. Role of hormones in mammary cancer initiation and progression. *J. Mammary Gland Biol. Neoplasia* 1998, 3, 49-61.
[17] Russo J, Russo IH. The role of estrogen in the initiation of breast cancer. *J. Steroid Biochem. Mol. Biol.* 2006, 102, 89-96.
[18] Pelekanou V, Leclercq G. Recent insights into the effect of natural and environmental estrogens on mammary development and carcinogenesis. *Int. J. Dev. Biol.* 2011, 55(7-9), 869-878.
[19] Germain D. Estrogen carcinogenesis in breast cancer. *Endocrinol. Metab. Clin. North. Am.* 2011, 40(3), 473-484.
[20] Howell A, Clarke RB, Anderson E. Oestrogens, Beatson and endocrine therapy. *Endocr. Relat. Cancer* 1997, 4, 371-380.
[21] Preston-Martin S, Pike MC, Ross RK, Jones PA, Henderson BE. Increased cell division as a cause of human cancer. *Cancer Res.* 1990, 50, 7415-7421.
[22] Yue W, Santen RJ, Wang JP, *et al.* Genotoxic metabolites of estradiol in breast: potential mechanism of estradiol induced carcinogenesis. *J. Steroid Biochem. Mol. Biol.* 2003, 86, 477-486.
[23] Simpson ER. Role of aromatase in sex steroid action. *J. Mol. Endocrinol.* 2000, 25, 149-156.

[24] Landeghem AA, Poortman J, Nabuurs M, Thijssen JH. Endogenous concentration and subcellular distribution of estrogens in normal and malignant human breast tissue. *Cancer Res.* 1985, 45, 2900-2906.
[25] Yue W, Wang JP, Hamilton CJ, Demers LM, Santen RJ. *In situ* aromatization enhances breast tumor estradiol levels and cellular proliferation. *Cancer Res.* 1998, 58, 927-932.
[26] Sasano H, Suzuki T, Nakata T, Moriya T. New development in intracrinology of breast carcinoma. *Breast Cancer* 2006, 13, 129-136.
[27] Pasqualini JR. The selective estrogen enzyme modulators in breast cancer: a review. *Biochim. Biophys. Acta* 2004, 1654, 123-143.
[28] Pasqualini JR, Chetrite GS. Recent insight on the control of enzymes involved in estrogen formation and transformation in human breast cancer. *J. Steroid Biochem. Mol. Biol.* 2005, 93, 221-236.
[29] Conley A, Hinshelwood M. Mammalian aromatases. *Reproduction* 2001, 121, 685-695.
[30] Santen RJ, Harvey HA. Use of aromatase inhibitors in breast carcinoma. *Endocr. Relat. Cancer* 1999, 6, 75-92.
[31] Suzuki T, Miki Y, Nakamura Y, *et al.* Sex steroid-producing enzymes in human breast cancer. *Endocr. Relat. Cancer* 2005, 12, 701-720.
[32] Suzuki T, Miki Y, Nakata T, *et al.* Steroid sulfatase and estrogen sulfotransferase in normal human tissue and breast cancer. *J. Steroid Biochem. Mol. Biol.* 2003, 86, 449-454.
[33] Wong ZW, Ellis MJ. First-line endocrine treatment of breast cancer: aromatase inhibitor or antioestrogen?. *Br. J. Cancer* 2004, 90, 20-25.
[34] Bush NJ. Advances in hormonal therapy for breast cancer. *Semin. Oncol. Nurs.* 2007, 23, 46-54.
[35] Obiorah I, Jordan VC. Progress in endocrine approaches to the treatment and prevention of breast cancer. *Maturitas* 2011, 70(4), 315-321.
[36] Lerner AB, Case JD, Takahashi Y, Lee TH, Mori W. Isolation of melatonin, the pineal gland factor that lightens melanocytes. *J. Amer. Chem. Soc.* 1958, 80, 2587.
[37] Vanecek J. Cellular mechanisms of melatonin action. *Physiol. Rev.* 1998, 78, 687-721.
[38] Becker-Andre M, Wiesenberg I, Schaeren-Wiemers N, *et al.* Pineal gland hormone melatonin binds and activates an orphan of the nuclear receptor superfamily. *J. Biol. Chem.* 1994, 269, 28531-28534.
[39] Anton-Tay F, Martínez I, Tovar R, Benitez-King G. Modulation of the subcellular distribution of calmodulin by melatonin in MDCK cells. *J. Pineal Res.* 1998, 24, 35-42.
[40] Arendt J. Role of the pineal gland and melatonin in seasonal reproductive function in mammals. *Oxf. Rev. Reprod. Biol.* 1986, 8, 266-320.
[41] Malpaux B, Migaud M, Tricoire H, Chemineau P. Biology of mammalian photoperiodism and the critical role of the pineal gland and melatonin. *J. Biol. Rhythms* 2001, 16, 336-347.
[42] Dubocovich ML, Rivera-Bermudez MA, Gerdin MJ, Masana MI. Molecular pharmacology, regulation and function of mammalian melatonin receptors. *Front. Biosci.* 2003, 8, 1093-1108.
[43] Yellon SM, Foster DL. Melatonin rhythms time photoperiod-induced puberty in the female lamb. *Endocrinology* 1986, 119, 44-49.
[44] Kauppila A, Kivela A, Pakarinen A, Vakkuri O. Inverse seasonal relationship between melatonin and ovarian activity in humans in a region with a strong seasonal contrast in luminosity. *J. Clin. Endocrinol. Metab.* 1987, 65, 823-828.

[45] Luboshitzky R, Lavie P. Melatonin and sex hormone interrelationships-a review. *J. Pediatr. Endocrinol. Metab.* 1999, 12, 355-362.

[46] Woo MM, Tai CJ, Kang SK, Nathwani PS, Pang SF, Leung PC. Direct action of melatonin in human granulosa-luteal cells. *J. Clin. Endocr. Metab.* 2001, 86, 4789-4797.

[47] Webley GE, Luck MR. Melatonin directly stimulates the secretion of progesterone by human and bovine granulosa cells *in vitro*. *J. Reprod. Fertil.* 1986, 78, 711-717.

[48] Cohen M, Lippman M, Chabner B. Role of pineal gland in aetiology and treatment of breast cancer. *Lancet* 1978, 2, 814-816.

[49] Blask DE, Brainard GC, Dauchy RT, *et al.* Melatonin-depleted blood from premenopausal women exposed to light at night stimulates growth of human breast cancer xenografts in nude rats. *Cancer Res.* 2005, 65, 11174-11184.

[50] Tamarkin L, Danforth DN, Lichter A, *et al.* Decreased nocturnal plasma melatonin peak in patients with estrogen receptor positive breast cancer. *Science* 1982, 216, 1003-1005.

[51] Maestroni JM, Conti A. Melatonin in human breast cancer tissue: association with nuclear grade and estrogen receptor status. *Lab. Invest.* 1996, 75, 557-561.

[52] Bartsch C, Bartsch H, Jain AK, Laumas KR, Wetterberg L. Urinary melatonin levels in human breast cancer patients. *J. Neural Transm.* 1981, 52, 281-294.

[53] Coleman MP, Reiter RJ. Breast cancer, blindness and melatonin. *Eur. J. Cancer* 1992, 28, 501-503.

[54] Verkasalo PK, Pukkala E, Stevens RG, Ojamo M, Rudanko SL. Inverse association between breast cancer incidence and degree of visual impairment in Finland. *Br. J. Cancer* 1999, 80, 1459-1460.

[55] Hrushesky W. Tumor cronobiology. *J. Control Release* 2001, 74, 27-30.

[56] Cos S, Mediavilla MD, Martínez-Campa C, González A, Alonso-González C, Sánchez-Barceló EJ. Exposure to light at night increases the growth of DMBA-induced mammary adenocarcinomas in rats. *Cancer Lett.* 2006, 235, 266-271.

[57] Blask DE, Hill SM. Effects of melatonin on cancer: studies on MCF-7 human breast cancer cells in culture. *J. Neural Transm. (Suppl)* 1986, 21, 433-449.

[58] Hill SM, Spriggs LL, Simon MA, Muraoka H, Blask DE. The growth inhibitory action of melatonin on human breast cancer cells is linked to the estrogen response system. *Cancer Lett.* 1992, 64, 249-256.

[59] Cos S, Fernández F, Sánchez-Barceló EJ. Melatonin inhibits DNA synthesis in MCF-7 human breast cancer cells *in vitro*. *Life Sci.* 1996, 58, 2447-2453.

[60] Molis TM, Walters MR, Hill SM. Melatonin modulation of estrogen receptor expression in MCF-7 human breast cancer cells. *Int. J. Oncol.* 1993, 3, 687-694.

[61] Cos S, Blask DE. Melatonin modulates growth factor activity in MCF-7 human breast cancer cells. *J. Pineal Res.* 1994, 17, 25-32.

[62] Molis TM, Spriggs LL, Jupiter Y, Hill SM. Melatonin modulation of estrogen-regulated proteins, growth factors and proto-oncogenes in human breast cancer. *J. Pineal Res.* 1995, 18, 93-103.

[63] Yuan L, Collins AR, Dai J, Dubocovich ML, Hill SM. MT-1 melatonin receptor overexpression enhances the growth suppressive effect of melatonin in human breast cancer cells. *Mol. Cell Endocrinol.* 2002, 192, 147-156.

[64] Cos S, Fernández R, Güezmes A, Sánchez-Barceló EJ. Influence of melatonin on invasive and metastatic properties of MCF-7 human breast cancer cells. *Cancer Res.* 1998, 58, 4383!4390.

[65] Soule HD, Vazquez J, Long A, Albert S, Brennan MJ. A human cell line from a pleural effusion derived from a breast carcinoma. *J. Natl. Cancer Inst.* 1973, 51, 1409-1412.

[66] Ram PT, Dai J, Yuan L, *et al.* Involvement of the MT-1 melatonin receptor in human breast cancer. *Cancer Lett.* 2002, 179, 141-150.

[67] Cos S, Martínez-Campa C, Mediavilla MD, Sánchez-Barceló EJ. Melatonin modulates aromatase activity in MCF-7 human breast cancer cells. *J. Pineal Res.* 2005, 38, 136-142.

[68] González A, Martínez-Campa C, Mediavilla MD, *et al.* Effects of MT_1 melatonin receptor overexpression on the aromatase-suppressive effect of melatonin in MCF-7 human breast cancer cells. *Oncol. Rep.* 2007, 17, 947-955.

[69] Cos S, González A, Güezmes A, *et al.* Melatonin inhibits the growth of DMBA-induced mammary tumors by decreasing the local biosynthesis of estrogens through the modulation of aromatase activity. *Int. J. Cancer* 2006, 118, 274-278.

[70] Martínez-Campa C, González A, Mediavilla MD, Alonso-González C, Sánchez-Barceló EJ, Cos S. Melatonin enhances the inhibitory effect of aminoglutethimide on aromatase activity in MCF-7 human breast cancer cells. *Breast Cancer Res. Treat.* 2005, 94, 249-254.

[71] Kao YC, Okubo T, Sun XZ, Chen S. Induction of aromatase expression by aminoglutethimide, an aromatase inhibitor that is used to treat breast cancer in postmenopausal women. *Anticancer Res.* 1999, 19, 2049-2056.

[72] González A, Martínez-Campa C, Mediavilla MD, Alonso-González C, Sánchez-Barceló EJ, Cos S. Inhibitory effects of pharmacological doses of melatonin on aromatase activity and expresión in rat glioma cells. *Br. J. Cancer* 2007, 97, 755-760.

[73] Bulun SE, Lin Z, Imir G, *et al.* Regulation of aromatase expression in estrogen-responsive breast and uterine disease: from bench to treatment. *Pharmacol. Rev.* 2005, 57, 359-383.

[74] Bulun SE, Sebastian S, Takayama K, Suzuki T, Sasano H, Shozu M. The human CYP 19 (aromatase p450) gene: update on physiologic roles and genomic organization of promoters. *J. Steroid Biochem. Mol. Biol.* 2003, 86, 219-224.

[75] Díaz-Cruz ES, Shapiro CL, Brueggemeier RW. Cyclooxygenase inhibitors suppress aromatase expression and activity in breast cancer cells. *J. Clin. Endocrinol. Metab* 2005, 90, 2563-2570.

[76] Prosperi JR, Robertson FM. Cyclooxygenase-2 directly regulates gene expression of P450 Cyp19 aromatase promoter regions pII, pI.3 and pI.7 and estradiol production in human breast tumor cells. *Prostag. Oth. Lipid M* 2006, 81, 55-70.

[77] Martínez-Campa C, González A, Mediavilla MD, *et al.* Melatonin inhibits aromatase promoter expression by regulating cyclooxygenases expression and activity in breast cáncer cells. *Br. J. Cancer* 2009, 101, 1613-1619.

[78] Wang J, Xiao X, Zhang Y, *et al.* Simultaneous modulation of COX-2, p300, Akt, and Apaf-1 signaling by melatonin to inhibit proliferation and induce apoptosis in breast cancer cells. *J. Pineal Res.* 2012, doi: 10.1111/j.1600-079X.2012.00973.x.

[79] Purohit A, Newman SP, Reed MJ. The role of cytokines in regulating estrogen synthesis: implications for the etiology of breast cancer. *Breast Cancer Res.* 2002, 4, 65-69.

[80] Alvarez-García V, González A, Alonso-González C, Martínez-Campa C, Cos S. Melatonin interferes in the desmoplastic reaction in breast cancer by regulating cytokine production. *J. Pineal Res.* 2012, 52, 282-290.

[81] Meng LI, Zhou J, Sasano H, Suzuki T, Zeitoun KM, Bulun SE. Tumor necrosis factor α and interleukin 11 secreted by malignant breast epitelial cells inhibit adipocyte differentiation by selectively down-regulating CCAAT/enhancer binding protein α and

peroxisome proliferator-activated receptor γ: mechasnism of desmoplastic reaction. *Cancer Res.* 2001, 61, 2250-2255.

[82] Bulun SE, Chen D, Lu M, *et al.* Aromatase excess in cancers of breast, endometrium and ovary. *J. Steroid Biochem. Mol. Biol.* 2007, 106, 81-96.

[83] Knower KC, To SQ, Takagi K, *et al.* Melatonin suppresses aromatase expression and activity in breast cancer associated fibroblasts. *Breast Cancer Res. Treat.* 2012, 132, 765-771.

[84] González A, Alvarez-García V, Martínez-Campa C, Alonso-González C, Cos S. Melatonin promotes differentiation of 3T3-L1 fibroblasts. *J. Pineal Res.* 2012, 52, 12-20.

[85] Harada N, Sasano H, Murakami H, Ohkuma T, Nagura H, Takagi Y. Localized expression of aromatase in human vascular tissues. *Circ. Res.* 1999, 84, 1285-1291.

[86] Mukherjee TK, Dinh H, Chaudhuri G, Nathan L. Testosterone attenuates expression of vascular cell adhesion molecule-1 by conversion to estradiol by aromatase in endothelial cells: implications in atherosclerosis. *Proc. Nat. Acad. Sci. USA* 2002, 6, 4055-4060.

[87] Cos S, González A, Alvarez-García V, Martínez-Campa C, Alonso-González C. Selective estrogen enzyme modulator actions of melatonin in breast cancer. In BIT's 4th Annual World Cancer Congress-2011-Breast Cancer Conference, Guangzhou: China 2011; pp. 137.

[88] Santner SJ, Rosen H, Osawa Y, Santen RJ. Additive effects of aminoglutethimide, testololactone, and 4-hydroxyandrostenedione as inhibitors of aromatase. *J. Steroid Biochem.* 1984, 20, 1239-1242.

[89] González A, Cos S, Martínez-Campa C, *et al.* Selective estrogen enzime modulator (SEEM) actions of melatonin in human breast cancer cells. *J. Pineal Res.* 2008, 45, 86-92.

[90] González A, Álvarez-García V, Martínez-Campa C, *et al. In vivo* inhibition of the estrogen sulfatase enzyme and growth of DMBA-induced mammary tumors by melatonin. *Curr. Cancer Drug Tar.* 2010, 10, 279-286.

[91] Evans TR, Rowlands MG, Luqmani YA, Chander SK, Coombes RC. Detection of breast cancer-associated estrone sulfatase in breast cancer biopsies and cell lines using polymerase chain reaction. *J. Steroid Biochem. Mol. Biol.* 1993, 46, 195-201.

[92] González A, Martínez-Campa C, Mediavilla MD, *et al.* Inhibitory effects of melatonin on sulfatase and 17β-hydroxysteroid dehydrogenase activity and expression in glioma cells. *Oncol. Rep.* 2010, 23, 1173-1178.

[93] Fournier S, Brihmat F, Durand JC, *et al.* Estradiol 17β-hydroxysteroid dehydrogenases, a marker of breast cancer hormone dependency. *Cancer Res.* 1985, 45, 2895-2899.

[94] Maitra SK, Ray AK. Role of light in the mediation of acute effects of a single afternoon melatonin injection on steroidogenic activity of testis in the rat. *J. Biosci.* 2000, 25, 253-256.

[95] Frungieri MB, Mayerhofer A, Zitta K, Pignataro OP, Calandra RS, González-Calvar SI. Direct effect of melatonin on Syrian hamster testes: melatonin subtype 1a receptors, inhibition of androgen production, and interaction with the local corticotropin-releasing hormone system. *Endocrinology* 2005, 146, 1541-1552.

Send Orders of Reprints at bspsaif@emirates.net.ae
238 *Advances in Cancer Drug Targets, Vol. 1,* 2013, 238-263

CHAPTER 8

Targeting Cancer and Neuropathy with Histone Deacetylase Inhibitors

V. Rodriguez-Menendez, L. Tremolizzo and G. Cavaletti*

Department of Neuroscience and Biomedical Technologies, University of Milano-Bicocca, Italy

Abstract: Histone deacetylase inhibitors (HDACi) belong to a novel class of drugs able to act on the epigenome, indirectly remodeling the spatial conformation of the chromatin: by increasing histone acetylation these drugs ultimately promote the detachment of DNA from the nucleosome octamer, thereby allowing transcription factors access to the double helix. Such a mechanism of action is of particular interest in the field of cancer treatment, as the reactivation of silenced tumor suppressor genes may be considered as being an important target at which to aim; indeed, it is currently believed that dysregulation of the epigenome plays a major role in cancer. Interestingly, some of the compounds belonging to the HDACi family have additional therapeutic properties, as in the case of valproate that may ameliorate neuropathic pain in animal models and in patients. Conceivably, this is a noteworthy observation, since peripheral neuropathy is a potentially severe side effect of several classes of anticancer agents, such as platinum-derived drugs, antitubulins or protesome inhibitors, limiting effective treatment of the underlying cancer. Based on these data, in this review we will argue that, with respect to other anticancer agents available nowadays, HDACi might offer the advantage not only of targeting the neoplastic disorder, but also of preventing peripheral neuropathies, possibly displaying a complementary mechanism of action.

Keywords: Cisplatin, neuropathy, cancer, histones, valproic acid, neuroprotection.

EPIGENETIC REGULATION OF GENE EXPRESSION

The classic nucleosome structure comprises 147 base pairs of double-stranded DNA wrapped around a histonic core formed by two copies of each of the H2, H2A, H3 and H4 histone proteins [1]. However, the complex mechanisms and governing dynamics that modulate the conformation, and even the composition,

***Address correspondence to G. Cavaletti:** University of Milano-Bicocca, Department of Neuroscience and Biomedical Technologies, *Via* Cadore 48, 20052 Monza (MI), Italy; Tel: +39-02.6448.8114; Fax: +39-02.6448.8250; E-mail: guido.cavaletti@unimib.it

Atta-ur-Rahman (Ed)

of such a structure, as well as all the participating players, are all still objects of study in an attempt to understand the "epigenetic code" that rules the mechanisms of transcription, both in physiological and pathological conditions.

Post-translational modifications of histone tails (N-terminal domain), such as acetylation, methylation or phosphorylation, contribute to changing the configuration of the nucleosomes, thereby rendering DNA more or less accessible to transcription factors and other regulatory molecules (co-repressors, co-activators). On one hand, the acetylation and phosphorylation modifications seem to contribute to reducing the positive charge of histones thereby altering their electrostatic interactions with the DNA and relaxing the nucleosome structure in order to give access to transcription factors or other remodeling chromatin complexes [2]. On the other hand, the modification of the histone tails seems to also have the purpose of acting as a "code" that can be recognized by specific domains present in proteins or complexes, such as the PHD finger of the ING family proteins that recognizes specific methylated lysine patterns, then recruiting additional chromatin remodeling enzymes such as HATs (histone acetyltransferases) and HDACs (histone deacetylases) [3, 4]. Also, mobilization of nucleosomes along the DNA is possible and depends on the binding, through the tandem chromo domain of the Chd1 protein (an ATP-dependent remodeling enzyme), to the tri-methylated H3K4 [5, 6]. H3K4me3 is associated with active transcription and is also directly bound by the tandem Tudor domains of the histone demethylase known as JMJD2. In general, methylation of H3K9, H3K27, or H4K20 tends to inactivate chromatin, whereas methylation of H3K4, H3K36, H3K79, and H3R17 seems to promote gene transcription [7]. Furthermore, methylation reactions govern gene transcription not only through the involvement of chromatin-associated proteins but also by direct targeting of CpG islands present in numerous gene promoter regions: when the content of 5-methyl cytosine residues within these regions reaches a critical threshold, the expression rate of the cognate gene is reduced and silencing may occur. Both levels of transcriptional control, *i.e.* histone tail modification and DNA methylation, seem to be closely related in a complex manner as demonstrated by several studies [8]. For example, it has been shown that the inhibition of histone deacetylation in mouse brain by peripheral administration of an HDAC inhibitor is able to promote DNA demethylation, thus synergistically enhancing target gene expression [9].

Moreover, in the last decade the discovery of histone protein variants seems to have opened up a new whole field of heightened interest in epigenetic regulation. There have been reported multiple histone variants with alternative amino acid sequences, with new sequences or even amino acid deletion and, therefore, they are likely to have different post-transcriptional modifications with respect to canonical histones. H2A and H3 variants are some of the most studied [10, 11]. For instance, the histone macroH2A contains an extended C-terminal domain (with respect to the classical H2A) whose function is still unknown. Interestingly, some of these variants appear to be concentrated in particular regions of the DNA, such as the histone macroH2A1 that is present throughout the inactive X chromosome [12]. These "new" histones endow their nucleosomes with distinct properties and different roles in transcription regulation with respect to canonical ones.

TARGETING HISTONE ACETYLATION WITH HDACi

Histone acetylation is probably one of the most studied histone tail modifications. While hyperacetylation of lysine residues promotes the open conformation of chromatin and, therefore, gene transcription, low levels of acetyl groups prevent the access and function of the transcription machinery. Histone acetyl transferases (HAT) and histone deacetylases (HDAC) are the enzymes that, with opposite functions, regulate the level of nucleosome acetylation.

18 different HDAC isoforms have been identified so far, and on the basis of their structure and functional characteristics they can be classified into four different groups. Class I comprises mainly nuclear isoforms: HDAC-1, -2, -3 and -8 whereas Classes IIa (HDAC-4,-5,-7 and -9) and IIb (HDAC-6 and -10) are able to shuttle between nucleus and cytoplasm. Class III isoforms, called also "sirtuins" due to their homology with the yeast protein SIR2 (silent information regulator-2), require the presence of NAD+ for their activity, unlike Classes I and II that need Zn^{++} in their catalytic domain. Finally, the nuclear HDAC-11 is the only component of Class IV, and displays structural similarities both with some Class I and II HDAC isoforms.

HDACs are capable of forming multiprotein complexes either with transcription repressor activity or transcription activators where they play an important additional regulatory role in transcription. For instance, Class I HDACs are known to be part of the well-conserved complexes Sin3 (Switch intensive 3), NuRDs (nucleosome remodeling and deacetylating), Co-REST (Co-repressor of REST) and NCoR/SMRT which participate in various important cellular processes, such as cell cycle and cell differentiation [13, 14]. Finally, most of the HDAC isoforms regulate cell homeostasis targeting also numerous non-histone proteins including calmodulin, other HDACs, various transcription factors, or α-tubulin [15].

Interestingly, epigenetic dysregulation is nowadays considered as a major mechanism of cancer, and aberrant transcriptional silencing of genes *via* DNA methylation and post-translational modifications of the histones is a hallmark of cancer cells [16]. Multiple genes acting on key homeostatic processes regulating cell survival and replication might be silenced by epigenetic mechanisms and, notably, this transcriptional silencing has been shown to be potentially reversible by epigenome-modifying drugs, such as HDAC inhibitors (HDACi) [17-22]. The latter is a very interesting category of drugs that are able, by blocking HDAC activity, to induce histone hyperacetylation and, therefore, to change chromatin conformation and the expression of transcriptionally silenced genes. These genes include several targets involved in tumorigenesis processes, such as cell cycle regulatory genes (p21WAF1/CIP1 and p16INK4A), tumor suppressor genes (p53, VHL, p107, gelsolin), genes involved in differentiation (RARa and TGFb1), apoptotic genes (CD95 and CD95L), *etc.* Quite surprisingly, the biochemical structure of HDACi is extremely heterogeneous and these drugs have been classified into different groups, displaying diverse potencies (and side effects when used *in vivo*): short-chain fatty acids (VPA, valproic acid; phenylbutyric acid [23-26]), hydroxamic acids (trichostatin-A or TSA; suberoylanilide hydroxamic acid or SAHA; [25, 27, 28]), benzamides (entinostat, MS-275; sulpiride [25, 29, 30]), epoxides (depudecin [31]), and cyclic peptides (romidepsin or FK-228; apicidin [25, 32, 33]). Notwithstanding the numerous differences existing among these compounds, globally HDACi are extremely effective in inducing the expression of multiple genes. The existence of this data has sometimes been regarded as a major drawback to a complete understanding of HDACi anticancer activity due to a presumed lack of specificity but, at the same time, it clearly represents a strong point for these drugs since, in this way, more genes might be targeted at the same time in cancer cells where, conceivably, multiple pathways are dysregulated.

Valproate (VPA) is a short-chain fatty acid belonging to the HDACi family, and it is a major anti-epileptic and mood-stabilizing drug [34]. Among the possible mechanisms of action of VPA, a direct effect on the epigenome has been documented *in vitro* and *in vivo* [35, 36], both in peripheral tissues and in the central nervous system (CNS) [9, 37], with very interesting putative novel clinical applications. In fact, VPA's ability to induce the hyperacetylation of histones has been regarded as a promising anticancer drug strategy (see next section). Also the teratogenic effect of VPA seems to be linked to the ability of this drug to inhibit HDACs [35, 38]. VPA-mediated HDAC inhibitory action results in an increase in the acetylation of histone and non-histone proteins, particularly transcription factors, markedly affecting their function, and usually inducing (but sometimes suppressing) the expression levels of target genes [39, 40]. It has become apparent that VPA preferentially inhibits the catalytic activity of HDAC belonging to class I [35, 37]. In addition, VPA stimulates selective proteosomal degradation of HDAC 2 [41] and has been shown to induce *in vitro* replication-independent active DNA demethylation in a manner that is closely related to its ability to inhibit HDACs and appears to be mediated, at least in part, by the methyl binding protein MBD2 [42].

VPA AND CANCER TREATMENT

VPA was first synthesized by B.S. Burton in 1882 [43] during the search for new organic solvents. Several years later, Pierre and colleagues recognized VPA's antiepileptic activity when using it as solvent for new antiepileptic compounds on experimentally induced seizures [44]. Since then, VPA has been widely used in the treatment of epilepsy and new applications have been discovered over the years. Indeed, VPA is also used as a mood-stabilizer in bipolar disorders, as a prophylactic drug for migraine, and as an add-on agent to neuroleptic treatment in schizophrenia [45-47]. The toxicity associated with the clinical use of VPA is reasonably low and is generally represented by mild dyspepsia, weight gain, dysphoria, fatigue, dizziness, drowsiness, hair loss, headache, nausea, sedation and tremor. Moreover, VPA may impair liver function and, very occasionally, may cause thrombocytopenia and impairment of blood coagulation; also VPA teratogenicity is well recognized, neural tube defects (*e.g.* spina bifida) being among the major associated abnormalities.

The first clues regarding the anticancer activity of VPA were detected *in vitro* more than 10 years ago, when it was shown that VPA was able to induce differentiation, inhibit cell proliferation and increase apoptosis and immunogenicity, decreasing the angiogenic potency in tumor cells [48]. In the last eight years, several clinical trials have been conducted using VPA on patients affected by different types of cancers [49], even if VPA is probably more effective in acute myeloid leukemia (AML) and myelodysplastic syndromes (MDS) than in solid tumors; recently, VPA has been tested in multiple clinical settings by different groups with several positive results [23, 24, 50-56]. In these trials VPA has often been used either alone or in combination with other antineoplastic drugs or other types of cancer therapy, such as ionizing radiation, or adenoviral mediated cancer gene therapy, in these latter cases acting as a chemo- and radio-sensitizer [50, 57-60]. These clinical trials are based on several pre-clinical studies. For example, Karagiannis and colleagues [61] have reported that, when using *in vitro* ionizing radiation, pre-treatment of cells with VPA for 24 hours markedly enhanced radiation-induced cell-death and apoptosis in erythroleukemic K562 human cells. VPA has also been shown to increase the efficacy of adenoviral-mediated cancer gene therapy through CAR (Coxsackie Adenovirus Receptor) upregulation [62]. Moreover, other reports suggest that VPA's ability to acetylate non-histone proteins such as tubulin may enhance the cytostatic and cytotoxic effects of Paclitaxel, as observed in two different anaplastic thyroid carcinoma cell lines (CAL-62 and ARO) [63]. The mechanism underlying this effect is probably based on the inhibition of HDAC-6 activity which leads to tubulin hyper-acetylation [63].

Although it has not yet been clearly established, it is likely that VPA's antitumoral action has its origin in its capacity to induce chromatin changes such as DNA hypomethylation and histone hyperacetylation. Furthermore, various clinical trials have confirmed that VPA synergistically enhances the antitumoral effects of other compounds [50, 51, 58, 64]. For example, the use of all-trans retinoic acid (ATRA) in patients with AML or high-risk MDS in combination with VPA and 5-azacitidine (5-AZA, a hypomethylating agent) was safe and clinically effective [50]. Bug and colleagues [65] observed that treatment with VPA in combination with ATRA results in transient disease control in a subset of patients with AML that has evolved from MDS. The administration of VPA to AML patients treated with retinoids significantly increased the effects of these drugs and prolonged the period of leukemic responsiveness to retinoid treatment. Kuedgen and colleagues [51, 52] have demonstrated that VPA monotherapy is beneficial for patients with low-risk MDS, although no additional effect was observed when administered in combination with ATRA. Another phase 1/2 study in patients with advanced leukemia reported that combined therapy of decitabine and VPA was safe and active, inducing a transient reversal of p15 mRNA expression and gene methylation levels. In fact, pre-treatment p15 methylation was significantly lower in responders *versus* non-responders suggesting that patients with lower pretreatment p15 methylation levels may belong to a subset of patients with a higher probability of a good prognosis when treated with this type of therapy [64]. However, in a similar study Blum and colleagues [58] observed that, in 25 patients with AML, the addition of VPA to the therapy with decitabine led to encephalopathy at relatively low doses. In the case of non-hematological tumors, VPA seems to be effective in cases of chemotherapy-refractory tumors when this resistance is attributed to epigenetic aberrations. In fact, clinical benefit was observed in 12 out of 15 cancer patients (cervix, breast, lung, testis, and ovarian) that underwent different chemotherapy regimens (including cisplatin, carboplatin, paclitaxel, vinorelbine, gemcitabine, pemetrexed, topotecan, doxorubicin, cyclophosphamide and anastrozole) when pre-treated for one week with VPA and hydralazine. The therapeutic effect was accompanied by a reduction in global DNA methylation, histone deacetylase activity and promoter demethylation (RARβ promoter demethylation in 2 patients with ovarian cancer and 1 with lung cancer; DAPK promoter demethylation in a patient with ovarian cancer) [66]. VPA was also effective in neuroblastoma tumor cells resistant to cisplatin and vincristine [67]. Such resistance involves an elevated adhesion of these cells to the endothelial cell monolayer, probably due to a downregulation of the adhesion receptor Neural Cell Adhesion Molecule (NCAM). In this study, VPA induced the upregulation of NCAM surface expression and blocked the adhesion of the tumor cells resistant to the antineoplastic drugs, thereby blocking the invasive processes. Moreover, in anthracycline-resistant solid tumors, Münster and colleagues [68] showed an interesting antitumoral activity with the combination of epirubicin (a topoisomerase II inhibitor) and VPA.

Despite all these encouraging results, some detrimental effects of VPA have also been reported in cancer patients. For instance, Atmaca and colleagues [69] reported in patients with refractory advanced cancer that VPA induced cognitive impairment. Moreover, another recent study reported that VPA and SAHA (Vorinostat, another HDACi much more potent than VPA) may induce a modest but irreversible increase in chemotherapy resistance in human colon cancer cells by stepwise drug exposure. The generated sub-lines resulted resistant to HDACi but not to anticancer agents of the non-HDACi-type [70].

PERIPHERAL NEUROPATHY AS A CRITICAL LIMITING FACTOR IN ANTICANCER TREATMENT

"Peripheral neuropathy" (PN) is a wide term used to designate any disease affecting the peripheral nerves. Peripheral nerve disorders are relatively common conditions affecting 2-3% of the general population, but the incidence may increase up to 8% with advancing age. They may be limited to only one nerve ("mononeuropathies"), or several nerves in a random fashion ("multineuropathies" or "mononeuritis multiplex"), or they may affect the nerves in a symmetrical way, generally with a distal-to-proximal gradient of involvement ("polyneuropathies"). PN may be inherited (such as Charcot-Marie-Tooth disease and related disorders) or acquired. Patients with PN may present with altered sensation and pain perception, weakness, or autonomic symptoms, depending on the affected nerve fiber type. Interestingly, peripheral nerves exhibit only a few distinct pathologic reactions to various injuries or diseases: Wallerian degeneration, axonal degeneration, and segmental demyelination. The specific mechanisms by which the various disorders affecting peripheral nerve induce these pathologic changes are largely unknown. Acquired PN can have a variety of origins: immune-mediated (Guillain-Barrè syndrome, *etc.*), infective (HIV, Epstein-Barr virus, *etc.*), iatrogenic, vitamin-related (pyridoxine intoxication, vitamin E or riboflavin deficiency), or idiopathic, *i.e.* without a recognizable cause [71].

Many compounds and drugs can be neurotoxic and produce iatrogenic PN, as is the case with several antineoplastic agents (*i.e.* platinum-derivatives, suramin, thalidomide, antitubulin agents, proteasome-inhibitors). These neurotoxic effects can appear immediately during or shortly after the administration of the drug, depending on both the target and site of the neurotoxic action. Remarkably, chemotherapy-induced PN (CIPN) is a serious and limiting side effect of the treatment in patients affected by tumors. In all cases, CIPN can significantly interfere with normal functions and critically compromise the quality of life of treated patients [72, 73]. The severity of damage due to the chemotherapy treatment depends on the drug, the duration of administration and the cumulative dose applied. The peripheral nervous system (PNS) has a great capacity for regeneration following injury. This occurs only if the cell body has been spared from the damage and the system is given enough time without treatment for the repair to be achieved. Depending on the dosage and agent used, symptoms resolve completely in some cases. Unfortunately, in most instances CIPN is only partially reversible and in the worst cases the damage is irreversible.

Interestingly, epigenetic mechanisms have been found to play an important role in neuropathic pain. In general, DNA methylation, and therefore gene silencing, seem to be behind the mechanisms that trigger neuropathic pain in several animal models of nerve injury. The increases in DNA methylation and MeCP2 expression (methyl-CpG-binding protein 2) in the spinal cord that occur after chronic constriction injury are attenuated by the administration of a DNA methyl-transferase inhibitor, along with the animal perception of pain [74]. It has also been observed in dorsal root ganglia (DRG) that nerve injury silences the expression of the voltage-gated potassium channel $K_V4.3$ (highly present in C-fibers) by promoting the binding of the transcriptional suppressor NRSF [75, 76]. In addition, histone tail hyperacetylation has been found to be involved in the inflammatory mechanisms underlying neuropathic pain both in sciatic nerves and DRG [77, 78]. In contrast, the action of HDACs seem to be determinant for myelin repair mechanisms and for the correct myelination processes to take place both in the CNS and PNS; in fact, HDAC inhibitors may have a negative effect on the capacity of the nervous system to perform proper axon myelination [79-81].

In the following paragraph we will focus on Cisplatin-induced PN, since interesting data on the neuroprotective action of HDACi or of other histone hyper-acetylating strategies are available.

CISPLATIN-INDUCED PN AS A PARADIGM OF CIPN

Cisplatin (Cis-diamine-dichloro-platinum-(II), CDDP) is a chemotherapeutic drug used in first line treatment for metastatic ovarian and testicular cancers [82, 83], but also in several other malignancies. CDDP cytotoxicity was discovered by serendipity about forty years ago when Rosenberg and colleagues [84] used platinum electrodes to apply electromagnetic radiation to bacterial and mammalian cells in order to investigate the mechanisms involved in cell division. A marked inhibition of cell proliferation was observed and it was related to the platinum release into the culture medium. No more than seven years later, after some animal experimentation, the first patients were treated with CDDP. Since then, the nephrotoxicity of CDDP treatment has limited the use of this compound during cancer treatment [85]. However, among the platinum compounds with well-established clinical use, CDDP is also known to be the most severely neurotoxic [86], so that about 20% of patients are unable to complete a full course of CDDP therapy due to the development of a sensory neuropathy [72, 87]. As with all the other platinum drugs, CDDP is virtually unable to cross the intact blood-brain barrier that protects the CNS. On the other hand, CDDP binds avidly to plasma proteins and has easy access to the PNS where it preferentially affects the sensory nerves and accumulates in the primary sensory neurons (and probably satellite cells) of the dorsal root ganglia (DRG) inducing shrinkage of the nuclear and cytoplasmic compartments and cell death [87, 88]. The sensory CDDP-induced PN is predominantly characterized by symptoms resulting from the damage of large myelinated fibers, such as numbness and tingling, paresthesias of the upper and lower limbs, reduced vibration and position sense perception, reduced tendon reflexes and incoordination with gait disturbance [89]. After completion of CDDP chemotherapy only some patients have significant neurotoxic symptoms, whereas 3-4 months later the number is definitely higher. Resolution or amelioration of symptoms occurs in most of the patients over the next twelve months and, in cases with mild neuropathy, after several months a new cycle of CDDP treatment is possible [86]. Although the exact mechanism is not completely understood, most of the evidence reported in the literature points to the formation of DNA adducts as the major process behind CDDP-mediated cell toxicity. It has been demonstrated that this drug enters the cells and preferentially binds to GpG and ApG adjacent bases of the DNA, creating intra- and inter-strand crosslinks in rapidly dividing cell lines, such as cancer cells [90, 91]; however, this drug also causes problems in non-dividing cells, such as DRG neurons [92, 93]. In fact, these adducts cause distortions in DNA, including unwinding and bending, and are recognized by several cellular proteins [94], generally leading to apoptotic cell death [95]. Moreover, CDDP has been shown to induce alteration of nucleosome dynamics, therefore involving once more the epigenetic machinery activity [96]. Other mechanisms presumably involved in CDDP neurotoxicity include binding to cytoplasmic proteins, interaction with ion channels, damage to mitochondria, the arrest of the cell cycle in the G2 phase, inhibition of ATPase activity, and alteration of cellular transport systems; all these mechanisms eventually converge on common downstream death pathways such as apoptosis or necrosis [97, 98]. In order to study the toxicity mechanisms of CDDP and to investigate the putative neuroprotective action of different compounds, several *in vivo* and *in vitro* models have been well characterized. The animal models, in particular, provide a useful tool in this field of research because they are able to mimic most of the clinical and pathological changes observed in humans [88, 99-102]. Rats treated with a dose of CDDP comparable to that given to patients show marked weight loss, reflecting the presence of general toxicity. Moreover, it has been specifically demonstrated that in these animals CDDP damages both nerves and DRG. The nerve conduction velocity of the tail nerve in these animals is lower with respect to healthy rats and reflects changes in large myelinated fibers [100], whereas the decrease in density of the nerve fibers in skin biopsy gauges the damage to small-diameter fibers that might be affected early on in the CIPN course [103]. Morphological and morphometric changes have also been described in the sciatic and peroneal nerves, and in the DRG of these animals. Specifically at the level of the nerves, Wallerian-like degeneration and signs of axonopathy have been observed [100]. At the DRG neuronal level, the nucleolar, nuclear and cytoplasmic size is reduced, while the presence of nucleolar eccentricity and the number of multinucleolar nuclei increases three- to five-fold [100, 104-106]. Signs of apoptosis have also been described in the DRG neurons with a correlation between the percentage of apoptotic neurons and the cumulative dose of CDDP administered to the animals [107].

VPA IN CDDP-INDUCED PN: TWO BIRDS WITH ONE STONE?

Interestingly, besides the already described possible clinical applications, VPA has also been used to ameliorate the symptoms of various PNs [108, 109]. In fact, VPA has recently been shown to promote axonal regeneration and the recovery of motor functions in animal models of nerve injury [110]. Moreover, this drug has been successfully used in the management of patients affected by neuropathic pain syndromes, such as painful diabetic PN [111]. Notably, recent guidelines conjunctly published by the American Academy of Neurology, the American Association of Neuromuscular and Electrodiagnostic Medicine, and the American Academy of Physical Medicine and Rehabilitation indicate that VPA should be considered as a valuable option for treating painful diabetic PN [112]. Starting from this data we hypothesized a theraputic strategy focused on VPA, theoretically able to prevent the occurrence of CIPN and, at the same time, interacting in a complementary manner with the antitumoral activity of the main cancer treatments, such as CDDP. Consistently with this idea, we recently demonstrated that VPA administered in combination with CDDP promoted rat embryo DRG neuron survival [113]. Moreover, VPA co-administration induced in CDDP-treated Wistar rats an improvement in body weight, sensory nerve conduction velocity, and DRG morphometric analysis. This protective effect was paralleled by an increase in the immunoreactivity of histone H3 acetylation in DRG explants, suggesting that VPA might act through the inhibition of HDACs. In contrast, VPA was not able to rescue CDDP-induced CIPN in treated rats when it was administered after the onset of peripheral nerve damage, suggesting that this molecule acts in a preventive way, possibly modulating the expression of protective genes. In order to evaluate if HDAC inhibition might be a suitable strategy for treating CIPN, we also performed preliminary experiments using another more potent HDACi, SAHA (with a μM potency, *versus* VPA mM potency). Consistently with VPA data, SAHA administered to Wistar rats after CIPN induction was not able to rescue the animals. In conclusion, although the specific mechanism of action has not yet been elucidated, in CIPN VPA displays a promising neuroprotective action deserving further investigation since it might be coupled with a theoretically very interesting synergistic antineoplastic effect. Based on these observations, we hypothesize that VPA, and possibly, selected related compounds, might be useful in treating malignancies in combination with CDDP, at the same time reducing the risk of developing CIPN.

OTHER HISTONE HYPER-ACETYLATING STRATEGIES: ACETYL-L-CARNITINE

Further evidence for a possible neuroprotective role of hyper-acetylating strategies can be inferred from the pre-clinical results obtained with Acetyl-L-carnitine (ALC). ALC is an ester of the trimethylated amino acid, L-carnitine, synthesized in the human brain, liver, and kidney by the enzyme ALC-transferase. The functions of ALC include the transport of long-chain fatty acids into the mitochondria and of small-chain and medium-chain fatty acids out of them. This mechanism, among other effects, maintains normal coenzyme A levels in this organelle. ALC plays an important role in the acetyl-CoA metabolism, since it donates its acyl group to enhance acetyl-CoA synthesis and exerts a cholinomimetic effect thanks to their structure similarity; moreover, ALC facilitates mitochondrial oxidative metabolism [114-116]. Through these mechanisms, ALC has demonstrated that it possesses interesting properties, including neuroprotective and neurothrophic actions, antioxidant activity or stabilization of internal membranes. In fact, several clinical trials and research studies have reported that ALC may be of benefit in treating different neuropsychiatric diseases such as Alzheimer's disease [117-119], depression in the elderly [120], brain ischemia and reperfusion [121], cognitive impairment associated with alcoholism [122], and in several types of PN. Regarding this last clinical setting, ALC administration has been primarily studied in clinical trials in diabetic neuropathy [123, 124], and in antiretroviral-induced neuropathy [125-127] showing that this drug is well-tolerated and effective in alleviating PN symptoms, especially pain. In neuropathic diabetic patients ALC improves neurophysiologic parameters, nerve fiber regeneration, and vibratory perception [128]. In the past few years, in CIPN animal models induced by antineoplastic drug exposure (*i.e.* paclitaxel, vincristine, CDDP and oxaliplatin), ALC administration has shown neuroprotective and neurothrophic actions by promoting the recovery of nerve conduction velocity, the restoration of the mechanical nociceptive threshold, and analgesia without altering the antitumor properties of the antineoplastic drugs [129-134]. These results and the safety profile of ALC in other neuropathy types, have led to the effect of ALC being investigated in patients affected by Paclitaxel- and CDDP-induced CIPN [135], and these preliminary studies have confirmed the good tolerability and the possible efficacy of ALC. Even though the ALC mechanism of neuroprotection has not yet been fully elucidated, current evidence suggests that the epigenetic regulation of gene expression may be involved. In fact, it has recently been reported in an animal model of CIPN and in a model of X-fragile syndrome that ALC promotes histone acetylation, possibly acting as an acetyl group donor, modifying chromatin conformation, and thus changing the accessibility of the transcriptional machinery molecules to the gene promoters [130, 136]. In fact, mitochondrial ALC is known to enter into nuclei, where it is transformed into acetyl-CoA that is used as an acetyl group donor for histone acetylation reactions [137]. This mechanism could explain the increased mRNA and protein levels of Nerve Growth Factor (NGF) and ACh-transferase activity found in the CNS of aged rats, and in animal models of Alzheimer's disease and CIPN treated with ALC [130, 138, 139].

CONCLUSIONS

In this review we have pointed out the need for new neuroprotective strategies able to effectively target CIPN. In fact, CIPN represents a major problem in patients treated with anticancer drugs, severely impairing their quality of life, and frequently inducing drug administration withdrawal, with possible negative effects on the clinical outcome of cancer patients. Considering the vast choice of available putative neuroprotective molecules, here we considered the possibility of taking advantage of drugs already used in cancer therapy. HDACi, in fact, currently represent an interesting therapeutic option in cancer treatment and there are some theoretical reasons why they be able to achieve a neuroprotective action while acting synergistically with the main anticancer drugs. A "general" neuroprotective action has already been shown for HDACi in the CNS compartment, since some molecules belonging to this class of drugs are able to reduce both ischemic and toxin-induced brain damage in animal models [140-142]. Moreover, selected HDACi, such as SAHA or sodium butyrate, significantly ameliorate different Huntington's disease-related endophenotypes both *in vitro*, and in animal models of this disease [143, 144]. Furthermore, considering that a phenotypic modulation was observed following sodium butyrate administration in mouse models of spinal and bulbar muscular atrophy [145], a role in therapeutics for polyglutamine disorders has been previously proposed for HDACi [146]. Considering another disorder affecting motor neurons, such as amyotrophic lateral sclerosis, some contrasting evidence might suggest a beneficial effect of VPA and sodium butyrate in the transgenic SOD1 mouse model [147-149], while other authors have reported a failure of VPA in significantly extending the survival in this animal model as in patients [150, 151]. Nevertheless, our preliminary data indicate that, among HDACs, VPA might exert a promising neuroprotective effect also in the context of CDDP neurotoxicity, assessed both *in vitro* where it induces an increase in DRG neuron survival rate, and *in vivo* (when co-administered) where it prevents damage to large myelinated fibers and DRG neurons [113]. Unfortunately, this neuroprotective effect of VPA is not paralleled, as shown also for SAHA, by a therapeutic effect when it is administered following CDDP-PN induction. Moreover, although an increased histone H3 acetylation has been shown in rat DRG explants following VPA administration, we can only suggest that VPA-mediated HDAC inhibition is involved in neuroprotection, since a direct demonstration is still lacking, at least in the nervous system [152]. In fact, multiple mechanisms have already been proposed in an attempt to account for the different therapeutic properties of VPA [34]. Overall, the currently available body of evidence makes it possible to hypothesize that HDACi might be useful as a neuroprotectant, at least when used in combination with DNA-interacting antineoplastic drugs, such as CDDP and other platinum-derived drugs; further experiments, however, are certainly needed to definitely clarify this issue. Interestingly, the reasonable profile of the side effects of VPA might be worth considering for preventive administration in those subjects at high risk of developing CIPN, and future studies might be designed in order to identify this subpopulation of patients. For all these reasons, we suggest that future experiments will be able to determine if HDACi putative neuroprotective activity might be transferable into the clinical setting, paying special attention when designing the study to the possibility of observing decreased neurotoxicity following exposure to combination therapies. Hopefully, this might allow for the first time the design of new anticancer drug cocktails with the ambitious aim of killing "two birds with one stone" in cancer chemotherapy.

ACKNOWLEDGEMENTS

Guido Cavaletti received an unrestricted research grant in the field of antineoplastic drug-induced peripheral neuropathies from the Fondazione Banca del Monte di Lombardia.

CONFLICT OF INTEREST

The author(s) confirm that this chapter content has no conflict of interest.

DISCLOSURE

The chapter submitted for the eBook Series entitled **"Advances in Cancer Drug Targets, Volume 1"** is an update of our article in **Current Cancer Drug Targets, Volume 8, Issue 4, 2008,** with additional text and references.

LIST OF ABBREVIATIONS

ALC =Acetyl-L-carnitine

CDDP =Cis-diamine-dichloro-platinum-(II), or cisplatin

CIPN =chemotherapy-induced PN

CNS =central nervous system

DRG =dorsal root ganglia

HAT =histone acetyltransferase

HDAC =histone deacetylase

HDACi =HDAC inhibitors

NGF =nerve growth factor

PN =peripheral neuropathy

PNS =peripheral nervous system

SAHA =suberoylanilide hydroxamic acid

VPA =valproic acid, or valproate

REFERENCES

[1] Luger K, Mader AW, Richmond RK, Sargent DF, Richmond TJ. Crystal structure of the nucleosome core particle at 2.8 A resolution. Nature 1997; 389: 251-60.

[2] Kouzarides T. Chromatin modifications and their function. Cell 2007; 128: 693-705.

[3] Yun M, Wu J, Workman JL, Li B. Readers of histone modifications. Cell Res 2011; 21: 564-78.

[4] Champagne KS, Kutateladze TG. Structural insight into histone recognition by the ING PHD fingers. Curr Drug Targets 2009; 10: 432-41.

[5] Sims RJ, III, Chen CF, Santos-Rosa H, Kouzarides T, Patel SS, Reinberg D. Human but not yeast CHD1 binds directly and selectively to histone H3 methylated at lysine 4 *via* its tandem chromodomains. J Biol Chem 2005; 280: 41789-92.

[6] Patel A, McKnight JN, Genzor P, Bowman GD. Identification of residues in chromodomain helicase DNA-binding protein 1 (Chd1) required for coupling ATP hydrolysis to nucleosome sliding. J Biol Chem 2011; 286: 43984-93.

[7] Klose RJ, Zhang Y. Regulation of histone methylation by demethylimination and demethylation. Nat Rev Mol Cell Biol 2007; 8: 307-18.

[8] Milutinovic S, D'Alessio AC, Detich N, Szyf M. Valproate induces widespread epigenetic reprogramming which involves demethylation of specific genes. Carcinogenesis 2007; 28: 560-71.

[9] Tremolizzo L, Doueiri MS, Dong E, Grayson DR, Davis J, Pinna G, Tueting P, Rodriguez-Menendez V, Costa E, Guidotti A. Valproate corrects the schizophrenia-like epigenetic behavioral modifications induced by methionine in mice. Biol Psychiatry 2005; 57: 500-9.

[10] Ederveen TH, Mandemaker IK, Logie C. The human histone H3 complement anno 2011. Biochim Biophys Acta 2011; 1809: 577-86.

[11] Sarma K, Reinberg D. Histone variants meet their match. Nat Rev Mol Cell Biol 2005; 6: 139-49.

[12] Mietton F, Sengupta AK, Molla A, Picchi G, Barral S, Heliot L, Grange T, Wutz A, Dimitrov S. Weak but uniform enrichment of the histone variant macroH2A1 along the inactive X chromosome. Mol Cell Biol 2009; 29: 150-6.

[13] Hayakawa T, Nakayama J. Physiological roles of class I HDAC complex and histone demethylase. J Biomed Biotechnol 2011; 2011:129383.

[14] Spiegel S, Milstien S, Grant S. Endogenous modulators and pharmacological inhibitors of histone deacetylases in cancer therapy. Oncogene 2012; 31: 537-51.

[15] Seidel C, Schnekenburger M, Dicato M, Diederich M. Histone deacetylase modulators provided by Mother Nature. Genes Nutr 2012 Feb 12; Epub ahead of print.

[16] Baylin SB, Jones PA. A decade of exploring the cancer epigenome - biological and translational implications. Nat Rev Cancer 2011; 11: 726-34.

[17] Verbrugge I, Johnstone RW, Bots M. Promises and challenges of anticancer drugs that target the epigenome. Epigenomics 2011; 3: 547-65.

[18] Best JD, Carey N. Epigenetic opportunities and challenges in cancer. Drug Discov Today 2010; 15: 65-70.

[19] Elaut G, Rogiers V, Vanhaecke T. The pharmaceutical potential of histone deacetylase inhibitors. Curr Pharm Des 2007; 13: 2584-20.

[20] Villar-Garea A, Esteller M. DNA demethylating agents and chromatin-remodelling drugs: which, how and why? Curr Drug Metab 2003; 4: 11-31.

[21] Moradei O, Maroun CR, Paquin I, Vaisburg A. Histone deacetylase inhibitors: latest developments, trends and prospects. Curr Med Chem Anticancer Agents 2005; 5: 529-60.

[22] Santini V, Gozzini A, Ferrari G. Histone deacetylase inhibitors: molecular and biological activity as a premise to clinical application. Curr Drug Metab 2007; 8: 383-93.

[23] Mohammed TA, Holen KD, Jaskula-Sztul R, Mulkerin D, Lubner SJ, Schelman WR, Eickhoff J, Chen H, Loconte NK A pilot phase II study of valproic acid for treatment of low-grade neuroendocrine carcinoma. Oncologist 2011; 16: 835-43.

[24] Raffoux E, Cras A, Recher C, Boëlle PY, de Labarthe A, Turlure P, Marolleau JP, Reman O, Gardin C, Victor M, Maury S, Rousselot P, Malfuson JV, Maarek O, Daniel MT, Fenaux P, Degos L, Chomienne C, Chevret S, Dombret H. Phase 2 clinical trial of 5-azacitidine, valproic acid, and all-trans retinoic acid in patients with high-risk acute myeloid leukemia or myelodysplastic syndrome. Oncotarget 2010; 1: 34-42.

[25] Song SH, Han SW, Bang YJ. Epigenetic-based therapies in cancer: progress to date. Drugs 2011; 71: 2391-403.

[26] Davie JR. Inhibition of histone deacetylase activity by butyrate. J Nutr 2003; 133: 2485S-93S.

[27] Sato A. Vorinostat approved in Japan for treatment of cutaneous T-cell lymphomas: status and prospects. Onco Targets Ther 2012; 5: 67-75.

[28] Yoshida M, Kijima M, Akita M, Beppu T. Potent and specific inhibition of mammalian histone deacetylase both *in vivo* and *in vitro* by trichostatin A. J Biol Chem 1990; 265: 17174-9.

[29] Pili R, Salumbides B, Zhao M, Altiok S, Qian D, Zwiebel J, Carducci MA, Rudek MA. Phase I study of the histone deacetylase inhibitor entinostat in combination with 13-cis retinoic acid in patients with solid tumours. Br J Cancer 2012; 106: 77-84.

[30] Tremolizzo L, Rodriguez-Menendez V, DiFrancesco JC, Sala G, Galbussera A, Appollonio I, Ferrarese C. Huntington's disease and HDACi: would sulpiride and valproate be of therapeutic value? Med Hypotheses 2007; 69: 964-5.

[31] Kwon H.J, Owa T, Hassig, CA, Shimada J, Schreiber SL. Depudecin induces morphological reversion of transformed fibroblasts *via* the inhibition of histone deacetylase. Proc Natl Acad Sci USA 1998; 95: 3356-61.

[32] VanderMolen KM, McCulloch W, Pearce CJ, Oberlies NH. Romidepsin (Istodax, NSC 630176, FR901228, FK228, depsipeptide): a natural product recently approved for cutaneous T-cell lymphoma. J Antibiot (Tokyo) 2011; 64: 525-31.

[33] Han JW, Ahn SH, Park SH, Wang SY, Bae GU, Seo DW, Kwon HK, Hong S, Lee HY, Leev YW, Lee HW. Apicidin, a histone deacetylase inhibitor, inhibits proliferation of tumor cells *via* induction of p21WAF1/Cip1 and gelsolin. Cancer Res 2000; 60: 6068-74.

[34] Perucca E. Pharmacological and therapeutic properties of valproate: a summary after 35 years of clinical experience. CNS Drugs 2002; 16: 695-14.

[35] Phiel CJ, Zhang F, Huang EY, Guenther MG, Lazar MA, Klein PS. Histone deacetylase is a direct target of valproic acid, a potent anticonvulsant, mood stabilizer, and teratogen. J Biol Chem 2001; 276: 36734-41.

[36] Tremolizzo L, Carboni G, Ruzicka WB, Mitchell CP, Sugaya I, Tueting P, Sharma, R, Grayson DR, Costa E, Guidotti A. An epigenetic mouse model for molecular and behavioral neuropathologies related to schizophrenia vulnerability. Proc Natl Acad Sci USA 2002; 99: 17095-100.

[37] Göttlicher M, Minucci S, Zhu P, Kramer OH, Schimpf A, Giavara S, Sleeman JP, Lo Coco F, Nervi C, Pelicci PG, Heinzel T. Valproic acid defines a novel class of HDAC inhibitors inducing differentiation of transformed cells. Embo J 2001; 20: 6969-78.

[38] Göttlicher M. Valproic acid: an old drug newly discovered as inhibitor of histone deacetylases. Ann Hematol 2004; 83: 91-2.

[39] Kim MS, Kwon HJ, Lee YM, Baek JH, Jang JE, Lee SW, Moon EJ, Kim HS, Lee SK, Chung HY, Kim CW, Kim KW. Histone deacetylases induce angiogenesis by negative regulation of tumor suppressor genes. Nat Med 2001; 7: 437-43.

[40] Nair AR, Boersma LJ, Schiltz L, Chaudhry MA, Muschel RJ. Paradoxical effects of trichostatin A: inhibition of NF-Y-associated histone acetyltransferase activity, phosphorylation of hGCN5 and downregulation of cyclin A and B1 mRNA. Cancer Lett 2001; 166: 55-64.

[41] Krämer OH, Zhu P, Ostendorff HP, Golebiewski M, Tiefenbach J, Peters MA, Brill B, Groner B, Bach I, Heinzel T, Göttlicher M. The histone deacetylase inhibitor valproic acid selectively induces proteasomal degradation of HDAC2. EMBO J 2003; 22: 3411-20.

[42] Detich N, Bovenzi V, Szyf M. Valproate induces replication-independent active DNA demethylation. J Biol Chem 2003; 278: 27586-92.

[43] Burton BS. On the propyl derivatives and decomposition products of ethylacetoacetate. Am Chem J 1882; 3: 385-95.

[44] Meunier H, Carraz G, Neunier Y, Eymard P, Aimard M. [Pharmacodynamic properties of N-dipropylacetic acid]. Therapie 1963; 18: 435-8.

[45] Loscher W. Valproate: a reappraisal of its pharmacodynamic properties and mechanisms of action. Prog Neurobiol 1999; 58: 31-59.

[46] Michaelis M, Doerr HW, Cinatl J Jr. Valproic acid as anti-cancer drug. Curr Pharm Des 2007; 13: 3378-93.

[47] Bowden CL, Singh V. Valproate in bipolar disorder: 2000 onwards. Acta Psychiatr Scand 2005; 111: 13-20.

[48] Kostrouchová M, Kostrouch Z, Kostrouchová M. Valproic acid, a molecular lead to multiple regulatory pathways. Folia Biol (Praha) 2007; 53: 37-49.

[49] Hrebackova J, Hrabeta J, Eckschlager T. Valproic acid in the complex therapy of malignant tumors. Curr Drug Targets 2010; 11: 361-79.

[50] Soriano AO, Yang H, Faderl S, Estrov Z, Giles F, Ravandi F, Cortes J, Wierda WG, Ouzounian S, Quezada A, Pierce S, Estey EH, Issa JP, Kantarjian HM, Garcia-Manero G. Safety and clinical activity of the combination of 5-azacytidine, valproic acid, and all-trans retinoic acid in acute myeloid leukemia and myelodysplastic syndrome. Blood 2007; 110: 2302-8.

[51] Kuendgen A, Strupp C, Aivado M, Bernhardt A, Hildebrandt B, Haas R, Germing U, Gattermann N. Treatment of myelodysplastic syndromes with valproic acid alone or in combination with all-trans retinoic acid. Blood 2004; 104: 1266-9.

[52] Kuendgen A, Knipp S, Fox F, Strupp C, Hildebrandt B, Steidl C, Germing U, Haas R, Gattermann N. Results of a phase 2 study of valproic acid alone or in combination with all-trans retinoic acid in 75 patients with myelodysplastic syndrome and relapsed or refractory acute myeloid leukemia. Ann Hematol 2005; 84: 61-6.

[53] Kuendgen A, Schmid M, Schlenk R, Knipp S, Hildebrandt B, Steidl C, Germing U, Haas R, Dohner H, Gattermann N. The histone deacetylase (HDAC) inhibitor valproic acid as monotherapy or in combination with all-trans retinoic acid in patients with acute myeloid leukemia. Cancer 2006; 106: 112-9.

[54] Raffoux E, Chaibi P, Dombret H, Degos L. Valproic acid and all-trans retinoic acid for the treatment of elderly patients with acute myeloid leukemia. Haematologica 2005; 90: 986-8.

[55] Pilatrino C, Cilloni D, Messa E, Morotti A, Giugliano E, Pautasso M, Familiari U, Cappia S, Pelicci PG, Lo Coco F, Saglio G, Guerrasio A. Increase in platelet count in older, poor-risk patients with acute myeloid leukemia or myelodysplastic syndrome treated with valproic acid and all-trans retinoic acid. Cancer 2005; 104: 101-9.

[56] Cimino G, Lo-Coco F, Fenu S. Sequential valproic acid/alltrans retinoic acid treatment reprograms differentiation in refractory and high-risk acute myeloid leukemia. Cancer Res 2006; 66: 8903–11.

[57] Shoji M, Ninomiya I, Makino I, Kinoshita J, Nakamura K, Oyama K, Nakagawara H, Fujita H, Tajima H, Takamura H, Kitagawa H, Fushida S, Harada S, Fujimura T, Ohta T. Valproic acid, a histone deacetylase inhibitor, enhances radiosensitivity in esophageal squamous cell carcinoma. Int J Oncol 2012; 40: 2140-6.

[58] Blum W, Klisovic RB, Hackanson B, Liu Z, Liu S, Devine H, Vukosavljevic T, Huynh L, Lozanski G, Kefauver C, Plass C, Devine SM, Heerema, N.A, Murgo, A, Chan, K.K, Grever, M.R, Byrd, J.C, Marcucci, G. Phase I study of decitabine alone or in combination with valproic acid in acute myeloid leukemia. J Clin Oncol 2007; 25: 3884-91.

[59] Kuendgen A, Gattermann N. Valproic acid for the treatment of myeloid malignancies. Cancer 2007; 110: 943-54.

[60] Camphausen K, Tofilon PJ. Inhibition of histone deacetylation: a strategy for tumor radiosensitization. J Clin Oncol 2007; 25: 4051-6.

[61] Karagiannis TC, Kn H, El-Osta A. The epigenetic modifier, valproic acid, enhances radiation sensitivity. Epigenetics 2006; 1: 131-7.

[62] Segura-Pacheco B, Avalos B, Rangel E, Velazquez D, Cabrera G. HDAC inhibitor valproic acid upregulates CAR *in vitro* and *in vivo*. Genet Vaccines Ther 2007; 5: 10.

[63] Catalano MG, Poli R, Pugliese M, Fortunati N, Boccuzzi G. Valproic acid enhances tubulin acetylation and apoptotic activity of paclitaxel on anaplastic thyroid cancer cell lines. Endocr Relat Cancer 2007; 14: 839-45.

[64] Garcia-Manero G, Kantarjian HM, Sanchez-Gonzalez B, Yang H, Rosner G, Verstovsek S, Rytting M, Wierda WG, Ravandi F, Koller C, Xiao L, Faderl S, Estrov Z, Cortes J, O'brien S, Estey E, Bueso-Ramos C, Fiorentino J, Jabbour E, Issa JP. Phase 1/2 study of the combination of 5-aza-2'-deoxycytidine with valproic acid in patients with leukemia. Blood 2006; 108: 3271-9.

[65] Bug G, Schwarz K, Schoch C, Kampfmann M, Henschler R, Hoelzer D, Ottmann OG, Ruthardt M. Effect of histone deacetylase inhibitor valproic acid on progenitor cells of acute myeloid leukemia. Haematologica 2007; 92: 542-45.

[66] Candelaria M, Gallardo-Rincón D, Arce C, Cetina L, Aguilar-Ponce JL, Arrieta O, González-Fierro A, Chávez-Blanco A, de la Cruz-Hernández E, *et al.* A phase II study of epigenetic therapy with hydralazine and magnesium valproate to overcome chemotherapy resistance in refractory solid tumors. Ann Oncol 2007; 18: 1529-38.

[67] Blaheta RA, Michaelis M, Natsheh I, Hasenberg C, Weich E, Relja B, Jonas D, Doerr HW, Cinatl JJr. Valproic acid inhibits adhesion of vincristine- and cisplatin-resistant neuroblastoma tumor cells to endothelium. Br J Cancer 2007; 96: 1699-06.

[68] Münster P, Marchion D, Bicaku E, Schmitt M, Lee JH, DeConti R, Simon G, Fishman M, Minton S, Garrett C, Chiappori A, Lush R, Sullivan D, Daud A. Phase I trial of histone deacetylase inhibition by valproic acid followed by the topoisomerase II inhibitor epirubicin in advanced solid tumors: a clinical and translational study. J Clin Oncol 2007; 25: 1979-85.

[69] Atmaca A, Al-Batran SE, Maurer A, Neumann A, Heinzel T, Hentsch B, Schwarz SE, Hövelmann S, Göttlicher M, Knuth A, Jäger E. Valproic acid (VPA) in patients with refractory advanced cancer: a dose escalating phase I clinical trial. Br J Cancer 2007; 97: 177-82.

[70] Fedier A, Dedes KJ, Imesch P, Von Bueren AO, Fink D. The histone deacetylase inhibitors suberoylanilide hydroxamic (Vorinostat) and valproic acid induce irreversible and MDR1-independent resistance in human colon cancer cells. Int J Oncol 2007; 31: 633-41.

[71] Sghirlanzoni A, Pareyson D, Lauria G. Sensory neuron diseases. Lancet Neurol 2005; 4: 349-61.

[72] Quasthoff S, Hartung HP. Chemotherapy-induced peripheral neuropathy. J Neurol 2002; 249: 9-17.

[73] Windebank AJ. Chemotherapeutic neuropathy. Curr Opin Neurol 1999; 12: 565-71.

[74] Wang Y, Liu C, Guo QL, Yan JQ, Zhu XY, Huang CS, Zou WY. Intrathecal 5-azacytidine inhibits global DNA methylation and methyl- CpG-binding protein 2 expression and alleviates neuropathic pain in rats following chronic constriction injury. Brain Res 2011; 1418: 64-9.

[75] Uchida H, Ma L, Ueda H. Epigenetic gene silencing underlies C-fiber dysfunctions in neuropathic pain. J Neurosci 2010; 30: 4806-14.

[76] Uchida H, Sasaki K, Ma L, Ueda H. Neuron-restrictive silencer factor causes epigenetic silencing of Kv4.3 gene after peripheral nerve injury. Neuroscience. 2010; 166:1-4.

[77] Kiguchi N, Kobayashi Y, Maeda T, Fukazawa Y, Tohya K, Kimura M, Kishioka S. Epigenetic augmentation of the macrophage inflammatory protein 2/C-X-C chemokine receptor type 2 axis through histone H3 acetylation in injured peripheral nerves elicits neuropathic pain. J Pharmacol Exp Ther 2012; 340: 577-87.

[78] Chiechio S, Zammataro M, Morales ME, Busceti CL, Drago F, Gereau RW 4th, Copani A, Nicoletti F. Epigenetic modulation of mGlu2 receptors by histone deacetylase inhibitors in the treatment of inflammatory pain. Mol Pharmacol 2009; 75: 1014-20.

[79] Popko B. Epigenetic control of myelin repair. Nat Neurosci 2008; 11: 987-8.

[80] Jacob C, Lebrun-Julien F, Suter U. How histone deacetylases control myelination. Mol Neurobiol 2011; 44: 303-12.

[81] Pereira JA, Lebrun-Julien F, Suter U. Molecular mechanisms regulating myelination in the peripheral nervous system. Trends Neurosci 2012; 35: 123-34.

[82] Ocean AJ, Vahdat LT. Chemotherapy-induced peripheral neuropathy: pathogenesis and emerging therapies. Support Care Cancer 2004; 12: 619-25.

[83] Peltier AC, Russell JW. Recent advances in drug-induced neuropathies. Curr Opin Neurol 2002; 15: 633-8.

[84] Rosenberg, B, Vancamp L, Krigas T. Inhibition of cell division in escherichia coli by electrolysis products from a platinum electrode. Nature. 1965; 205: 698-9.

[85] Kelland L. The resurgence of platinum-based cancer chemotherapy. Nat Rev Cancer 2007; 7: 573-84.

[86] Cavaletti G, Marmiroli P. Chemotherapy-induced peripheral neurotoxicity. Expert Opin Drug Saf 2004; 3: 535-46.

[87] McDonald ES, Randon KR, Knight A, Windebank AJ. Cisplatin preferentially binds to DNA in dorsal root ganglion neurons *in vitro* and *in vivo*: a potential mechanism for neurotoxicity. Neurobiol Dis 2005; 18: 305-13.

[88] Barajon I, Bersani M, Quartu M, Del Fiacco M, Cavaletti G, Holst JJ, Tredici G. Neuropeptides and morphological changes in cisplatin-induced dorsal root ganglion neuronopathy. Exp Neurol 1996; 138: 93-04.

[89] Mollman, JE. Cisplatin neurotoxicity. N Engl J Med 1990; 322: 126-7.

[90] Baik MH, Friesner RA, Lippard SJ. Theoretical study of cisplatin binding to purine bases: why does cisplatin prefer guanine over adenine? J Am Chem Soc 2003; 125: 14082-92.

[91] Huang H, Zhu L, Reid BR, Drobny, G.P, Hopkins, P.B. Solution structure of a cisplatin-induced DNA interstrand cross-link. Scienc. 1995; 270: 1842-45.

[92] Meijer C, de Vries EG, Marmiroli P, Tredici G, Frattola L, Cavaletti G. Cisplatin-induced DNA-platination in experimental dorsal root ganglia neuronopathy. Neurotoxicology 1999; 20: 883-7.

[93] Dzagnidze A, Katsarava, Z, Makhalova J, Liedert B, Yoon MS, Kaube H, Limmroth V, Thomale J. Repair capacity for platinum-DNA adducts determines the severity of cisplatin-induced peripheral neuropathy. J Neurosci 2007; 27: 9451-7.

[94] Chaney SG, Campbell SL, Temple B, Bassett E, Wu Y, Faldu M. Protein interactions with platinum-DNA adducts: from structure to function. J Inorg Biochem 2004; 98: 1551-9.

[95] Eastman A. Activation of programmed cell death by anticancer agents: cisplatin as a model system. Cancer Cells 1990; 2: 275-80.

[96] Wu B, Davey CA. Platinum drug adduct formation in the nucleosome core alters nucleosome mobility but not positioning. Chem Biol 2008; 15: 1023-8.

[97] Scott RH, Woods AJ, Lacey,MJ, Fernando D, Crawford JH, Andrews PL. An electrophysiological investigation of the effects of cisplatin and the protective actions of dexamethasone on cultured dorsal root ganglion neurons from neonatal rats. Naunyn Schmiedebergs Arch Pharmacol 1995; 352: 247-55.

[98] Carozzi VA, Marmiroli P, Cavaletti G. The role of oxidative stress and anti-oxidant treatment in platinum-induced peripheral neurotoxicity. Curr Cancer Drug Targets 2010; 10: 670-82.

[99] Cece R, Petruccioli MG, Cavaletti G, Barajon I, Tredici G. An ultrastructural study of neuronal changes in dorsal root ganglia (DRG) of rats after chronic cisplatin administrations. Histol Histopathol 1995; 10: 837-45.

[100] Cavaletti G, Tredici G, Marmiroli,P, Petruccioli MG, Barajon I, Fabbrica D. Morphometric study of the sensory neuron and peripheral nerve changes induced by chronic cisplatin (DDP) administration in rats. Acta Neuropathol (Berl) 1992; 84: 364-71.

[101] Malgrange B, Delree P, Rigo JM, Baron H, Moonen G. Image analysis of neuritic regeneration by adult rat dorsal root ganglion neurons in culture: quantification of the neurotoxicity of anticancer agents and of its prevention by nerve growth factor or basic fibroblast growth factor but not brain-derived neurotrophic factor or neurotrophin-3. J Neurosci Methods 1994; 53: 111-22.

[102] Hayakawa K, Sobue G, Itoh T, Mitsuma T. Nerve growth factor prevents neurotoxic effects of cisplatin, vincristine and taxol, on adult rat sympathetic ganglion explants *in vitro*. Life Sci 1994; 55: 519-25.

[103] Lauria G, Lombardi R, Borgna M, Penza P, Bianchi R, Savino C, Canta A, Nicolini G, Marmiroli, P, Cavaletti G. Intraepidermal nerve fibre density in rat foodpad: neuropathologic-neurophysiologic correlation. J Peripher Nerv Syst 2005; 10: 199-205.

[104] Schmidt Y, Unger JW, Bartke I, Reiter R. Effect of nerve growth factor on peptide neurons in dorsal root ganglia after taxol or cisplatin treatment and in diabetic (db/db) mice. Exp Neurol 1995; 132: 16-23.

[105] ter Laak MP, Hamers FP, Kirk CJ, Gispen WH. rhGGF2 protects against cisplatin-induced neuropathy in the rat. J Neurosci Res 2000; 60: 237-44.

[106] Holmes J, Stanko J, Varchenko M, Ding H, Madden VJ, Bagnell CR, Wyrick SD, Chaney SG. Comparative neurotoxicity of oxaliplatin, cisplatin, and ormaplatin in a Wistar rat model. Toxicol Sci 1998; 46: 342-51.

[107] Fischer SJ, McDonald ES, Gross L, Windebank AJ. Alterations in cell cycle regulation underlie cisplatin induced apoptosis of dorsal root ganglion neurons *in vivo*. Neurobiol Dis 2001; 8: 1027-35.

[108] Kochar DK, Rawat N, Agrawal RP, Vyas A, Beniwal, R, Kochar SK, Garg P. Sodium valproate for painful diabetic neuropathy: a randomized double-blind placebo-controlled study. QJM 2004; 97: 33-8.

[109] Tremont-Lukats IW, Megeff C, Backonja MM. Anticonvulsants for neuropathic pain syndromes: mechanisms of action and place in therapy. Drugs 2000; 60: 1029-52.

[110] Cui SS, Yang CP, Bowen, RC, Bai O, Li XM, Jiang W, Zhang X. Valproic acid enhances axonal regeneration and recovery of motor function after sciatic nerve axotomy in adult rats. Brain Res 2003; 975: 229-36.

[111] Zilliox L, Russell JW. Treatment of diabetic sensory polyneuropathy. Curr Treat Options Neurol. 2011; 13: 143-59.

[112] Bril V, England J, Franklin GM, Backonja M, Cohen J, Del Toro D, Feldman E, Iverson DJ, Perkins B, Russell JW, Zochodne D; American Academy of Neurology; American Association of Neuromuscular and Electrodiagnostic Medicine; American Academy of Physical Medicine and Rehabilitation. Evidence-based guideline: Treatment of painful diabetic neuropathy: report of the American Academy of Neurology, the American Association of Neuromuscular and Electrodiagnostic Medicine, and the American Academy of Physical Medicine and Rehabilitation. Neurology. 2011; 76: 1758-65.

[113] Rodriguez-Menendez V, Gilardini A, Bossi M, Canta A, Oggioni N, Carozzi V, Tremolizzo L, Cavaletti G. Valproate protective effects on cisplatin-induced peripheral neuropathy: an *in vitro* and *in vivo* study. Anticancer Research 2008; 28: 335-42.

[114] Fritz IB. Carnitine and its role in fatty acid metabolism. Adv. Lipid Res 1963; 1: 285-334.

[115] Bremer J. The role of carnitine in intracellular metabolism. J Clin Chem Clin Bioche 1990; 28: 297-01.

[116] Furlong JH. Acetyl-L-carnitine: metabolism and applications in clinical practice. Alter Med Rev 1996; 1: 85-93.

[117] Montgomery SA, Thal LJ, Amrein R. Meta-analysis of double blind randomized controlled clinical trials of acetyl-L-carnitine *versus* placebo in the treatment of mild cognitive impairment and mild Alzheimer's disease. Int Clin Psychopharmacol 2003; 18: 61-71.

[118] Abdul HM, Calabrese V, Calvani M, Butterfield DA. Acetyl-L-carnitine-induced up-regulation of heat shock proteins protects cortical neurons against amyloid-beta peptide 1-42-mediated oxidative stress and neurotoxicity: implications for Alzheimer's disease. J Neurosci Res 2006; 84: 398-08.

[119] Bianchetti A, Rozzini R, Trabucchi M. Effects of acetyl-L-carnitine in Alzheimer's disease patients unresponsive to acetylcholinesterase inhibitors. Curr Med Res Opin 2003; 19: 350-3.

[120] Pettegrew JW, Levine J, Gershon S, Stanley JA, Servan-Schreiber D, Panchalingam K, McClure RJ. 31P-MRS study of acetyl-L-carnitine treatment in geriatric depression: preliminary results. Bipolar Disord 2002; 4: 61-6.

[121] Xie J, Zeng Q, Wang L. The protective effect of L-carnitine on ischemia-reperfusion heart. J Huazhong Univ Sci Technolog Med Sci 2006; 26: 188-91.

[122] Tempesta E, Troncon R, Janiri L, Colusso L, Riscica P, Saraceni G, Gesmundo E, Calvani M, Benedetti N, Pola P. Role of acetyl-L-carnitine in the treatment of cognitive deficit in chronic alcoholism. Int J Clin Pharmacol Res 1990; 10: 101-7.

[123] De Grandis D, Minardi C. Acetyl-L-carnitine (levacecarnine) in the treatment of diabetic neuropathy. A long-term randomized, double-blind, placebo-controlled study. Drugs R.D 2002; 3: 223-31.

[124] Sima AA. Acetyl-L-carnitine in diabetic polyneuropathy: experimental and clinical data. CNS Drugs 2007; 21: 13-23.

[125] Youle M, Osio M, ALCAR Study Group. A double-blind, parallel-group, placebo-controlled, multicentre study of acetyl L-carnitine in the symptomatic treatment of antiretroviral toxic neuropathy in patients with HIV-1 infection. HIV Med 2007; 8: 241-50.

[126] Herzmann C, Johnson MA, Youle M. Long-term effect of acetyl-L-carnitine for antiretroviral toxic neuropathy. HIV Clin Trials 2005; 6: 344-50.

[127] Osio M, Muscia, F, Zampini L, Nascimbene C, Mailland E, Cargnel A, Mariani C. Acetyl-l-carnitine in the treatment of painful antiretroviral toxic neuropathy in human immunodeficiency virus patients: an open label study. J Peripher Nerv Syst 2006; 11: 72-6.

[128] Sim, AA, Calvani M, Mehra M, Amato A, Acetyl-L-Carnitine Study Group. Acetyl-L-carnitine improves pain, nerve regeneration, and vibratory perception in patients with chronic diabetic neuropathy: an analysis of two randomized placebo-controlled trials. Diabetes Care 2005; 28: 89-94.

[129] Ghirardi O, Lo Giudice P, Pisano C, Vertechy M, Bellucci A, Vesci L, Cundari S, Miloso M, Rigamonti LM, Nicolini G, Zanna C, Carminati P. Acetyl-L-Carnitine prevents and reverts experimental chronic neurotoxicity induced by oxaliplatin, without altering its antitumor properties. Anticancer Res 2005; 25: 2681-7.

[130] Pisano C, Pratesi G, Laccabue D, Zunino F, Lo Giudice P, Bellucci A, Pacifici L, Camerini B, Vesci L, Castorina M, Cicuzza S, Tredici G, Marmiroli P, Nicolini G, Galbiati S, Calvani M, Carminati P, Cavaletti G. Paclitaxel and Cisplatin-induced neurotoxicity: a protective role of acetyl-L-carnitine. Clin Cancer Res 2003; 9: 5756-67.

[131] Flatters SJ, Xiao WH, Bennett GJ. Acetyl-L-carnitine prevents and reduces paclitaxel-induced painful peripheral neuropathy. Neurosci Lett 2006; 397: 219-23.

[132] De Grandis D. Acetyl-L-carnitine treatment of chemotherapy/induced peripheral neuropathy: a short review. CNS Drugs 2007; 21: 39-43.
[133] Chiechio S, Copani A, Gereau RW 4th, Nicoletti F. Acetyl-L-carnitine in neuropathic pain: experimental data. CNS Drugs 2007; 21: 31-8.
[134] Head KA. Peripheral neuropathy: pathogenic mechanisms and alternative therapies. Altern Med Rev 2006; 11: 294-329.
[135] Maestri, A, De Pasquale Ceratti A, Cundari S, Zanna C, Cortesi E, Crino L. A pilot study on the effect of acetyl-L-carnitine in paclitaxel- and cisplatin- induced peripheral neuropathy. Tumori 2005; 91: 135-8.
[136] Tabolacci E, Pietrobono R, Moscato U, Oostra BA, Chiurazzi P, Neri G. Differential epigenetic modifications in the FMR1 gene of the fragile X syndrome after reactivating pharmacological treatments Eur J Hum Genet. 2005; 13: 641-8.
[137] Madiraju P, Pande SV, Prentki M, Madiraju SR. Mitochondrial acetylcarnitine provides acetyl groups for nuclear histone acetylation. Epigenetics 2009; 4: 399-403.
[138] Chauhan NB, Siegel GJ. Effect of PPF and ALCAR on the induction of NGF- and p75-mRNA and on APP processing in Tg257 brain. Neurochem Int 2003; 43: 225-33.
[139] Taglialatela G, Navarra D, Cruciani R, Ramacci, MT, Alema GS, Angelucci L. Acetyl-L-carnitine treatment increases nerve growth factor levels and choline acetyltransferase activity in the central nervous system of aged rats. Exp Gerontol 1994; 29: 55-66.
[140] Faraco G, Pancani T, Formentini L, Mascagni P, Fossati G, Leoni F, Moroni F, Chiarugi A. Pharmacological inhibition of histone deacetylases by suberoylanilide hydroxamic acid specifically alters gene expression and reduces ischemic injury in the mouse brain. Mol Pharmacol 2006; 70: 1876-84.
[141] Kim HJ, Rowe M, Ren M, Hong JS, Chen PS, Chuang DM. Histone deacetylase inhibitors exhibit anti-inflammatory and neuroprotective effects in a rat permanent ischemic model of stroke: multiple mechanisms of action. J Pharmacol Exp Ther 2007; 321: 892-01.
[142] Morland C, Boldingh KA, Iversen EG, Hassel B. Valproate is neuroprotective against malonate toxicity in rat striatum: an association with augmentation of high-affinity glutamate uptake. J Cereb Blood Flow Metab 2004; 24: 1226-34.
[143] Hockly E, Richon VM, Woodman B, Smith DL, Zhou X, Rosa E, Sathasivam K, Ghazi-Noori S, Mahal A, Lowden PA, Steffan JS, Marsh JL, Thompson LM, Lewis CM, Marks PA, Bates GP. Suberoylanilide hydroxamic acid, a histone deacetylase inhibitor, ameliorates motor deficits in a mouse model of Huntington's disease. Proc Natl Acad Sci USA 2003; 100: 2041-6.
[144] Sadri-Vakili G, Cha JH. Histone deacetylase inhibitors: a novel therapeutic approach to Huntington's disease (complex mechanism of neuronal death). Curr Alzheimer Res 2006; 3: 403-8.
[145] Minamiyama M, Katsuno M, Adachi H, Waza M, Sang C, Kobayashi Y, Tanaka F, Doyu M, Inukai A, Sobue G. Sodium butyrate ameliorates phenotypic expression in a transgenic mouse model of spinal and bulbar muscular atrophy. Hum Mol Genet 2004; 13: 1183-92.
[146] Butler R, Bates GP. Histone deacetylase inhibitors as therapeutics for polyglutamine disorders. Nat Rev Neurosci 2006; 7: 784-96.
[147] Sugai F, Yamamoto Y, Miyaguchi K, Zhou Z, Sumi H, Hamasaki T, Goto M, Sakoda S. Benefit of valproic acid in suppressing disease progression of ALS model mice. Eur J Neurosci 2004; 20: 3179-83.
[148] Ryu H, Smith K, Camelo SI, Carreras I, Lee J, Iglesias AH, Dangond F, Cormier KA, Cudkowicz ME, Brown RH Jr, Ferrante RJ. Sodium phenylbutyrate prolongs survival and

regulates expression of anti-apoptotic genes in transgenic amyotrophic lateral sclerosis mice. J Neurochem 2005; 93: 1087-98.

[149] Tremolizzo L, Rodriguez-Menendez V, Sala G, Di Francesco JC, Ferrarese C. Valproate and HDAC inhibition: a new epigenetic strategy to mitigate phenotypic severity in ALS? Amyotroph Lateral Scler Other Motor Neuron Disord 2005; 6: 185-6.

[150] Rouaux C, Panteleeva I, René F, Gonzalez de Aguilar JL, Echaniz-Laguna A, Dupuis L, Menger Y, Boutillier AL, Loeffler JP. Sodium valproate exerts neuroprotective effects *in vivo* through CREB-binding protein-dependent mechanisms but does not improve survival in an amyotrophic lateral sclerosis mouse model. J Neurosci 2007; 27: 5535-45.

[151] Piepers S, Veldink JH, de Jong SW, van der Tweel I, van der Pol WL, Uijtendaal EV, Schelhaas HJ, Scheffer H, de Visser M, de Jong JM, Wokke JH, Groeneveld GJ, van den Berg LH. Randomized sequential trial of valproic acid in amyotrophic lateral sclerosis. Ann Neurol. 2009; 66: 227-34.

[152] Tremolizzo L, Difrancesco JC, Rodriguez-Menendez V, Riva C, Conti E, Galimberti G, Ruffmann C, Ferrarese C. Valproate induces epigenetic modifications in lymphomonocytes from epileptic patients. Prog Neuropsychopharmacol Biol Psychiatry. 2012 May 11; Epub ahead of print.

INDEX

Atta-ur-Rahman (Ed)

B

D

F

H

I

Q

R

S

T

U

W

Y

Made in the USA
Las Vegas, NV
03 November 2026

57424370R00190